Chemical Peels
A Global Perspective

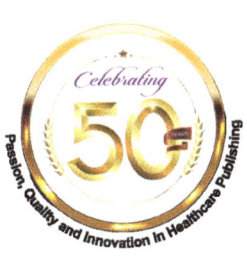

Chemical Peels
A Global Perspective

Editors

Rashmi Sarkar MD MNAMS
Professor of Dermatology, STD and Leprosy
Maulana Azad Medical College and
Lok Nayak Jai Prakash Narayan Hospital
New Delhi, India

Wendy E Roberts MD FAAD
Generational and Cosmetic Dermatology
Rancho Mirage, California, USA

Associate Editors

Sneha Ghunawat MD DNB
Consultant Dermatologist and Cosmetologist
Gurugram, Haryana, India

Ishad Aggarwal MBBS MD
Consultant Dermatologist
Kolkata, West Bengal, India

Zubin K Mandlewala MBBS
Surat Municipal Institute of Medical Education and Research
Surat, Gujarat, India

Foreword
Valerie D Callender

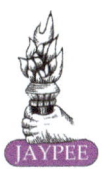

JAYPEE BROTHERS MEDICAL PUBLISHERS
The Health Sciences Publisher
New Delhi | London | Panama

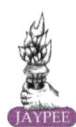 **Jaypee Brothers Medical Publishers (P) Ltd**

Headquarters

Jaypee Brothers Medical Publishers (P) Ltd
4838/24, Ansari Road, Daryaganj
New Delhi 110 002, India
Phone: +91-11-43574357
Fax: +91-11-43574314
Email: jaypee@jaypeebrothers.com

Overseas Offices

J.P. Medical Ltd
83 Victoria Street, London
SW1H 0HW (UK)
Phone: +44 20 3170 8910
Fax: +44 (0)20 3008 6180
Email: info@jpmedpub.com

Jaypee-Highlights Medical Publishers Inc
City of Knowledge, Bld. 235, 2nd Floor, Clayton
Panama City, Panama
Phone: +1 507-301-0496
Fax: +1 507-301-0499
Email: cservice@jphmedical.com

Jaypee Brothers Medical Publishers (P) Ltd
Bhotahity, Kathmandu, Nepal
Phone: +977-9741283608
Email: kathmandu@jaypeebrothers.com

Website: www.jaypeebrothers.com
Website: www.jaypeedigital.com

© 2019, Jaypee Brothers Medical Publishers

The views and opinions expressed in this book are solely those of the original contributor(s)/author(s) and do not necessarily represent those of editor(s) of the book.

All rights reserved. No part of this publication may be reproduced, stored or transmitted in any form or by any means, electronic, mechanical, photocopying, recording or otherwise, without the prior permission in writing of the publishers.

All brand names and product names used in this book are trade names, service marks, trademarks or registered trademarks of their respective owners. The publisher is not associated with any product or vendor mentioned in this book.

Medical knowledge and practice change constantly. This book is designed to provide accurate, authoritative information about the subject matter in question. However, readers are advised to check the most current information available on procedures included and check information from the manufacturer of each product to be administered, to verify the recommended dose, formula, method and duration of administration, adverse effects and contraindications. It is the responsibility of the practitioner to take all appropriate safety precautions. Neither the publisher nor the author(s)/editor(s) assume any liability for any injury and/or damage to persons or property arising from or related to use of material in this book.

This book is sold on the understanding that the publisher is not engaged in providing professional medical services. If such advice or services are required, the services of a competent medical professional should be sought.

Every effort has been made where necessary to contact holders of copyright to obtain permission to reproduce copyright material. If any have been inadvertently overlooked, the publisher will be pleased to make the necessary arrangements at the first opportunity. The **CD/DVD-ROM** (if any) provided in the sealed envelope with this book is complimentary and free of cost. **Not meant for sale.**

Inquiries for bulk sales may be solicited at: jaypee@jaypeebrothers.com

Chemical Peels: A Global Perspective / *Rashmi Sarkar, Wendy E Roberts*

First Edition: **2019**

ISBN: 978-93-5270-352-4

Dedicated to

I would like to dedicate it to my late father, Dr Asim Kumar Sarkar and my late mother, Mrs Chhobi Sarkar

Contributors

EDITORS

Rashmi Sarkar MD MNAMS
Professor of Dermatology, STD and Leprosy
Maulana Azad Medical College and
Lok Nayak Jai Prakash Narayan Hospital
New Delhi, India

Wendy E Roberts MD FAAD
Generational and Cosmetic Dermatology
Rancho Mirage, California, USA

ASSOCIATE EDITORS

Sneha Ghunawat MD DNB
Consultant Dermatologist and Cosmetologist
Gurugram, Haryana, India

Ishad Aggarwal MBBS MD
Consultant Dermatologist
Kolkata, West Bengal, India

Zubin K Mandlewala MBBS
Surat Municipal Institute of Medical Education and Research
Surat, Gujarat, India

CONTRIBUTING AUTHORS

Aarti Sarda MD
Consultant Dermatologist
Department of Dermatology
Wizderm Speciality Skin and Hair Clinic
Kolkata, West Bengal, India

Abhishek De MD
Associate Professor
Department of Dermatology
Calcutta National Medical College
Kolkata, West Bengal, India

Atula Gupta MBBS MD
Senior Consultant Dermatologist
Department of Dermatology
Skin Aid Clinic
Gurugram, Haryana, India

Borelli Claudia MD
Professor and Head
Unit of Aesthetic Dermatology
and Laser
Department of Dermatology
University Hospital Tübingen
Liebermeister, Germany

Carlos G Wambier MD PhD
Adjunct Professor
Department of Medicine
State University of Ponta Grossa
Ponta Grossa, Brazil

Doris Hexsel MD
Principal Investigator
Department, Brazilian Center for
Studies in Dermatology
Porto Alegre, RS, Brazil
Medical Director
Department
Hexsel Dermatology Clinic
Porto Alegre, RS and Rio de
Janeiro, RJ, Brazil

Fischer Sabrina MD
Medical Staff
Unit of Aesthetic Dermatology
and Laser
Department of Dermatology
University Hospital Tübingen
Liebermeister, Germany

Geraldine Jain MBBS DVD PhD
Consultant Dermatologist and
Laser Surgeon
Department of Dermatology
Punarnawah Medical and
Research Centre
Jaipur, Rajasthan, India

Gunjan Verma MD
Senior Resident
Department of Dermatology
and STD
Dr Ram Manohar Lohia Hospital
and PGIMER
New Delhi, India

Jacob R Stewart BS
Fourth Year Medical Student
Department of Dermatology
University of Texas Southwestern
Medical School
Dallas, Texas, USA

Jaishree Sharad MBBS DDV
FAAD
Medical Director
Department of Aesthetic
Dermatology
Skinfiniti Aesthetic Skin and
Laser Clinic
Mumbai, Maharashtra, India

Kachiu C Lee MD MPH
Assistant Professor
Department of Dermatology
Brown University
Providence, Rhode Island,
United States

Kaveri Korgavkar MD
Dermatology Resident
Department of Dermatology
Brown University
Providence, Rhode Island,
United States

Lark G Guss MD MSc
Dermatologist, Mohs Surgeon
Mohs Surgery and Dermatology
Center Scripps Clinic
La Jolla, California, USA

Latika Arya MD
Consultant Dermatologist
L A Skin and Aesthetic Clinic
New Delhi, India

Manmit K Hora MD
Consultant Dermatologist
Department of Dermatology
Max Smart Super Speciality
Hospital
New Delhi, India

Meenaz Khoja DDV
Consultant Dermatologist
Department of Dermato-
Cosmetology
GMF Ruby Hall Clinic and MMF
Joshi Hospital
Pune, Maharashtra, India

Monica B Dassi MBBS DVD
FCPS PGDHHM
Head
Department of Dermatology
and Cosmetology
Artemis Hospital
Gurugram, Haryana, India

Mukta Sachdev MD
Senior Consultant
Dermatologist
Medical Director
Department of Dermatology
MS Skin Centre
Bangalore, Karnataka, India
Head of Department
Department of Dermatology
Manipal Hospital
Bengaluru, Karnataka, India

Nicole A Negbenebor MD
Dermatology Resident
Department of Dermatology
Brown University
Providence, Rhode Island,
United States

Nisha V Parmar MD
Consultant Dermatologist
Aster Medical Center
Dubai, United Arab Emirates

Peter P Rullan MD
Private Practice
Department of Cosmetic
Dermatology
Dermatology Institute
Chula Vista, California, USA

Contributors

Rachana Shilpakar MD
Consultant Dermatologist
Department of Dermatology
MS Skin Centre
Bengaluru, Karnataka, India

Sahar MF Ghannam MD PhD
Consultant Dermatologist and Cosmetic Dermatologist
Associate Professor of Dermatology and Venereology
Alex University
Alexandria, Egypt

Sakshi Srivastava MD
Executive Consultant
Department of Dermatology and Aesthetic Medicine
Jaypee Hospital
Noida, Uttar Pradesh, India

Seaver L Soon MD
Staff Physician, Division of Dermatology and Dermatologic Surgery, Scripps Clinic
La Jolla, California, USA

Seemal R Desai MD
Founder and Medical Director
Innovative Dermatology
PA Clinical Assistant Professor
Department of Dermatology
University of Texas Southwestern Medical Center
Dallas, Texas, USA

Shankila Mittal MD DNB
Senior Resident
Department of Dermatology
VMMC and Associated Safdarjung Hospital
New Delhi, India

Shehnaz Z Arsiwala MD DDV
Founder and Managing Director
Renewderm
Honorary Consultant Saifee Hospital and Prince Aly Khan Hospital
Mumbai, Maharashtra, India

Sidharth Sonthalia MBBS (Hons) MD DNB MNAMS FISD
Founder, CEO and Medical Director
Medical Director and Senior Consultant Dermatologist
Dermatosurgeon and Trichologist
Skinnocence: The Skin Clinic and Research Centre
Gurugram, Haryana, India

Sonali Langar MD Diploma American Academy of Aesthetic Medicine
Consultant Dermatologist
Department of Dermatology
Apollo Hospital
Noida, Uttar Pradesh, India

Sourabh Jain MBBS MD
Senior Resident
Department of Dermatology
All India Institute of Medical Sciences
Bhopal, Madhya Pradesh, India

Sumit Sethi MBBS MD DNB
Consultant Dermatologist
Dermastation-The Skin Clinic
New Delhi, India

Surabhi Sinha MBBS MD DNB MNAMS
Department of Dermatology and STD
Dr Ram Manohar Lohia Hospital and PGIMER
New Delhi, India

Foreword

Chemical Peels: A Global Perspective (1st edition) is a comprehensive textbook on the art and science of chemical peels. Professor Rashmi Sarkar and Dr Wendy Roberts, both respected leaders in the field of Dermatology and pioneers in the World of Chemical Peels, have edited this textbook, while bringing together experts from around the world. Each author, with their own unique perspective, preferred chemical peeling agent, and individualized approach to the patient, have provided the reader with an overview of chemical peel selection, indications for peeling, proper techniques, risks, potential complications and just as importantly, an assortment of clinical pearls. This textbook is especially beneficial to practitioners who treat darker skin types (Fitzpatrick IV–VI) and the authors share their wisdom and experience in addressing some of the challenges in treating this diverse population. In addition, this textbook on Chemical Peels is an important reference for the established clinician and residents. I am honored to write this foreword on this invaluable contribution to the dermatology literature and commend Professor Sarkar and Dr Roberts on their scholarship, insight, knowledge and dedication to this very important topic.

Valerie D Callender MD FAAD
Professor of Dermatology
Howard University, Washington, DC, USA
Medical Director
Callender Dermatology and Cosmetic Center
Glenn Dale, MD, USA

Preface

All of us, who like chemical peeling, also bond together. That is what we believe and it is of no surprise that although we met as friends, realized that we both had an interest in chemical peeling. No doubt, it is one of the oldest procedures in Dermatology and Plastic Surgery, but the fact that many of us believe in it, shows that it works well. This book has been on the wishlist but took some time to coming out due to the large number of chapters which addresses the different peels, different indications, as well as different skin types and ethnicities. The idea was to create a book which would have everything from history to combination peels and I hope we did it!

We hope the patient's, benefit by your reading the book and you incorporate pearls in your practice. We would like to have our boys, Abhik and Jonah look back at this book with pride. We would like to thank all our global experts and young authors for their enthusiastically contribution for this book. We also thank Dr Neeraj Choudhary (Senior Acquisition Editor, Corporate) and Ms Himani Pandey (Development Editor) at Jaypee Brothers Medical Publishers Pvt Ltd for managing this project well. We would love to get your feedback.

Rashmi Sarkar MD MNAMS
Wendy E Roberts MD FAAD

Contents

1. **The History of Chemical Peels** — 1
   Rashmi Sarkar, Zubin K Mandlewala

2. **Histology of the Skin and Wound Healing** — 5
   Lark G Guss, Seaver L Soon

3. **Definition and Classification of Chemical Peels** — 14
   Doris Hexsel, Carlos G Wambier

4. **Basic Chemistry and Technical Variables while Applying Peels** — 22
   Rashmi Sarkar, Sneha Ghunawat

5. **Priming, Prepeel and Postpeel Care** — 27
   Rashmi Sarkar, Sneha Ghunawat

6. **Patient Assessment and Counseling** — 30
   Sneha Ghunawat, Rashmi Sarkar

7. **Glycolic Acid Peels** — 37
   Shankila Mittal, Rashmi Sarkar, Sneha Ghunawat

8. **Procedure of Glycolic Acid Peel** — 50
   Sumit Sethi

9. **Salicylic Acid Peels** — 59
   Surabhi Sinha, Rashmi Sarkar

10. **Trichloroacetic Acid Peels** — 64
    Jaishree Sharad

11. **Lactic Acid Peels** — 72
    Surabhi Sinha, Gunjan Verma

12. **Mandelic Acid Peels** — 78
    Seemal R Desai, Jacob R Stewart

13. **Pyruvic Acid Peel** — 82
    Ishad Aggarwal

14. **Jessner's and Resorcinol Peels** — 86
    Sonali Langar

15.	Tretinoin and Retinol Peels Latika Arya	96
16.	Phytic Acid Peel Rashmi Sarkar, Sneha Ghunawat	102
17.	Medium-depth Peeling with Special Consideration to Ethnic Skin Sidharth Sonthalia	108
18.	Phenol Peels and Its Modifications for Skin of Color Sidharth Sonthalia	122
19.	Medium-depth Peels Fischer Sabrina, Borelli Claudia	131
20.	Deep Peels: A Review of Chemical Peels for All Skin Types Peter P Rullan	141
21.	Sequential Peels Aarti Sarda, Abhishek De	158
22.	Yellow Peels Shehnaz Z Arsiwala	163
23.	Arginine Peel Ishad Aggarwal, Manmit K Hora	170
24.	Ferulac Peel Aarti Sarda, Abhishek De	174
25.	Combination Peels Rashmi Sarkar, Zubin K Mandlewala	180
26.	Proprietary Peels Mukta Sachdev, Rachana Shilpakar	192
27.	Combination Therapy: Chemical Peels with Other Technologies Mukta Sachdev, Rachana Shilpakar	203
28.	Chemical Peels in Melasma Sahar MF Ghannam, Zubin K Mandlewala, Rashmi Sarkar	209
29.	Chemical Peels for the Treatment of Postinflammatory Hyperpigmentation Nisha V Parmar, Rashmi Sarkar	218
30.	Chemical Peels for Acne and Acne Scars in Dark Skin Monica B Dassi	223
31.	Special Scenario: Peels for Photoaging Sonali Langar	239

32.	Special Scenario: Chemical Peeling in Sensitive Skin *Surabhi Sinha*	248
33.	Party Peels *Atula Gupta*	252
34.	Extra-facial Peeling *Meenaz Khoja, Sourabh Jain*	259
35.	Home-based Peeling Systems *Ishad Aggarwal, Manmit K Hora*	270
36.	Innovations with Chemical Peels in Dark Skin *Geraldine Jain*	274
37.	Chemical Peels in Dark Skinned Patients: Asian and African Skin *Nicole A Negbenebor, Kaveri Korgavkar, Kachiu C Lee*	286
38.	Chemical Peels in Ethnic Skin: Latin American Skin *Carlos G Wambier*	297
39.	Complications of Chemical Peels and How to Deal with Them *Shehnaz Z Arsiwala*	302
40.	Recent Advances in Treatment with Chemical Peels *Sakshi Srivastava, Sidharth Sonthalia*	309
41.	Chemical Peel Pearls *Wendy E Roberts*	318
	Appendix	321
Index		323

The History of Chemical Peels

Rashmi Sarkar, Zubin K Mandlewala

INTRODUCTION

Chemical peeling, also termed as chemexfoliation, is a skin-resurfacing procedure wherein a chemical agent is applied in a controlled manner to cause destruction of layer(s) of the skin. The desired depth of the wound is constituted by the concentration of the peeling agent and by the dermatological condition for which it is being utilized. The damage is thus repaired in a natural manner through the mechanism of wound healing, whereby, there is stimulation of cell renewal and regeneration of a healthier skin.

HISTORICAL ASPECTS

The use of chemical peels dates back to the time of Queen Cleopatra (69–30 BC), who ruled ancient Egypt for nearly three decades. Legend has it that for purposes of beautification of her skin, Cleopatra bathed in sour donkey milk (Fig. 1), which contains a generous amount of lactic acid [an alpha-hydroxy acid (AHA)]. It was understood that donkey milk renders the skin more delicate, preserves its whiteness and erases facial wrinkles.[1] With high lactose ratios and low fat content, donkey milk is the closest known milk to human breast milk. French leader Napoleon Bonaparte's sister, Pauline (1780–1825 AD), was also reported to have used donkey milk for her skin's health care.[1] Much before the advent of Botox and lasers, ancient Egyptians fancied the use of animal oils, alabaster (a translucent form of gypsum/calcite) and salt for enhancing appearance and textural changes to the skin. The Greeks, Romans and the French used soured milk, fermented grape juice (containing tartaric acid) and lemon extract (containing citric acid) to clarify their skin. Greek women would notably make poultices of lime, mustard and sulfur to rejuvenate their skin. Turkish women would intentionally singe their skin with fire

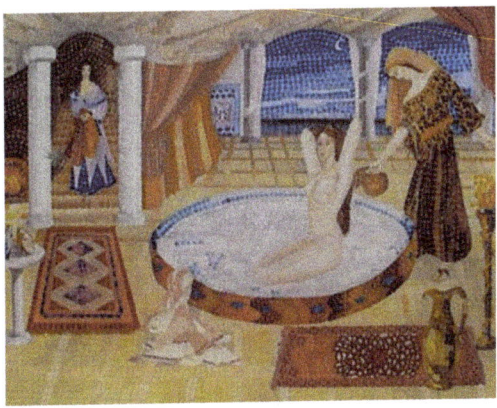

FIG. 1: Ancient Egyptians bathed in sour donkey milk for beautifying the skin.

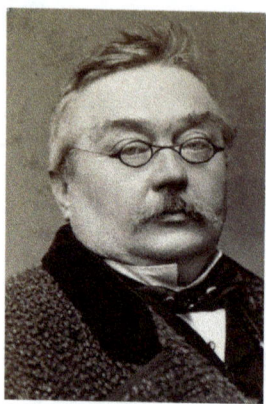

FIG. 2: Ferdinand Ritter von Hebra.

to achieve exfoliation of the skin. Hungarian Gypsies were reportedly the first ethnicity to use phenol for deep chemical peels, passing down their secret chemical recipe to further generations. According to historians, Indian women mixed urine with pumice for skin rejuvenation.

Modern times saw the rise of many physicians with their respective contributions towards chemical peels. Austrian dermatologist, Ferdinand von Hebra (Fig. 2), is credited for being the first dermatologist to use chemical peels. In the mid-1800s, Dr Hebra treated freckles and melasma with various exfoliative substances.[2] Apart from that, he also documented the use of croton oil as a chemical peel.[3] In 1882, German dermatologist PG Unna formulated a paste containing zinc oxide, resorcinol, ichthammol and petrolatum. "Unna's paste" was applied for 3 days and thereby promoted rejuvenation of skin that was wrinkled from irregular pigmentation and actinic keratosis.[4] Dr Unna is also credited as being one of the first physicians to utilize trichloroacetic acid (TCA) as a peeling agent. The 1900s were a period when many physicians used phenol peels and their research thus provided the framework for future dermatologists to build upon. In 1903, British dermatologist George Mackee began using phenol peels for acne scarring (Table 1). Dr Mackee, along with his associate Dr Karp, would later publish an article in 1952, which happened to be the first attempt by any dermatologist to correlate the histology of chemical peeling with clinical results.[5] Phenol solutions even found place in warfare, wherein, gunpowder burns of the face were treated with various concentrations of phenol.[6] In 1927, HO Bames, a Los Angeles based plastic surgeon, used phenol covered with adhesive plaster for deep face peeling.[7] The importance of Dr "Bames" work lies in the fact that he lay emphasis of dividing the facial

TABLE 1: Timeline of phenol-based peels

Physician and year(s)	Phenol-based work
Fox, 1871	Phenol for freckles
Unna, 1882	Salicylic acid, resorcinol, phenol and TCA
Saalfeld, 1892	Lime and phenol for freckles
Fox, 1905	Phenol for freckles
Mackee and Karp, 1903–1952	Histological aspects of scarring post phenol
Eller, 1941	Phenol, salicylic acid combinations and CO_2 snow peels
Brown, 1960	Buffered phenol and histological aspects
Baker and Gordon, 1961	Phenol mixed with water, hexachlorophene and croton oil as a deep peeling agent

Source: Brody HJ, Monheit GD, Resnik SS, et al. A history of chemical peeling. Dermatol Surg. 2000;26:405-9.

peel into halves separated by a week's time to avoid phenol poisoning or nephritis.[7] This fact was again re-emphasized by Dr Joseph Eller in 1941; wherein he detailed the dangers of renal phenol toxicity as well as degreasing the skin prior to application of the peeling agent.[8] In the 1950s, Max Jessner, an American submarine doctor wanted to prepare an antiseptic for mariners and to stop infection spreading among the crew during voyages. Using what he had at hand, he created a unique solution comprising resorcinol, lactic acid and salicylic acid.[9] After facial application, the mariners' relatives were stunned to see their fresh and radiant faces. Interestingly, the crew had been using his magical solution as an aftershave lotion. In 1960, Samuel Ayres, an American dermatologist, studied extensively the utility of TCA as an agent for actinic damage. In 1961, Baker and Gordon, plastic surgeons by profession, developed a formula containing 55% phenol mixed with water, hexachlorophene and croton oil as a deep peeling agent for skin rejuvenation that is still in use today. Overall, the 1960s and 1970s saw the use of various concentrations of TCA along with other procedures for skin rejuvenation. American dermatologist James Stagnone followed TCA peels with dermabrasion and thereby coined the term "chemabrasion".[10] The term "medium-depth" peel was coined in 1986 by Harold Brody and Chenault Hailey, when they used solid carbon dioxide followed by TCA.[11] Eugene Van Scott and RJ Yu are credited for their research on AHAs and their subsequent use as superficial peeling agents.[12] Of note, glycolic acid, derived from sugarcane, was widely used in the 1990s in every part of the world. Even today, lower concentrations of glycolic acid have found their place in every dermatologist's office because of their beneficial safety profile. Not only do they mildly exfoliate the skin, they also enhance the penetration of certain home care products, producing a brighter, smoother and more even-toned skin. Another benefit is that there is no real downtime associated with AHAs; serving commonly as a "lunch time" procedure for most working patients. Mandelic acid, another AHA, is derived from bitter almonds and has relatively the same properties as glycolic acid but has less penetration and irritation potential overall. Similarly salicylic acid, a beta-hydroxy acid (BHA), has been widely used over the past 30 years especially for comedonal and inflammatory acne. Derived from the bark of the willow tree, salicylic acid has traditionally been used as a remedy for pain, inflammation and fever.

CONCLUSION

From the times of the ancient Egyptians to that acne patient being treated this very day in a dermatologist's office, chemical peels have served as an essential utility in the armamentarium of therapeutic procedures. In ancient days, peels were relatively deeper and thereby less controlled, thus producing more side effects; whereas now peels are formulated and applied in such ways so as to cause least discomfort, yet providing optimum results to the patient. Nowadays, due to the ever-growing demand of anti-aging procedures, many peels have served as an important tool for reducing wrinkles and evening of one's skin tone. With the advent of many new formulations and the dedicated research to go along with it, the future of chemical peels is certainly a "bright" one indeed.

REFERENCES

1. Ancient Foods. (2015). Donkey milk: ancient elixir of life experiences modern-day resurgence. [online] Available from https://ancientfoods.wordpress.com/2015/02/01/donkey-milk-ancient-elixir-of-life-experiences-modern-day-resurgence/ [Accessed March 2018].
2. Hebra F, Kaposi M. On Diseases of the Skin. London: New Sydenham Society; 1874. pp. 22-3.

3. Skin Care Guide. History of Chemical Peels. [online] Available from http://www.skincareguide.com/article/chemical-peels/history-of-chemical-peels. [Accessed March 2018].
4. Letessier SM. Chemical peel with resorcinol. In: Roenigk RK, Roenigk HH, (Eds). Dermatologic Surgery. New York: Marcel Dekker; 1989. p. 1017.
5. Mackee GM, Karp FL. The treatment of post acne scars with phenol. Br J Dermatol. 1952;64:456-9.
6. Brody HJ, Monheit GD, Resnik SS, et al. A history of chemical peeling. Dermatol Surg. 2000;26:405-9.
7. Bames HO. Truth and fallacies of face peeling and face lifting. Med J Rec. 1927;126:86-7.
8. Eller JJ, Wolff S. Skin peeling and scarification. JAMA. 1941;116:934-8.
9. Cosmetology. (2014). Jessner Pee. [online] Available from http://cosmetology-info.com/15/Jessner-Peel/ [Accessed March 2018].
10. Stagnone JJ. Chemabrasion, a combined technique of chemical peeling and dermabrasion. J Dermatol Surg Oncol. 1977;3:217.
11. Brody HJ, Hailey CW. Medium depth chemical peeling of the skin: a variation of superficial chemosurgery. J Dermatol Surg Oncol. 1986;12:1268.
12. Van Scott EJ, Yu RJ. Hyperkeratinization, corneocyte cohesion and alpha hydroxy acids. J Am Acad Dermatol 1984;11:867-79.

CHAPTER 2

Histology of the Skin and Wound Healing

Lark G Guss, Seaver L Soon

INTRODUCTION

Many properties of the normal healing response have been exploited to improve the cosmetic appearance of the skin. Experiments using various agents have contributed to the development of a depth-dependent algorithm to guide appropriate agent selection for a desired outcome. For concerns pertaining to pigmentation and texture of the superficial layers of the skin, a chemical peel reaching the epidermis or superficial dermis would be desirable. Whereas, if the goal is to treat deeper rhytides, dyschromias and scarring, peels extending up to the mid-dermis should certainly be considered.

WOUND HEALING OVERVIEW

Epithelial cells lining the epidermal appendages such as hair follicles, sebaceous glands and apocrine glands continuously regenerate normal skin and participate in normal wound healing. Within 24 hours after wounding, inflammatory mediators such as fibronectin, laminin and platelet-derived growth factors trigger keratinocytes to migrate over the wound bed matrix. Soon after, epithelial cells along the epidermal appendages and wound edges begin to regenerate the overlying epidermis. This process is often completed within 7–10 days.[1,2]

Dermal regeneration occurs following deeper wounds and the process may take several months to complete.[1] The reticular dermis lacks keratinocytes and thus relies on fibroblasts to synthesize collagen during the wound repair process. Two to three days following wounding, granulation tissue begins to form with the onset of angiogenesis through migrating endothelial cells and collagen replacing the fibronectin matrix. Over the following months, collagen type III and subsequently type I orient parallel to the epidermis.[2] If the fibroblasts become overstimulated during a chemical peel, scarring may occur.[3]

Superficial Peels

Agents used for light or superficial peels encompass chemicals that cause peeling of either part or the entirety of the epidermis. The most common agents are the alpha-hydroxy acids (AHAs or fruit acids), beta-hydroxy acids (BHAs), trichloroacetic acid (TCA) 10–35% and combination solutions, such as Jessner's solution. For superficial peels, the acidity of the solutions causes keratinocyte discohesion, leading to exfoliation.[1,4] Although many of the above described acids are most commonly used as "superficial" peeling agents, repeat applications, increased duration (in the case of glycolic acid), pressure and volume of application may cause the peel to extend into the dermis. For example, when studied on eyelid skin, 20% TCA causes necrosis of the upper 30% of the epidermis while a 50% TCA followed by a second 50% TCA peel causes necrosis into the papillary dermis.[5] Decreasing the pH of acidic peeling solutions also increases the depth of the peel with a higher potential for crusting and necrosis.[6]

Salicylic acid is a BHA with several supplementary mechanisms of action as a superficial peel. The acidity causes epidermolysis, but the acid also acts as a keratolytic and comedolytic agent to enhance penetration of other components which may be included in the solution, as it does in Jessner's solution.[7] Trichloroacetic acid precipitates epidermal proteins to cause individual cell necrosis in addition to separation of the keratinocytes themselves.[7] Unlike the AHAs, both salicylic acid and TCA do not require a neutralizing solution and terminate their peeling action independently.

In addition to epidermal exfoliation and subsequent epidermal thickening, histologic studies with superficial peels have shown effects into the dermis. Abdel-Motaleb et al. treated 10 patients with a weekly 30% salicylic acid peel for 6 weeks. Postauricular skin biopsied 1 week prior to treatment and 1 week following the completion of all six treatments demonstrated a statistically significant increase in epidermal thickness seen on hematoxylin and eosin sections. Deeper dermal papillae, increased inflammation surrounding sebaceous glands, and an increase in percentage area of collagen fibers in the papillary and upper reticular dermis were observed (Figs. 1A and B). Additionally, Orcein-stained sections showed an increase in the percentage area of elastic fibers in the dermis (Fig. 1C). The study also investigated

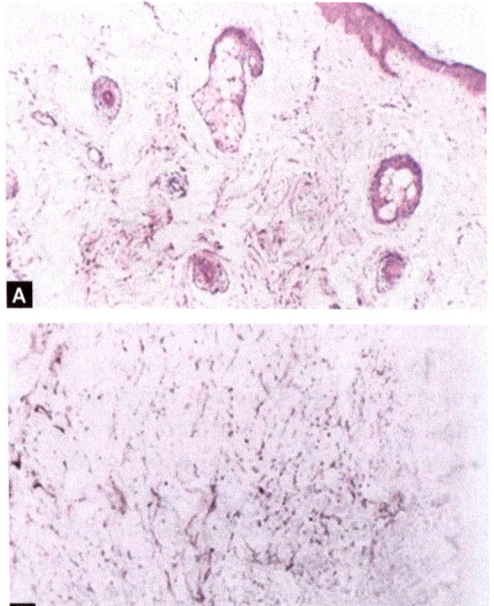

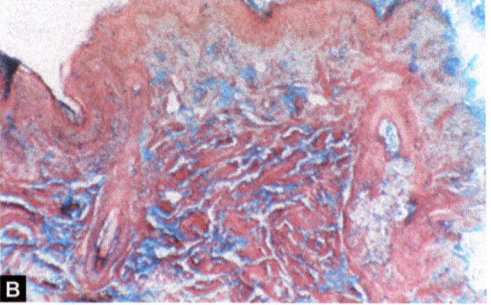

FIG. 1: A, Hematoxylin and eosin-stained photomicrograph of postauricular skin treated with salicylic acid 30% solution showing increased epidermal thickness when compared to control (not pictured) and increased inflammation surrounding sebaceous glands; **B,** Masson trichrome staining of a photomicrograph of salicylic acid 30% solution treated skin showing scattered networks of collagen fibers throughout the papillary, upper reticular, and deep reticular dermis; **C,** Orcein-stained photomicrograph of salicylic acid 30% solution treated skin showing elastic fibers diffusely throughout the papillary, upper reticular, and deep reticular dermis.

the effects of microdermabrasion on an additional ten patients and found that the epidermal thickness and collagen fibers again increased, though the collagen fibers formed patchy small networks rather than forming the more diffuse pattern seen in the salicylic acid-treated patients. The elastic fibers also appeared to have decreased in the microdermabrasion skin versus control skin.[8]

A similar outcome was observed when 17 patients' forearms were treated with either 25% lactic acid, 25% glycolic, or 25% citric acid for several months (an average of 6 months); biopsies after only 3 months showed an increase in epidermal cell layers and granular cell layers. The papillary dermis was thicker, with increased acid mucopolysaccharides, improved quality of elastic fibers and increased density of collagen.[9]

Similar results were seen when patients were treated weekly for 2 months with 70% glycolic acid peels or Jessner's solution peels (resorcinol 14 g, salicylic acid 14 g and lactic acid 14 g in a sufficient quantity of ethanol 95% to make 100 mL of solution). Following treatment, there was a statistically significant increase in epidermal thickness, inflammatory cell counts, fibroblast counts and density of collagen fibers. Dermal microvessel density, measured by staining with CD34 and CD31, was also increased following both peeling agents.[10] The authors hypothesized that despite superficial peeling agents not reaching into the dermis, the activation of fibroblasts triggered by the superficial wounding leads to collagen proliferation and inflammatory angiogenesis. Wound healing in superficial peels, thus, not only results in epidermal regeneration, but also exhibits superficial dermal effects including increased collagen, elastin and mucopolysaccharide density.

Medium Peels

Medium-depth peels penetrate through the epidermis and cause wounding into the papillary dermis, often with deeper, indirect effects into the upper reticular dermis. Though increasing the concentration or the number of applications of a single peeling agent, such as TCA, increases the depth of insult, the degree of epidermal and dermal injury was inconsistent.[4] Pioneering work by Harold Brody investigated an effective way to consistently wound the epidermis and allow for penetration of lower concentrations of TCA to reach the papillary dermis without causing unpredictable adverse effects.[11,12] As a result, medium-depth peels are now routinely performed as a two-step process, with initial application of an epidermolytic agent such as solid CO_2 followed by a 35% solution of TCA. A white frost is used as a clinical endpoint correlating with keratocoagulation or protein denaturation of keratin histologically.[12]

The degree of wounding and the chronology of subsequent healing were studied by biopsies of one patient taken prior to the peel, at day 5, day 30 and finally at day 90. After 5 days, the epidermis was necrotic and substantial edema was seen in the papillary and upper reticular dermis. The depth of the peel's effects was further substantiated by elastic and mucin stains, which showed disruption of elastic fibers and loss of glycosaminoglycans. A lymphocytic infiltrate was observed, reaching the level of the sebaceous gland. By 1 month post-procedure, the epidermis and papillary dermis had regenerated, although the reticular dermis continued to show collagen homogenization. By 3 months, the elastotic fibers had organized into a band below a papillary dermal grenz zone of renewed collagen and elastin. Stronger mucin staining (Fig. 2) was noted in the dermis correlating with glycosaminoglycan density compared to baseline (Fig. 3). A second patient with biopsies taken prior to the procedure and an additional biopsy performed 120 days later confirmed the long-term histologic effects of an expanded papillary dermis with more organized collagen when compared to baseline.[12]

Similar histologic effects were observed with other medium-depth peel combinations, such as 70% glycolic acid + TCA 35% and Jessner's solution + TCA 35%. Coleman et al. treated patients first with a 2-minute application of 70% glycolic acid followed by application of 35% TCA. Biopsies were performed at 24 hours, followed by additional biopsies at 1, 2 and 3 months. Twenty four hours following the peel, epidermal pallor was noted with smudging and homogenization of the collagen seen in the papillary and upper reticular dermis. By 2 months, the epidermis had thickened and the upper dermis had expanded with an increase of collagen bundles, which continued to be

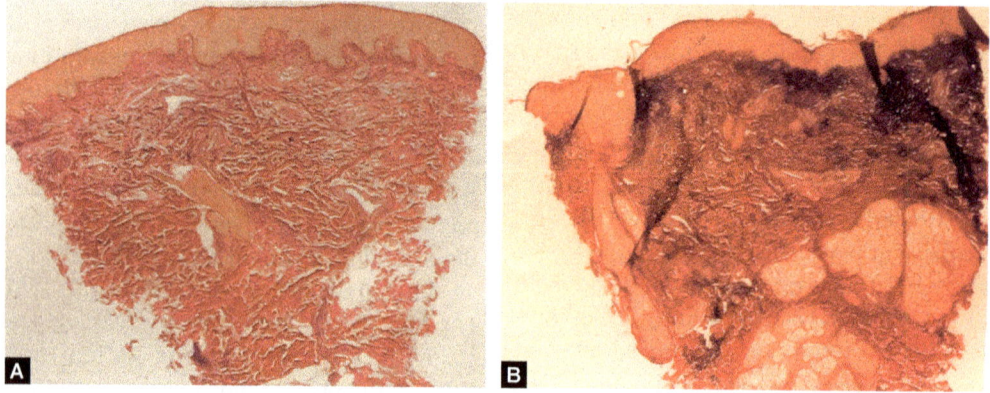

FIG. 2: Relative to baseline, at day 90, medium-depth chemical peeling using solid CO_2 and trichloroacetic acid (TCA) 35% exhibits increased dermal glycosaminoglycan density by colloidal iron stain.

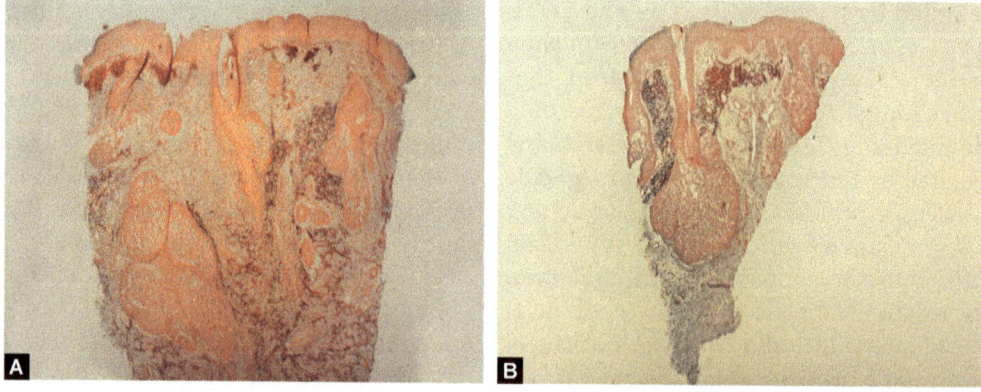

FIG. 3: Relative to baseline, at day 90, medium-depth chemical peeling using solid CO_2 and trichloroacetic acid (TCA) 35% exhibits increased a papillary dermal grenz zone of neocollagen which appears to replace and overlie the solar elastosis observed at baseline.

visible 3 months postprocedure. Notably, the expanded papillary dermis found following the combination glycolic acid or TCA peel was not as dramatic as that found following the combination of carbon dioxide or TCA peel and thus may not injure the dermis as deeply.[13] Monheit studied the effects of combination peels using Jessner's solution prior to 35% TCA and found similar results. Histologic analysis showed discohesion of the keratinocytes by Jessner's solution, which was hypothesized to allow for deeper and more even penetration of the TCA.[14]

Comparison of Wound Healing in Different Medium-depth Chemical Peels

Further studies compare the histologic effects of different peel combinations. Two patients were treated in a split face study with Jessner's solution on one side and solid CO_2 on the other. For the second patient, 35% TCA was applied immediately following the first agent. Two additional applications of 35% TCA were then applied to the second patient over a different area of skin for 10 minutes after the last application. For the first patient treated only with a superficial peel, biopsies taken on day 2 showed minimal epidermal edema on the Jessner's treated side and complete epidermal necrosis and pronounced dermal edema on the CO_2 treated side; clinically correlating with minimal erythema and swelling on the Jessner's side and severe erythema and crusting seen on the CO_2 side. By day 7, the epidermis on both sides had regenerated to the prepeel thickness and staining of the tissue showed no difference in elastic tissue when compared to biopsies taken prior to the peel. However, the patient treated with a medium-depth peel of Jessner's solution and a single application of TCA showed epidermal necrosis and minimal papillary dermal edema by day 3. The skin treated with Jessner's solution and three applications of TCA also showed epidermal necrosis but with a more significant amount of papillary dermal edema and a dermal lymphocytic infiltrate. The contralateral face treated with CO_2 prior to TCA had similar results but with disruption of collagen fibers and edema extending into the reticular dermis. Three months following the peel, histologic sections showed a hyperplastic epidermis and organized parallel collagen fibers in the upper reticular dermis on both sides of the face. Staining for elastic fibers following the medium-depth peel also showed a densely staining elastotic band following the triple application of TCA after either Jessner's solution or CO_2. The difference between one and three applications of TCA shows greater epidermal hyperplasia and deeper elastotic band associated with greater number of applications. Thus, it appears that though the initial wounding is deeper with the CO_2 or TCA peel, the final differences 90 days following the peel are likely not clinically significant.[11]

The role for glycolic acid as an initial agent in a medium-depth peel has also been investigated. In one large case series, 13 male patients were treated with a split-face protocol with 70% glycolic acid on one side and Jessner's solution on the other, followed by 35% TCA. Clinically, the investigators found that the facial sides undergoing glycolic acid applications demonstrated a greater benefit with regard to actinic keratoses. Both peels were equally efficacious in lightening lentigines, though neither peel had any significant effect on rhytides. Histologically, epidermal regeneration was noted at 7 days in both groups and a hyperplastic epidermis with an expanded papillary dermis was seen by 60 days in both groups as well. More newly developed elastic fibers were seen following treatment with glycolic acid, though surprisingly, more neovascularization and fibrosis was seen in biopsies treated with Jessner's solution. Thus, the authors concluded that glycolic acid may have allowed for slightly deeper penetration of TCA in their study, although a heavier coat of Jessner's would likely have negated the difference, and the two agents were very similar in their clinical results.[15]

Lastly, Johnson et al. studied the histologic correlation of clinical outcomes of Obagi's modified TCA solution. Twenty patients pretreated for 1 month with a combination of 0.1% tretinoin, 4% hydroquinone and 7% lactic acid, underwent 41.7% TCA peel diluted with 10% glycerin using saponin as a surfactant. By using glycerin to slow the kinetics of TCA, the operator may control the level of peeling more accurately using clinical cues to indicate depth. Following the initial application, an "epidermal sliding" or coarse wrinkling is described, which combined with a light white frosting and strong pink background, indicates TCA penetration to the papillary dermis. Biopsies taken 5 minutes after the clinical endpoint showed a normal epidermis and some mild endothelial swelling and edema in the papillary dermis. No involvement of the reticular dermis was noted after 2 days. At 6 weeks, the papillary dermis failed to show any continued changes from baseline. A second application leads to uniform solid white frosting and a firm texture to the skin with edema and protein coagulation. The biopsy displayed features suggesting complete loss of stratum corneum and most of the stratum granulosum. By 2 days, approximately one-third of the reticular dermis showed involvement, and at 6 weeks, a new layer of collagen was noted in the upper reticular dermis. Following the final layer, the skin would lose its pink hue and thus become more gray/yellow due to mid-dermal involvement. Five minutes following the gray hue and 2 days later, biopsies showed vascular coagulation down to the level of the deep vascular plexus. At 6 weeks, a new fibrillar collagen layer was noted throughout almost the entire thickness of the reticular dermis.[16] Medium-depth peels using TCA 35%, preceded by solid CO_2, Jessner's and 70% glycolic acid, or the modified TCA 41.7% with glycerin, have comparable histologic effects eventuating in renewed papillary and upper reticular dermal components.

Deep Peels

By extending the depth of wounding to the reticular dermis, deep chemical peels improve deep rhytides and may also achieve skin tightening. Similar to the effects seen in medium peels, the papillary dermis and upper reticular dermis regenerate with realignment of new collagen without evidence of contracture. However, deep peels also reach down to the deeper reticular dermis which undergoes healing through a scarring process.[17] Phenol combined with croton oil is the prototypical deep peeling agent originally described by Baker and Gordon in 1961. Phenol was diluted to approximately 50% or 55% with croton oil and liquid soap which allowed for penetration of the phenol-croton oil solution. Following the peel, the skin first demonstrated an inflammatory and coagulation phase over 12–24 hours with the epidermis separating from the dermis. The skin then transitions to a re-epithelialization phase from day 3 to day 14 as the brightly red exposed dermis fades to a dull pink. The final fibroplastic phase continued for 3–4 months following the peel with neocollagenesis and neoangiogenesis.[4,18]

Application of phenol in combination with croton oil causes complete keratocoagulation and increased papillary dermal thickness but the most important effect was the fibrosis occurring deep in the dermis.[19] This observation was confirmed in murine models. One study examined the effects of Baker's phenol-croton oil solution on the dorsum of mice exposed to chronic ultraviolet B irradiation. By day 60 postpeel, mice treated with phenol-croton oil showed a significant increase in dermal thickness and reorganization of collagen in both the papillary and reticular dermis. Furthermore, clumped elastotic masses noted in the control photoaged group were replaced by reorganized elastic fibers in the dermis of the mice in the treatment group.[20]

To further define the independent effects of phenol, Hetter found that at least 35% phenol was required to cause even mild keratolysis. No dermal effect was noted with even an increase to 50% phenol resulting in only a mild dermal effect. It was only when the concentration of phenol was increased to 88% that upper dermal wounding could be identified. However, the addition of croton oil relatively increased the depth of injury, healing time and clinical outcome when compared with phenol alone.[21] Like Obagi's findings with TCA, Hetter postulated that multiple applications of a peeling agent resulted in far greater penetration than simply increasing the concentration of phenol. Stone then confirmed that with the addition of croton oil, the number of applications needed to reach a specific depth on biopsy could be significantly lowered.[22] These studies confirm that croton oil is the principal wounding agent in deep peels. The dermal fibrosis with deep chemical peeling is persistent. Baker also commented on the dermal scar in his original paper and subsequently found the same scar still present in patients 13 years after their peel.[23,24] Face lift specimens obtained up to 20 years following a phenol peel additionally demonstrated a continued dense network of elastic fibers in a band of regenerated collagen that was not seen in the areas of unpeeled skin (Fig. 4).[25]

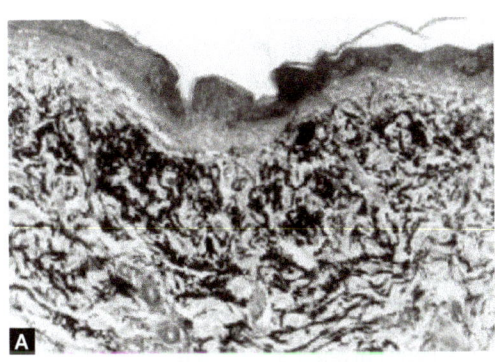
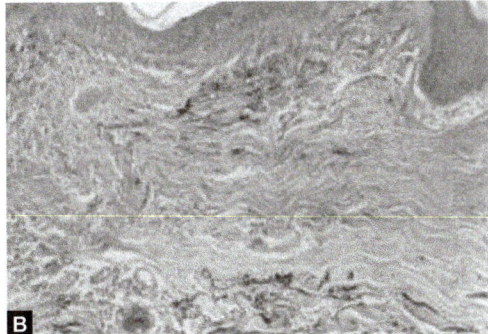
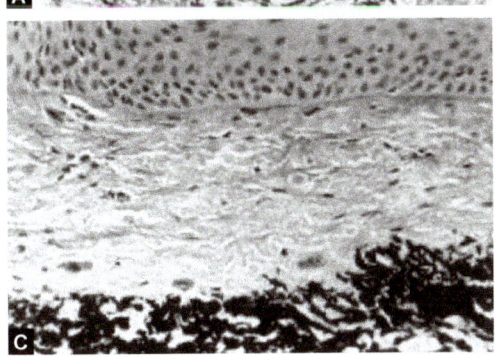

FIG. 4: **A,** Control skin specimen with significant actinic damage and solar elastosis; **B,** Skin biopsied 14 years following a Baker–Gordon 50% phenol peel in the same patient with a wide band of parallel collagen bundles and intermixed elastic fibers; and **C,** Second patient 4 years following a Baker–Gordon 50% phenol peel with a distinct collagen band above the elastotic dermis below.

In conclusion, deep peels as obtained with phenol-croton oil exhibit long lasting papillary and reticular dermal fibroplasia and reorganization of elastic fibers.

SPECIAL CIRCUMSTANCES

Retinoids

As re-epithelialization begins with appendageal structures, the face has a particular ability to heal quickly given the high concentration of sebaceous glands. Thus, it has been assumed that peels following isotretinoin treatment, with subsequent sebaceous atrophy, may be associated with greater risk of scarring due to impaired wound healing capacity. Although this may apply to medium and deep peels, a recent consensus statement contended that superficial peels are safe to perform even with concurrent isotretinoin therapy.[26]

Topical tretinoin prior to chemical peeling has been shown to hasten wound healing. Histologically, guinea pigs were used to demonstrate the effects of a topical retinoid prior to a chemical peel. Biopsies were obtained at baseline, 1 month following daily 0.1% tretinoin cream and several days post-50% TCA. One month following a topical retinoid (but prior to any peeling), the treated animals were noted to have 7–8 cell layers in the epidermis versus only 4–5 cell layers in the control group. Both control and treated biopsies appeared similar at days 1 and 3, but at day 7, the treated guinea pigs healed more quickly and had 1.5 times the amount of epidermal regeneration when compared to the control animals. At 6 weeks, epidermal regeneration had plateaued in both groups, however, the treated epidermis continued to have 8–9 cell layers versus only 4–5 cell layers in the control group. Thus, pretreatment of the skin with a topical retinoid appears to improve the results of a chemical peel.[27]

Postradiation Therapy

Wound healing of the skin relies extensively on migration of keratinocytes and regeneration of epithelial cells originating from appendageal structures. Radiated tissue associated with destruction of adnexal structures has an inherently decreased ability to heal. Thus, prior radiation therapy has been cited as a risk factor for scarring; a skin biopsy or examination for the presence of vellus hairs has been recommended prior to performing a chemical peel.[2] Limited reports of peeling following radiation are available in the literature, but one successful case of a deep perioral peel has been reported 3 years following radiation.[28]

CONCLUSION

By appropriating the skin's wound repair mechanisms, chemical peels can safely and effectively improve the appearance and texture of the skin. The histologic effects of chemical peels have been defined through studies in both animal models and human subjects. The understanding of the pathophysiology of wound healing in the skin allows the physician to select the appropriate chemical peel based on its known effects on skin wounding and repair.

REFERENCES

1. Clark E, Scerri L. Superficial and medium-depth chemical peels. Clin Dermatol. 2008;26(2):209-18.
2. Brody HJ. Chemical Peeling and Resurfacing. Baxtor S. (Ed.) St. Louis, Missouri: Mosby-Year Book; 1997. p. 240.
3. Deprez P. Textbook of Chemical Peels, Second Edition: Superficial, Medium, and Deep Peels in Cosmetic Practice, 2nd edition. Boca Raton, FL: CRC Press; 2016. p. 387.
4. Mangat DS, Tansavatdi K, Garlich P. Current chemical peels and other resurfacing techniques. Facial Plast Surg. 2011;27(1):35-49.
5. Dailey RA, Gray JF, Rubin MG, et al. Histopathologic changes of the eyelid skin following trichloroacetic

acid chemical peel. Ophthal Plast Reconstr Surg. 1998;14(1):9-12.
6. Becker FF, Langford FP, Rubin MG, et al. A histological comparison of 50% and 70% glycolic acid peels using solutions with various pHs. Dermatol Surg. 1996;22(5):463-5.
7. Fabbrocini G, De Padova MP, Tosti A. Chemical peels: what's new and what isn't new but still works well. Facial Plast Surg. 2009;25(5):329-36.
8. Abdel-Motaleb AA, Abu-Dief EE, Hussein MR. Dermal morphological changes following salicylic acid peeling and microdermabrasion. J Cosmet Dermatol. 2017;16(4):e9-14.
9. Ditre CM, Griffin TD, Murphy GF, et al. Effects of alpha-hydroxy acids on photoaged skin: a pilot clinical, histologic, and ultrastructural study. J Am Acad Dermatol. 1996;34(2 Pt 1):187-95.
10. Hussein MR, Ab-Deif EE, Abdel-Motaleb AA, et al. Chemical peeling and microdermabrasion of the skin: comparative immunohistological and ultrastructural studies. J Dermatol Sci. 2008;52(3):205-9.
11. Brody HJ. Variations and comparisons in medium-depth chemical peeling. J Dermatol Surg Oncol. 1989;15(9):953-63.
12. Brody HJ, Hailey CW. Medium-depth chemical peeling of the skin: a variation of superficial chemosurgery. J Dermatol Surg Oncol. 1986;12(12):1268-75.
13. Coleman WP 3rd, Futrell JM. The glycolic acid trichloroacetic acid peel. J Dermatol Surg Oncol. 1994;20(1):76-80.
14. Monheit GD. Medium-depth chemical peels. Dermatol Clin. 2001;19(3):413-25.
15. Tse Y, Ostad A, Lee HS, et al. A clinical and histologic evaluation of two medium-depth peels. Glycolic acid versus Jessner's trichloroacetic acid. Dermatol Surg. 1996;22(9):781-6.
16. Johnson JB, Ichinose H, Obagi ZE, et al. Obagi's modified trichloroacetic acid (TCA)-controlled variable-depth peel: a study of clinical signs correlating with histological findings. Ann Plast Surg. 1996;36(3):225-37.
17. Hayes DK, Berkland ME, Stambaugh KI. Dermal healing after local skin flaps and chemical peel. Arch Otolaryngol Head Neck Surg. 1990;116(7):794-7.
18. Monheit GD. Chemical peels. Skin Therapy Lett. 2004;9(2):6-11.
19. Brown AM, Kaplan LM, Brown ME. Phenol-induced histological skin changes: hazards, technique, and uses. Br J Plast Surg. 1960;13:158-69.
20. Butler PE, Gonzalez S, Randolph MA, et al. Quantitative and qualitative effects of chemical peeling on photo-aged skin: an experimental study. Plast Reconstr Surg. 2001;107(1):222-8.
21. Hetter GP. An examination of the phenol-croton oil peel: Part I. Dissecting the formula. Plast Reconstr Surg. 2000;105(1):227-39.
22. Stone PA, Lefer LG. Modified phenol chemical face peels: recognizing the role of application technique. Facial Plast Surg Clin North Am. 2001;9(3):351-76.
23. Baker TJ, Gordon HL. Chemical face peeling and dermabrasion. Surg Clin North Am. 1971;51(2):387-401.
24. Baker TJ, Gordon HL, Mosienko P, et al. Long-term histological study of skin after chemical face peeling. Plast Reconstr Surg. 1974;53(5):522-5.
25. Kligman AM, Baker TJ, Gordon HL. Long-term histologic follow-up of phenol face peels. Plast Reconstr Surg. 1985;75(5):652-9.
26. Spring LK, Krakowski AC, Alam M, et al. Isotretinoin and Timing of procedural interventions: a systematic review with consensus recommendations. JAMA Dermatol. 2017;153(8):802-9.
27. Vagotis FL, Brundage SR. Histologic study of dermabrasion and chemical peel in an animal model after pretreatment with Retin-A. Aesthetic Plast Surg. 1995;19(3):243-6.
28. Wolfe SA. Chemical face peeling following therapeutic irradiation. Plast Reconstr Surg. 1982;69(5):859-62.

CHAPTER 3

Definition and Classification of Chemical Peels

Doris Hexsel, Carlos G Wambier

INTRODUCTION

Chemical peels are a popular and well-known cosmetic procedure. They are probably among the first cosmetic procedures in history with reports since ancient times.[1] Currently, many exfoliating agents are available. Although it was believed that chemical peels could be replaced by laser/ablative technologies, they are still used routinely and have high efficacy rates.[2,3] Their efficacy in skilled hands and low cost of consumables have undisputed balance of cost-effectiveness. Therefore, chemical peels are still irreplaceable in the cosmetic surgery weaponry.

Chemical peels are chemical agents with keratolytic or caustic properties that cause ablation of skin layers. The use of these agents targets and damages specific layers of the epidermis and/or dermis leading to an accelerated exfoliation of the skin for either cosmetic or therapeutic purposes.

The usual classification of chemical peels is defined by the depth of penetration into the skin, which can be superficial, medium or deep.[4] The success of the procedure depends much on the understanding of the chemical and biological characteristics of the agent applied and on the proper patient evaluation, selection and preparation.

DEFINITION

Chemical peels consist in the ablation of skin layers induced by the application of chemical agents with keratolytic or caustic effects. The objective of chemical peels is to damage specific layers of the epidermis and/or dermis leading to an accelerated exfoliation of the skin. The ablated skin is thus spontaneously eliminated over the days after the procedure and subsequent regeneration of tissues occur with the induction of repair mechanisms.

Chemical peels are used either for cosmetic or therapeutic purposes. Indications include pigmentary disorders such as melasma, post-inflammatory hyperpigmentation (PIH), freckles and lentigines; epidermal growths such as seborrheic keratoses, actinic keratoses and sebaceous hyperplasia among others; acne and acne scars; superficial scars; photoaging changes; wrinkles and textural alterations can be treated with this procedure.[5-12] The histologic depth of a lesion or the condition to be treated defines the particular peel to be utilized for a desired outcome.

Definition and Classification of Chemical Peels

CLASSIFICATION

Chemical peels are usually classified by the depth of penetration into the skin as shown in table 1. In general, the depth of the chemical peel is directly proportional to the discomfort during and after the procedure, the need for sedation, the healing time, the rate of the potential side effects, the need for training and the clinical results.[2]

Very Superficial Chemical Peels

Very superficial chemical peels cause minimal exfoliation of the skin as they target only the stratum corneum. The most commonly used agents are:

- Salicylic acid 20-30% in ethanol or 30% in polyethyleno glycol (PEG)
- Glycolic acid 30-50% applied briefly (1-5 minutes)
- Jessner's solution, 1-3 coats
- Modified Jessner's solution (Fig. 1)
- Resorcinol 20-30%, applied briefly (5-10 minutes)

TABLE 1: Classification of chemical peels according to the depth[4]

Depth of the peel	Target skin layer
Very superficial	Destruction of the stratum corneum without creating a wound below the stratum granulosum
Superficial	Destruction of part or all of the epidermis, anywhere from the stratum granulosum to the basal cell layer
Medium	Destruction of the epidermis and part or all of the papillary dermis
Deep	Destruction of the epidermis and papillary dermis, extending into the reticular dermis

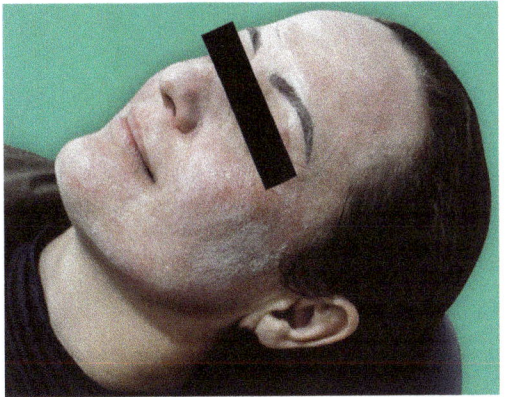

FIG. 1: Very superficial peels with 4 coats of modified Jessner's solution. Pseudofrosting from crystallization of salicylic acid from the evaporation of ethanol. Clinical endpoint: diffuse, even erythema.

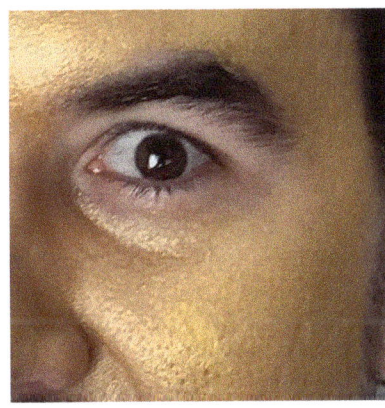

FIG. 2: Superficial 5% retinoic acid in a "gold peel", containing also melatonin and Curcuma longa extract for additional anti-inflammatory and antioxidant properties.

- Trichloroacetic acid (TCA) 10-20%, 1 coat
- Retinoic acid 3-5%, for 4-6 hours (Figs. 2 and 3)
- Mandelic acid 30-40%.

Previous priming is not required in fair skinned patients but one should do it in dark skinned patients. Usually, these peels require a series of 3-6 sessions every 7-30 days to achieve results. There is not much downtime with very superficial chemical peels and thus patients can resume day-to-day activities with

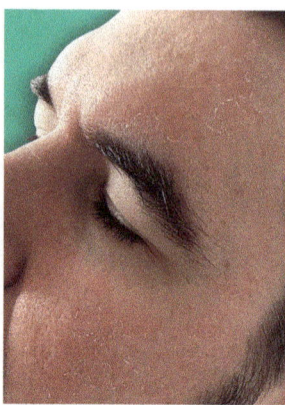

FIG. 3: Patient with mild scaling 3 days after a superficial peeling with 5% retinoic acid in the "gold peel", containing also melatonin and Curcuma longa extract for additional anti-inflammatory and anti-oxidant properties.

immediate effect. The common indications wherein very superficial chemical peels are utilized are: melasma, solar lentigines, acne and PIH.[13]

Superficial Chemical Peels

Superficial chemical peels produce an ablation anywhere between the stratum granulosum and the basal cell layer. The epidermis becomes thinner and its regeneration is caused by multiplication of the epidermal cells. In the superficial dermis, mild inflammation stimulates fibroblastic activity and thereby neocollagenesis signaling to fibroblasts and some new collagen synthesis. The most commonly used agents are:
- Glycolic acid 50–70%, until erythema
- Jessner's solution, more than 4 coats
- Modified Jessner's solution more than 4 coats
- TCA 20–35%
- Pyruvic acid 40–50%
- *Combination peels*: Salicylic acid 30% + TCA 20%
- Jessner's + TCA 20%
- Resorcinol 40–50%, applied for 30–60 minutes.

For superficial peels to produce desired effects, it is important to prepare the skin with a mild topical primer for at least 14 days, such as 0.1% adapalene, 0.01–0.05% retinoic acid, 10% glycolic acid or 15–20% azelaic acid. Like the very superficial peels, these are also performed in a series of 3–6 sessions every 15–30 days and do not require downtime (Fig. 3). Superficial peels are the most commonly performed chemical peels, and promote a "refreshed and rejuvenated look of skin". The increase in epidermal turnover improves skin color, texture and reduces comedones. This occurs faster than that which occurs through oral or topical therapies (Fig. 4). The common indications wherein superficial chemical peels are utilized are: photoaging, skin texture, acne, actinic keratoses, superficial dyschromias, solar lentigines, melasma, PIH and irregular tanning.[2,3,13]

Medium-depth Chemical Peels

The medium-depth chemical peels cause necrosis of all the epidermis and part or all of the papillary dermis. The regeneration of skin is mainly from cells of the hair follicles, which are present deeper than the areas destroyed by the peeling process. New layers of epidermis are formed and synthesis of collagen is stimulated. The most commonly used agents are:
- Jessner's solution + TCA 35%
- Modified Jessner's solution + TCA 35%
- Glycolic acid 70% + TCA 35%
- Solid carbon dioxide slush + TCA 35%
- *Alternatives in disuse*: TCA 50%, pyruvic acid >60%, pure phenol 88%.

In the case of medium-depth peels, priming is advised for regular and fast penetration of TCA. Since medium-depth peels are prone to cause PIH, in susceptible individuals, the use of bleaching agents, such as hydroquinone, in association with retinoic acid and a corticosteroid is advisable

Definition and Classification of Chemical Peels

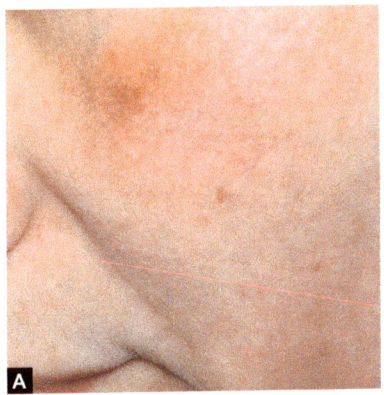
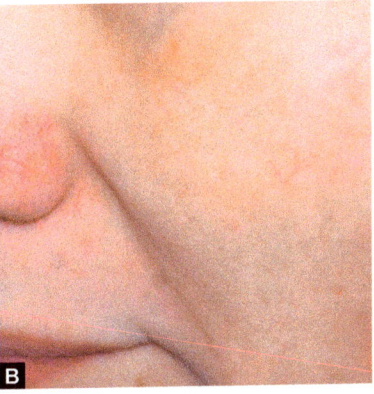

FIG. 4: A patient presenting with postinflammatory hyperpigmentation and melasma. **A,** Before; **B,** 14 days after one superficial peel with modified Jessner's solution.

(explained in subsequent chapters). In individuals with fair skin and without melasma, topical retinoids are enough. Priming works best if prescribed for over 30 days, and stopped 72–48 hours before the scheduled date of the peel. A single session is performed at 6–12 months intervals. These peels cause edema for the first 24–48 hours, with mild tenderness. After the first 48 hours, the skin turns dark and dry, until thick brown-black scales fall off (Fig. 5). Some patients are able to work with tinted sunscreen and moisturizers if the peel is performed before weekend, but most need to be absent from work because of the dark mask for at least 7 days (Fig. 6). Medium-depth chemical peels are mainly used to treat melasma, moderate photoaging, actinic keratosis (Fig. 7), lentigines, fine lines and wrinkles, PIH and superficial atrophic scars.[3,13] Wrinkles and acne scars display only a slight improvement with medium-depth chemical peels.[2]

Deep Chemical Peels

The necrosis caused by deep chemical peels can reach up to the mid-reticular dermis. Although, necrosis itself isn't the most important factor in terms of the eventual effects with deep peels. The main chemical

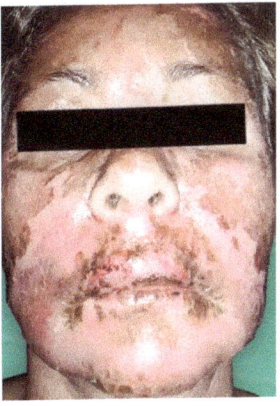

FIG. 5: Five days post procedure of a combination of medium-depth peel of sequential modified Jessner's solution, followed by 35% trichloroacetic acid and deep chemical peel performed in the perioral area with Hetter's 1.6% croton oil in 35% phenol.

agent that makes deep chemical peels so different to dermabrasion, ablative lasers and microneedling is the direct action of phorbol esters in the protein synthesis and stem cell stimulation.[14-16] Even though some degree of focal apoptosis is inevitable, the overall rejuvenating effect is quite appreciable with deep peels. Generally, the epidermal architecture returns to normal, while the dermal layers may display a collagen band

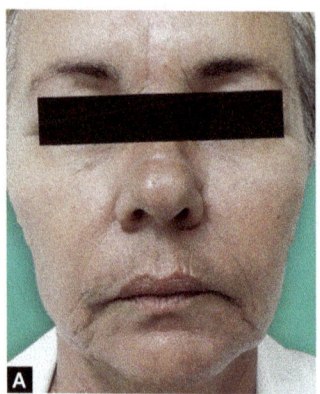
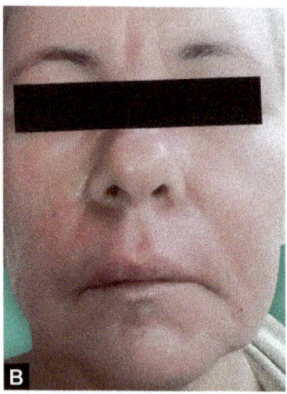

FIG. 6: **A,** Patient before a medium-depth peel with modified Jessner's solution, followed by 35% trichloroacetic acid, combined with a deep peel in the perioral area with Hetter's 1.6% croton oil in 35% phenol; **B,** Three months after the procedure, fine wrinkles, lentigines, and diffuse melanosis are no longer present.

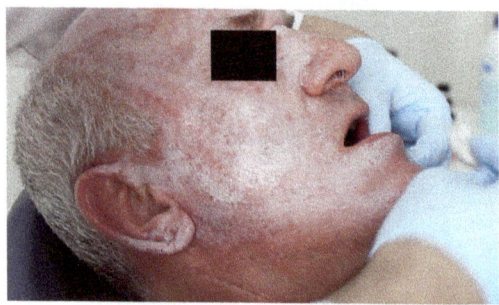

FIG. 7: Medium-depth chemical peel with Jessner's solution followed by 35% trichloroacetic acid (illustrated), performed in a patient presenting with actinic keratosis and actinic cheilitis.

up to 2-3 mm thick. In the dermis, a new subepidermal band of collagen and a band 2-3 mm thick appears. It is located above the dermis where elastosis occurs, the part of the dermis unaffected by peeling. These modifications can be observed up to 20 years after phenol peeling.[17] In general, it is believed that the skin that underwent treatment with deep peeling is less susceptible to skin cancer.[18] Although occlusion is believed to increase penetration and to enhance results, this assumption lacks support from scientific data and is not performed by many specialists, who prefer simple ointments, such as Vaseline®.[19,20]

Croton oil, a deep peel causes an intense inflammatory reaction with heat-like pain caused by the swelling that usually peaks 3 hours post peeling and lasts up to 12 hours. Pain is controlled with opiates, nonsteroidal anti-inflammatory drugs, cold wind, water mist or saline compresses. The resulting edema reaches its peak and pain disappears on the following day. Edema usually lasts 72 hours. After the third day, it is common to observe purulent exudate, yellow crust formation and eschars (Fig. 8). The facial skin is usually completely healed in 7-10 days. After that, intense erythema reaches its peak 14 days after the procedure and takes 2-4 months to fade. The rejuvenation process continues until erythema persists.

The most commonly used agents are:
- Hetter's formulas (0.4-1.6% croton oil in 33-35% phenol) (Figs. 5, 6, 8 to 10)[21]
- Baker-Gordon's formula (2.1% croton oil in 50% phenol).

Definition and Classification of Chemical Peels

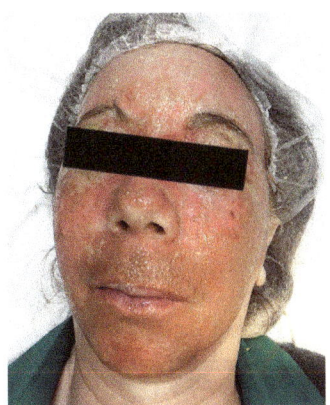

FIG. 8: Patient presenting with purulent exudate, yellow crusts and erythema 5 days after a deep chemical peel with Hetter's 1.6% croton oil in 35% phenol.

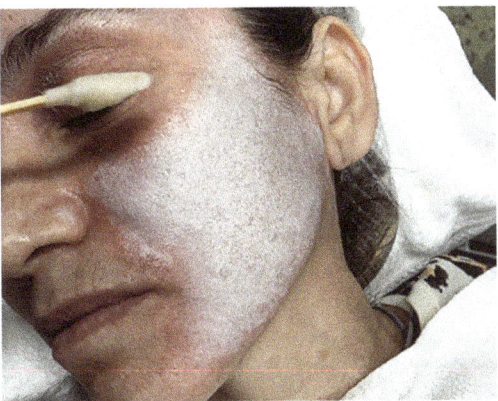

FIG. 9: Deep peeling with Hetter's croton oil 1.6% in 35% phenol, in a patient presenting with severe acne scarring and moderate photoaging.

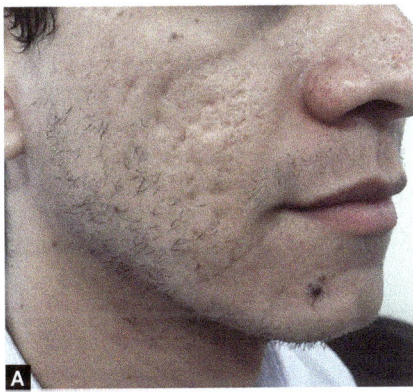
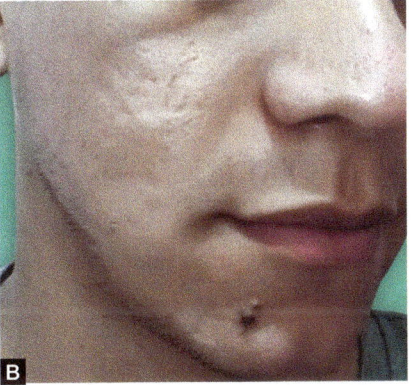

FIG. 10: A patient presenting with severe acne scarring. **A,** Before; **B,** 6 months after a deep peel with Hetter's croton oil 1.2% in 35% phenol.

Although priming is usually not necessary for deep peels, adapalene or retinoic acid generally improve penetration of the formula with increased uniformity of results. Sometimes, a smaller amount of the chemical agent is used to complete the procedure. Adequate priming is likely to reduce the time taken for the epidermis to heal completely. Usually, only a single session is performed, yet, a few patients with very thick/oily skin, may require an additional treatment. As results are long lasting, the procedure may be repeated after 6 months, if necessary. As these peels can cause significant downtime, it is advisable for patients to abstain from routine outdoor activities for atleast a week. Deep chemical peels are mainly indicated in— severe photoaging, dermal-type melasma, PIH, dyschromia, fine and coarse wrinkles, premalignant skin tumors and acne scars (Fig. 10).[2,3]

Although very effective, deep chemical peels are not as frequently performed as medium-depth and superficial peels. As deep peels may warrant a thoroughness in comprehending/managing the likelihood of side effects (e.g., cardiovascular toxicity), they should only be utilized by experienced hands. Postpeel, it is imperative that the treating physician clinically examine the patient routinely during the first week itself. Full-face procedures must be performed under multiparameter monitoring (in ICU facilities), with intravenous access for hyperhydration. The surgeon must be prepared to deal with arrhythmias and to control anxiety, blood pressure and pain. Deep peels are not performed in dark-skin types (V–VI) because of the high risk of hypertrophic scars and irregular pigmentation. Inhalation of phenol fumes during the procedure is an important concern for the physicians and staff. The authors recommend to perform the procedure in rooms equipped with air exhaustion and to wear activated charcoal masks during the peels.

CHEMICAL PEEL DEPTH

The peel classification mentioned above is routinely followed by many physicians, yet, it is important to note that there are many variables that can alter postpeel wound depth. These can be related to the chemical agent itself, to the technique, or to the patient (Table 2).[4,22,23] All these factors should be taken into account when performing the chemical peel as they will directly interfere in the depth of the peel and consequently in its outcomes. The choice of a particular agent primarily relies on the skin condition/disorder for which it is applied.

CONCLUSION

Chemical peels are best classified according to their depth of wounding. Many agents available in formulations with varying concentrations and also the techinque

TABLE 2: Factors affecting the depth of chemical peels[4,22,23]

	Variables
Chemical agent	• Agent nature • Agent concentration • Volume applied
The technique	• Number of coats • Pressure • Applicator used (brush, cotton ball, cotton-tipped applicator, and gauze) • Thickness of the layer applied • Saturation of the applicator • Degree of buffering (when applicable) • Occlusion • Exposure time • Frequency
The patient	• Type of skin (seborrheic, sebaceous gland density, and sun-damaged) • Integrity of epidermal barrier and presence of subclinical lesions (microtraumas) • Previous use of priming agents and other exfoliants • Cleansing and degreasing the skin before the peel • Anatomical location of the peel

implented, allow physicians to individualize peel protocols for a particular patient. Their versatility and effectiveness serve as a major utility for physicians in treating numerous skin conditions.

TAKE HOME POINTS

- Chemical peels may be more effective than ablative technology
- Unmatched cost-effectiveness as a cosmetic treatment
- Versatile and easy to combine with other treatments.

REFERENCES

1. Brody HJ, Monheit GD, Resnik SS, et al. A history of chemical peeling. Dermatol Surg. 2000;26(5):405-9.
2. Landau M. Chemical peels. Clin Dermatol. 2008;26(2):200-8.
3. Fisher TC, Perosino E, Poli F, et al. Chemical peels in aesthetic dermatology: an update 2009. J Eur Acad Dermatol Venereol. 2010;24(3):281-92.
4. Rubin MG. Manual of Chemical Peels. Philadelphia: JB Lippincott; 1992. pp. 17-25.
5. Khunger N; IADVL Task Force. Standard guidelines of care for chemical peels. Indian J Dermatol Venereol Leprol. 2008;74 Suppl:S5-12.
6. Rendon MI, Berson DS, Cohen JL, et al. Evidence and considerations in the application of chemical peels in skin disorders and aesthetic resurfacing. J Clin Aesthet Dermatol. 2010;3(7):32-43.
7. Sarkar R, Garg V, Bansal S, et al. Comparative evaluation of efficacy and tolerability of glycolic acid, salicylic mandelic acid, and phytic acid combination peels in melasma. Dermatol Surg. 2016;42(3):384-91.
8. Sarkar R, Parmar NV, Kapoor S. Treatment of post-inflammatory hyperpigmentation with a combination of glycolic acid peels and a topical regimen in dark-skinned patients: a comparative study. Dermatol Surg. 2017;43(4):566-73.
9. Fabi SG, Goldman MP. Hand rejuvenation: a review and our experience. Dermatol Surg. 2012;38(7 Pt 2):1112-27.
10. Ghersetich I, Brazzini B, Peris K, et al. Pyruvic acid peels for the treatment of photoaging. Dermatol Surg. 2004;30(1):32-6.
11. Abdel Meguid AM, Elaziz Ahmed Attallah DA, Omar H. Trichloroacetic acid versus salicylic acid in the treatment of acne vulgaris in dark-skinned patients. Dermatol Surg. 2015;41(12):1398-404.
12. Puri N. Efficacy of Modified Jessner's Peel and 20% TCA Versus 20% TCA Peel Alone for the Treatment of Acne Scars. J Cutan Aesthet Surg. 2015;8(1):42-5.
13. Salam A, Dadzie OE, Galadari H. Chemical peeling in ethnic skin: an update. Br J Dermatol. 2013;169 Suppl 3:82-90.
14. Bensimon RH. Croton oil peels. Aesthet Surg J. 2008;28(1):33-45.
15. Larson DL, Karmo F, Hetter GP. Phenol-Croton Oil Peel: Establishing an Animal Model for Scientific Investigation. Aesthetic Surg J. 2009;29(1):47-53.
16. Wambier CG, Brody HJ, Hetter GP. Comments: Hemiface comparative study of two phenol peels (Baker-Gordon and Hetter formulas) for the correction of facial rhytids. Surg Cosmet Dermatol. 2017;9(2):109-1.
17. Brown AM, Kaplan LM, Brown ME. Phenol induced histological skin changes: hazards, technique, and uses. Br J Plast Surg. 1960;13:158-69.
18. Baker TJ. Is the phenol-croton oil peel safe? Plast Reconstr Surg. 2003;112(1):353-4.
19. Stuzin JM, Baker TJ, Gordon HL. Chemical peel: a change in the routine. Ann Plast Surg. 1989;23(2):166-9.
20. Wambier CG, de Freitas FP. Combining Phenol-Croton Oil Peel. In: Issa MCA, Tamura B (Eds). Chemical and Physical Procedures. Cham: Springer International Publishing; 2017. pp. 1-13.
21. Hetter GP. An examination of the phenol-croton oil peel: part IV. Face peel results with different concentrations of phenol and croton oil. Plast Reconstr Surg. 2000;105(3):1061-83.
22. Landau M, Ghannam SF. Chemical peels. In: Robinson JK, Hanke CW, Siegel DM, Fratila A (Eds). Surgery of the Skin: Procedural Dermatology, 3rd edition. Philadelphia: Saunders Elsevier; 2015. pp. 393-408.
23. Matarasso SL, Glogau RG. Chemical face peels. Dermatol Clin. 1991;9(1):131-50.

Basic Chemistry and Technical Variables while Applying Peels

Rashmi Sarkar, Sneha Ghunawat

INTRODUCTION

Chemical peels are commonly used in the dermatology practice. These are compounds that act by their acidic properties and metabolic interactions to produce desired effects on the skin. For a proper understanding of chemical peels, it is of utmost importance to have an in-depth knowledge of the basic concepts in chemistry that govern these molecules.

This chapter covers elementary concepts of chemistry that help to understand the possible mechanism and interactions of these peeling agents on the skin. It also gives a brief overview of the different peel formulations as well as the factors that govern peel penetration.

ACIDS

Chemical peels are acidic molecules and thus, in order to understand their functioning, it is important to have an idea regarding the concepts of chemistry pertaining to acids. However, not all the effects of the chemical peels are attributed to the acidity of the molecule. Other properties such as metabolic and toxic effects of the chemicals also play a role. Essentially, three theories have been described in relation to the concept of acidity.

1. *Arrhenius acid*: It is a substance that when dissolved in water increases the concentration of hydronium ions. Similarly, an Arrhenius base is a molecule that increases the concentration of hydroxide ion in the aqueous solution
2. *Bronsted acid*: It is a substance that denotes a proton, while Bronsted base is a molecule that accepts a proton. This is the most widely used definition for acid–base reactions
3. *Lewis acid*: A Lewis acid is a substance that accepts a pair of electrons from another molecule.[1]

Acid Dissociation Constant—Ka

In solution, there exists equilibrium between the acid and its conjugate base. The equilibrium constant K measures the equilibrium concentration of the molecules in the solution.

$$HA \rightarrow H^+ + A^-$$

$$Ka = \frac{[H^+][A^-]}{[HA]}$$

HA represents an acid, while A^- is the conjugate base.

Strength of an acid is measured by the equilibrium constant also known as acid dissociation or acid ionization constant (Ka).

Basic Chemistry and Technical Variables while Applying Peels

Acids with a higher Ka are stronger acids than those with a lower Ka, regardless of the fact that it is an Arrhenius acid or Bronsted acid.[2] As the range of Ka is broad, a more frequently used constant is pKa (pKa = –log10 Ka). Stronger acids have stronger pKa than weak acids. Experimentally determined pKa at 25°C is widely used as references in text.

pH

Hydronium ion concentration is an important characteristic of a solution. Since it is a small number, to avoid use of exponentials in the expression, it is defined as pH (Table 1).

$$pH = -\log [H_3O^{1+}]$$

Low pH implies a high hydronium ion concentration, while a high pH implies a low hydronium ion concentration. Neutral pH is defined as pH = –log (1.0 × 10^{-7}) = 7.0.[3]

Monoprotic Acid

These compounds donate one proton per molecule following ionization. They contain one carboxyl group and are commonly called as monocarboxylic acid. Examples of organic acids in this category are acetic acid, lactic acid and glycolic acid.

Polyprotic Acid

These compounds donate more than one proton per molecule. Depending on the potential to donate protons, they can further be divided into diprotic (two potential protons to donate) and triprotic acid (three potential protons to donate). These dissociate depending on the pH of the media.

Each dissociation has its own dissociation constant (the first one being greater than the second). A triprotic acid can undergo three dissociations with three different dissociation constants (first being higher than the second, which is higher than the third). It successively loses three protons to form the ion. An example of organic triprotic acid is citric acid.

Buffer Solution

A buffer solution is a solution consisting of a weak acid and its conjugate base or a weak base and its conjugate acid. Such a solution resists pH change when small amount of acid or base is added to it. Such solutions are a means of keeping the pH constant and have wide range of utility. An example of buffer solution in the human body is blood. It has a buffer of carbonic acid and bicarbonate to maintain pH 7.35-7.45. Buffers are vital for the functioning of the body and are necessary inside the body for the proper functioning of the various enzyme systems.[4,5]

Buffer capacity of a solution is a quantitative measure of the resistance of the buffer solution to change in pH on addition of hydroxide ions. The property of the buffer solution to resist change in pH finds many uses in the biochemical process. A solution with maximum buffer capacity for a particular pH has a pKa equal to the pH.

Neutralization

Neutralization is a reaction wherein acid and base react to form salt and water. Neutralization of chemical peels is achieved by either applying cold water or neutralizing agents such as bicarbonate spray.

In a partially neutralized solution, reversible reaction between acid and base yields unneutralized acid and salt. The resulting solution has a less free acid and higher pH than an unneutralized solution.

TABLE 1: pH value of a solution and its type

Solution's pH	Solution type
pH <7	Acidic
pH = 7	Neutral
pH >7	Basic

In partially neutralized formulations, salt functions as a reservoir of acid that is available for second-phase penetration. Thus, partially neutralized solutions deliver the acid in a safer controlled manner when compared with free acid.[6]

CHOOSING PEEL FORMULATION

Many formulations exist for the various chemical peels available in the market. The chemical peels are usually procured in the raw form as crystals that are then dissolved in a particular vehicle. The choice of a particular vehicle can also play a role in the efficacy of a certain peel. For example, a gel-based peel slows the delivery of the active agent into the skin. Such formulations are desirous in patients with sensitive skin as it causes minimal irritation. In contrast, aqueous-based peels allow better bioavailability and thus cause greater desquamation.

Various peel formulations available are:
- *Free acid:* It refers to the non-neutralized solution of the acid. When such solution is applied to the skin, it has greater bioavailability and reactivity. It has a higher potential to cause erythema and related adverse effects
- *Partially neutralized:* It refers to a solution with combination of acid and base. Such solutions have pH higher than the ones containing free acids only
- *Buffered solution*: Such solutions contain equal molar concentration of acid and the conjugate base, so that the solution resists any change in the pH on addition of further acid or base
- *Esterified solution*: It refers to the peel solution ester compounds (formed by reaction of alcohol with acid). Such solutions are claimed to have less skin irritation.

While most of the chemical peeling agents work on the principle of acidity, many produce the desired effects due to their metabolic activities. One such example is the alpha-hydroxy acids (AHAs namely- lactic, glycolic and mandelic). When used at lower concentrations, they primarily act via a metabolic action decreasing the cohesion of corneocytes; while at higher concentrations, their effect is primarily based on their acidity. Some chemicals such as phenol and resorcinol act as protoplasmic poisons. They cause protein denaturation and enzyme inactivation. They also modify the permeability of the cell membrane, leading to cell death.

Alpha-hydroxy Acid

They are a class of compounds that contain carboxyl and hydroxyl acid on adjacent carbon. AHAs are either naturally occurring or synthetic. They are obtained from natural sources such as sugarcane (glycolic acid), citrus fruits (citric acid), sour milk (lactic acid), apples (malic acid) and grape wine (tartaric acid). They find a wide number of applications in cosmetic dermatology helping improve the appearance of the skin and reduce signs of aging.[7]
- *Aliphatic:*
  - Glycolic acid
  - Lactic acid
  - Tartaric acid
  - Malic acid.
- *Aromatic:*
  - Mandelic acid.

Alpha-hydroxy acids are weak acids. Their effect on the skin is concentration dependent. At low concentration, they induce skin exfoliation by decreasing corneocyte cohesion. AHAs play a role in the keratinization process by affecting the formation of the stratum corneum. They also interfere with the action of enzymes that add sulfate and phosphate groups to corneocytes. This leads to an increase in the cohesion between cells causing them to exfoliate. This action is attributed to their metabolic effects. At higher concentrations, they produce epidermolysis.[8] Glycolic acid has the smallest size and thus penetrates the skin much more rapidly than other AHAs. It is used extensively in photodamaged skin by increasing skin thickness, collagen and mucopolysaccharide synthesis.[9]

When used at pH greater than the pKa, they essentially function as moisturizers. This is due to the neutralization of the hydroxy acid molecule to create a salt, which has a more moisturizing effect. At pH less than or equal to the pKa, their acidic form is predominant causing skin exfoliation. AHAs are generally safer and free from any significant adverse effects. Common side effects include skin irritation and redness. The incidence is dependent on the concentration of the acid used, length of application as well as the pH of the solution.

Beta-hydroxy Acid Peel

Beta-hydroxy acids (BHAs) are lipophilic compounds that penetrate the pilosebaceous units. Salicylic acid is a lipid soluble BHA with anti-inflammatory and anesthetic effects. It is a crystalline carboxyl acid and chemically known as 2-hydroxybenzoic acid. It has exfoliative and comedolytic activity. It is prepared by treating sodium phenolate with carbon at high temperature and pressure. Acidification with sulfuric acid gives salicylic acid.[10]

Trichloroacetic Acid

Trichloroacetic acid (TCA) is obtained as hygroscopic, anhydrous white crystals. Because of the hygroscopic nature of the molecule, it has to be stored in a cool and dry environment. Its molecular structure resembles glycolic acid. It is a much stronger acid with lowest pKa among all the acids used currently. The clinical effects of TCA are predominantly due to acidity of the molecule. When applied to the skin, it leads to coagulation of skin proteins. Its action is proportional to the concentration and amount of acid applied.[11] The visual changes that are seen following TCA application indicate the degree of coagulation.

Phenol

Phenol, also called as phenic acid or hydroxybenzene, is an aromatic alcohol. It is a weak acid with pKa 9-9.5. It has a hydroxyl group directly attached to the carbon atom in the benzene ring. It has a melting point of 41°C and boiling point of 182°C. It is soluble in ethanol and ether.[12]

A detailed knowledge of the chemical peels, points out that acidity of the peeling agents is not the only mechanism of action responsible for the clinical effects. They also induce metabolic effects on cell synthesis and structure, in particular the AHAs peels and retinoic acid peels. Chemicals that exert mainly caustic effects include phenol and resorcinol. Thus, a better understanding of the chemical properties of the chemical peels aids in optimum use while minimizing the side effects.

TECHNICAL VARIABLES WHILE APPLYING PEELS

Factors that affect peel penetration include the following:
- *Chemical peel used*: Chemical peels have been classified according to the depth of penetration as superficial, medium and deep chemical peels. Choice of the peel is of utmost importance as this will influence the depth of penetration of the molecule. Medium and deep peels are to be avoided in dark-skinned patients as they carry risk of postinflammatory hyperpigmentation[13]

- *Concentration of the peel used*: Increasing concentration of the molecule also influences the depth of penetration. Glycolic acid at low concentration of 5–10% has action limited to the topmost layer of the skin and can be used daily by most people. At medium concentration of 10–50%, it causes temporary skin smoothening and dyscohesion between keratinocytes. At even higher concentration of 50–70%, it causes splitting between the cells and can even function as a medium-depth peel[14]
- *Technique of application*: The dermatologist should standardize his/her method of application of the chemical peel. Factors such as the pressure applied, has profound effect on the depth of penetration of the peel
- *Number of coats applied*: More number of coats increases the concentration and eventually the peel depth
- *Prior skin priming*: Prior priming of the skin aids in uniform penetration of the chemical peel. Retinoids have been shown to reduce the thickness of the skin, allowing better penetration[15]
- *Prepeel preparation*: Degreasing the skin with acetone allows uniform peel penetration by defatting the skin
- *Skin type*: Sensitive skin such as that damaged by previous topical steroid use or with concomitant rosacea is more prone to chemical burn following chemical peeling due to increased penetration of these agents in the already thinned skin
- *Duration of contact with the peel*: Peels that do not self-neutralize such as glycolic acid, have increased penetration with time
- *Anatomic site of the peel*: Sensitive areas, such as around the eyes and mouth, are more prone to post peel burn due to the thin skin in these anatomical locations.

CONCLUSION

It is important for all peelers to know the technical variables of their chemical peels to attain a successful outcome. For a beginner, it is best to start with a monopeel with a lower concentration and then build up to a higher concentrations gradually.

REFERENCES

1. Henderson L. Concerning the relationship between the strength of acids and their capacity to preserve neutrality. Am J Physiol. 1908;21(4):173-9.
2. Kortum G, Vogel W, Andrussow K. Dissociation constants of organic acids in aqueous solution. London: Butterworths; 1961.
3. Perrin DD. Dissociation constants of inorganic acids. London: Butterworths; 1969.
4. Hornby M, Peach JM. Foundations of organic chemistry. Oxford: Oxford University Press; 1991.
5. Howard P, Meylan W. Handbook of Physical Properties of Organic Chemicals. Boca Raton: CRC/Lewis Publishers; 1997.
6. Pavia DL, Lampman GM, Kriz GS. Organic chemistry. Mason, OH: South-Western Cengage Learning; 2004.
7. According to Vancouver style Van Scott EJ, Yu RJ. Alpha hydroxy acids: therapeutic potentials. Can J Dermatol. 1989;1:108-12.
8. According to Vancouver Style Van Scott EJ, Yu RJ. Control of keratinization with alphahydroxy acids and related compounds: (I. Topical treatment of ichthyotic disorders.). Arch Dermatol. 1974;110:586-90.
9. Bernstein EF, Underhill CB, Lakkakorpi J, et al. Citric acid increases viable epidermal thickness and glycosaminoglycan content of sun-damaged skin. Dermatol Surg. 1997;23:689-94.
10. Imayama S, Ueda S, Isoda M. Histologic changes in the skin of hairless mice following peeling with salicylic acid. Arch Dermatol. 2000;136:1390-5.
11. Monhet GD. The Jessner's-trichloroacetic acid peel. An enhanced medium-depth chemical peel. Dermatol Clin. 1995;13:277-83.
12. Brown AM, Kaplan LM, Brown ME. Phenol induced histological skin changes: hazards, techniques and users. Br J Plast Surg. 1960;13:158.
13. Litton C, Trinidad G. Complications of chemical face peeling as evaluated by a questionnaire. Plast Reconstr Surg. 1981;67:738-44.
14. Ditre CM. Glycolic acid peels. Dermatol Ther. 2000;13:165-72.
15. Khunger N, Sarkar R, Jain RK. Tretinoin peels versus glycolic acid peels in the treatment of melasma in dark-skinned patients. Dermatol Surg. 2004;30:756-60.

Priming, Prepeel and Postpeel Care

Rashmi Sarkar, Sneha Ghunawat

INTRODUCTION

Skin priming can be divided into two phases—(1) pretreatment; (2) preparation.

The aim of the above two phases is to thin the epidermal barrier, to achieve uniform penetration of the active agent, to accelerate the healing process and thereby reduce post-operative complications. It also aids in assessing patient compliance and tolerance to the pre and postpeel regimen. Priming also helps prepare the patient mentally for the procedure. Regular use of the pretreatment medications enforces the habits necessary for safe and efficacious postpeel healing. Agents used in the pretreatment phase include hydroquinone, tretinoin, salicylic acid, kojic acid, retinol, glycolic acid, azelaic acid and lactic acid.[1] These agents are to be accompanied by the use of a broad spectrum sunscreen (ultraviolet A or ultraviolet B) with minimum sun protection factor (SPF) of 30. Sunscreen reduces background hyperpigmentation and the risk of postpeel hyperpigmentation. Adequately primed skin will frost uniformly and rapidly as compared to unprimed skin. The goal of the preparation phase is to ensure even application of the peeling agent, achieve the desired depth of penetration and to reduce patient pain and discomfort.[2]

Priming of the skin with topical agents is to be done at least 2–4 weeks before the procedure. The topical agents used in priming of the skin before a peel are listed below.

Hydroquinone

Hydroquinone 2–4% cream is used for skin priming in dark-skinned individuals. Higher concentration is generally employed in light-skinned individuals. Hydroquinone is an inhibitor of the enzyme tyrosinase and acts by inhibiting melanin production. It helps to decrease the risk of postinflammatory hyperpigmentation as well as maintain the results of the peel.[3]

Tretinoin

Tretinoin accelerates epidermal proliferation. Concentrations ranging from 0.025–0.05% is used in patients with darker skin while a concentration of 0.1% is used in fair-skinned patients. It decreases the thickness of the stratum corneum and corneocyte adhesion, redistributes epidermal melanin and stimulates new collagen production.[4] Tretinoin is to be discontinued several days prior to the procedure. It is resumed postprocedure once the skin peeling and irritation subsides.

In a study by Nanda et al. comparing the efficacy of 2% hydroquinone versus 0.025% tretinoin as priming agents with 20–30% trichloroacetic acid (TCA) peels concluded that the group receiving hydroquinone showed significantly better results at 12–24 weeks and during maintenance compared to the one on hydroquinone.[5] In another study by Garg et al., results were better in the group receiving 2% hydroquinone at 3, 6 and 12 months compared to 0.025% tretinoin and glycolic acid peel alone.[6] Even after stopping the chemical peeling, the maintenance of the results was better in the hydroquinone group.

Since tretinoin also causes epidermal thinning, it leads to increased peel penetration, thus increasing the chances of postinflammatory hyperpigmentation in dark-skinned individuals. It may also lead to new pigment production by inducing inflammation, thus further increasing the risk of postinflammatory pigmentation. This leads to the conclusion that tretinoin use as a priming agent may carry a risk of postinflammatory hyperpigmentation, especially in the dark-skinned patients.

Glycolic Acid

Glycolic acid is used in a concentration of 8–10% in the prepeel period to prime the skin. It acts by its exfoliative effect. At low concentration, it reduces keratinocyte adhesion; at higher concentrations, superficial to deep peeling can be expected.[7] Pretreatment for 2–3 weeks helps to thin the epidermis and prepare it for the peel. In patients with hyperkeratotic lesions such as actinic keratosis, it helps to increase penetration of the peeling agent. Glycolic acid, however, does not have much effect on the incidence of postinflammatory hyperpigmentation.[8]

Others

Other agents such as salicylic acid, kojic acid, lactic acid, arbutin, licorice etc., also can be used in the prepeel priming phase.

PREPEEL CARE

- *Degreasing agents:* Alcohol, acetone or a combination of these is used to degrease the skin prior to the peel. The amount, force of application and the time of application have an impact on the depth and uniformity of the peel
- *Topical anesthetics:* The purpose of using topical anesthetics is in the pain control as well as skin hydration. The improved skin hydration aids in uniform peeling
- *Fluorescent additives:* Acids with florescent additives such as fluorescein sodium or salicylic acid with Wood's lamp visualization ensures even coverage of the treated areas. It helps to avoid the skip areas. Glycolic acid compounded with fluorescein sodium is commercially available.[9] It requires a windowless or tightly shuttered room, in order to be of value. Although, it is not used in routine practice
- *Depth-enhancing agents:* Jessner's solution, glycolic acid and solid CO_2 promote even penetration of the acid and facilitate uniformity of the depth. These agents have proven to be effective when combined with TCA to give a more reproducible peel.

POSTPEEL CARE

Postpeel care is of utmost importance to the patient, as much as the prepeel care and the steps of peeling. Proper instructions in this period help to decrease the incidence of complications such as postinflammatory hyperpigmentation.

- *Broad-spectrum sunscreen:* Use of a broad-spectrum sunscreen having a minimum SPF of 30 is to be applied by the patient every 3-4 hourly. It blocks the effect of ultraviolet rays on the healing skin and reduces the incidence of pigmentation
- *Bland moisturizer:* Use of bland moisturizers in the postpeel period decreases skin dryness and sensitivity. Fragrance-free products carry minimal risk of contact allergic reactions
- *Mild cleansers:* Mild soap-free cleansers are recommended during the postpeel phase. They help to reduce the incidence of drying and contact sensitization
- *Cool water or ice compresses:* Cooling of the skin in the immediate postpeel period helps to soothe the skin
- *Avoid scratching:* Strict advice against scratching of skin should be given to all patients. Scratching induces skin trauma and increasing local inflammation giving rise to risk of postinflammatory hyperpigmentation. Moisturizers and antihistamines will help.

TAKE HOME POINTS

- Skin priming is done at least 2-4 weeks prior to the procedure
- Multiple benefits of skin priming include:
  - Rapid and uniform peel penetration
  - Rapid wound healing and re-epithelialization
  - Reduce the risk of postprocedure complications such as postinflammatory hyperpigmentation.
- Priming enforces the habit of postpeel care and mentally prepares the patient for the procedure
- Tretinoin carries a risk of postinflammatory hyperpigmentaion in dark-skinned individuals.

REFERENCES

1. Rubin MG. What are skin peels? In: Winters SR, James M, Caputo GR (Eds). Manual of Chemical Peels: Superficial and Medium Depth, 1st edition. Philadelphia: JB Lippincott Co.; 1995. pp. 17-25.
2. Monheit GD, Kayal JD. Chemical peeling. In: Nouri K, Leal Khouri S (Eds). Techniques in Dermatologic Surgery, 1st edition. St. Louis: Mosby; 2004. pp. 233-44.
3. Monheit G. Commentary. Efficacy of hydroquinone (2%) versus tretinoin (0.025%) as adjunct topical agents for chemical peeling in patients of melasma. Dermatol Surg. 2004;30:385-9.
4. Khunger N, Sarkar R, Jain RK. Tretinoin peels versus glycolic acid peels in the treatment of melasma in dark-skinned patients. Dermatol Surg. 2004;30:756-60.
5. Nanda S, Grover C, Reddy BS. Efficacy of hydroquinone (2%) versus tretinoin (0.025%) as adjunct topical agents for chemical peeling in patients of melasma. Dermatol Surg. 2004;30:385-9.
6. Garg VK, Sarkar R, Agarwal R. Comparative evaluation of beneficiary effects of priming agents (2% hydroquinone and 0.025% retinoic acid) in the treatment of melasma with glycolic acid peels. Dermatol Surg. 2008;34.1032-40.
7. Murad H, Shamban AT, Premo PS. The use of glycolic acid as a peeling agent. Dermatol Clin. 1995;13(2): 285-307.
8. Tung RC, Bergfeld WF, Vidimos AT, et al. Alpha-hydroxy acid-based cosmetic procedures. Guidelines for patient management. Am J Clin Dermatol. 2000;1(2): 81-8.
9. Sharad J. Glycolic acid peel therapy – a current review. Clin Cosmet Investig Dermatol. 2013;6:281-8.

6
CHAPTER

Patient Assessment and Counseling

Sneha Ghunawat, Rashmi Sarkar

INTRODUCTION

Chemical peeling is a procedure done very commonly in the dermatology office. Although the procedure is safe and does not cause much problems, yet, some complications can even occur under expert hands. Most of the complications can be prevented by carefully selecting the patients, proper patient counseling and good pre- and postpeel care of the patients. Some of the points to consider while selecting patients for chemical peel are highlighted in this chapter.

Chemical peel is a method of inducing a controlled wound to the skin thereby further inducing the process of collagen remodelling leading to an improvement in skin texture. Based on the level of the wound, they can be classified into superficial (penetrate up to epidermis), medium (epidermis, papillary dermis and upper reticular dermis) and deep peel (mid-reticular dermis). The correct peel for a patient is dependent on the indication for which it is being done.

HISTORY

To minimize complications, it is of utmost importance to choose patients wisely. This process includes extensive history and careful clinical examination. Important points to be elicitated in the history include history of infections such as herpes simplex virus, human immunodeficiency virus (HIV) status, previous procedures resulting in keloid formation, past or present history of isotretinoin use history of concurrent intake of photosensitizing drugs, previous X-ray therapy, history of nicotine use, and past history of facial surgeries. Patients with past history of recurrent outbreaks of herpes infection need to be started on prophylactic antivirals to prevent an outbreak of the infection. Patients infected with HIV virus are poor candidates for peeling as wound healing is slow in these individuals, increasing the risk of wound infection and scarring. The risk of delayed wound healing and subsequent scarring is also increased in candidates with recent (within 6 months of stopping the drug) history of isotretinoin intake.[1] But, this is more pertinent for medium-depth and deep peels. Some evidence in the literature points that isotretinoin inhibits wound healing. Eliciting good drug history is of utmost importance, and it may be a cause of untoward complications later. Use of photosensitizing drugs such as minocycline, amiodarone, thiazide, etc., increases the risk of pigmentary complications following the procedure. Exposure of the skin to X-ray radiation has been shown to destroy pilosebaceous glands resulting in poor epithelialization following the procedure. Patients with thick sebaceous skin can tolerate deeper peels well as compared with those having thinner and dryer skin.[2] Patients with history of atopy are more sensitive to peels. Candidates with history of smoking also qualify for increased risk and poor outcome following the peeling procedure due to decreased blood supply to the skin. Nicotine is a potent vasoconstrictor, and thus it is advisable to discontinue smoking at least 2 weeks before a deep peel. Patients who have recently undergone facial surgeries should wait for 6 months before taking a session of peeling as these procedures compromise the blood supply of the skin. Previous resurfacing procedures increase scarring potential following deep peels.

The most important discussion to have with the patient is regarding the realistic expectation. The treatment options, the healing time, risk of complications and anticipated results are to be discussed with the patient in detail. It is important to discuss with the patient the reason for choosing a particular peel, alternative treatment that is available and possible range of complications of the particular peel. It is a good idea to sit with the patient and discuss the problems of the patient as perceived by him or her. They may be given a mirror to point out the specific areas of concern. A well-educated patient must be able to understand the risk involved in the procedure as well as be able to identify the risk factors in his/her history and examination that pose an increased risk of complication. To make it simple for the patient, it is important to make them understand the four-peels classes, i.e., very superficial, superficial, medium-depth, and deep peels, and the expectant risks and results. Superficial peels are used in acne, pigmentary abnormalities and textural irregularities. They do not have a significant downtime and carry very low risk of complications. However, the noticeable improvement noted with these peels is minimal. This is important for the patient to understand as they might feel that the peel is not working. Medium-depth peels can be described as resulting in significant downtime and thus more risk of complications such as postinflammatory hyperpigmentation. These complications are, however, transient and possibility of more serious adverse events such as scarring and permanent pigmentary complication is remote. These peels, however, result in more noticeable improvement in the patient's condition. Deeper peels such as phenol carry increased risk of complications. Patients with darker skin are poor candidates for deep peels and and thus such peels are avoided in them. Patients planned for deep peels need to be evaluated for some more details before the procedure.[3,4] History of hypertrophic scarring, dark-skinned patients, underlying medical problems, recent facial surgeries and heavy smokers are at higher risk of developing complications and should be counseled against undergoing the procedure.

A good history is incomplete without mentioning the personal habits and home care regimen of the patient. Patients who habitually excoriate need to be identified before as this habit may lead to some unwanted results. It is imperative to note down all the topical medications that the patient has used and ones that he/she is currently using. Use of cleansing products, waxing, electrolysis, hair plucking, etc., done in immediate pre or postoperative period may adversely affect the outcome following the peel.[5] Simple scrubbing for removing makeup may lead to unexpected deeper peel penetration. The nature of the patients' occupation as well as his/her hobbies would aid the physician in gauging averagely the amount of time the patient is under the sun. Patients with a history of prolonged exposure in the sun are at risk of developing postinflammatory hyperpigmentation. Patient should also be asked about the use of sunscreen as a part of their routine skin care regimen. At this time, the importance of using a sunscreen after chemical peeling should be re-stressed to the patient. Use of a topical retinoid should be stopped at least 3 days before the chemical peel. Retinoids thin the skin and may adversely affect the outcome.[6] However, in the experience of the authors, stopping the retinoid even a day prior is relatively devoid of any untoward adverse events.

CLINICAL EXAMINATION

A thorough history is supplemented by careful examination by the physician to choose the appropriate treatment option. The most important factor in assessing the skin response to any peeling agent is the skin type of the patient and degree of photo damage. Glogau photoaging classification is used to assess the degree of photodamage (Box 1).[3] Patients with Glogau type I skin are likely to benefit from superficial peels while those with type IV skin benefit from deep peels. This classification is practical for use in the office setting. Another classification that is useful during prepeel assessment is Fitzpatrick's classification of sun-reactive skin types (Table 1). This classification helps to predict how patients' pigmentation will respond to a specific chemical peel. Patients with Fitzpatrick's skin type III-V have to be cautioned regarding the increased risk of postinflammatory hyperpigmentation. The physician should also note the oiliness of the skin before the peeling session begins. The skin that has an excessive activity of the sebaceous glands needs more thorough degreasing before the peeling. This increases the depth of penetration of the peel agent and also ensures uniform penetration.

BOX 1 Glogau classification of photoaging

Type I: No wrinkles
Early photoaging
- Mild pigmentary changes
- No keratosis
- Minimal wrinkles

Younger patient: 20s–30s
Minimal or no makeup

Type II: Wrinkles in motion
Early-to-moderate photoaging
- Early senile lentigines visible
- Keratosis palpable but not visible
- Parallel smile lines beginning to appear lateral to the mouth

Patient age: Late 30s or 40s
Usually wears some foundation

Type III: Wrinkles at rest
Advanced photoaging
- Obvious dyschromia
- Visible keratoses
- Wrinkles even when not moving

Patient age: 50s or older
Always wears heavy foundation

Type IV: Only wrinkles
Severe photoaging
- Yellow gray skin color
- Prior skin malignancies
- Wrinkled throughout, no normal skin

Patient age: 60s–70s
Cannot wear makeup – cakes and craks

TABLE 1: Fitzpatrick's classification of skin types

Skin type	Color	Reaction to first summer exposure
I	White	Always burn, never tan
II	White	Usually burn, tan with difficulty
III	White	Sometimes mild burn, tan average
IV	Moderate brown	Rarely burn, tan with ease
V	Dark brown	Very rarely burn, tan very easily
VI	Black	No burn, tan very easily

Patient Assessment and Counseling

> **BOX 2** Table postulating the contraindications for chemical peels
>
> **Absolute**
> - History of hypertrophic or keloidal scarring
> - Recent facial surgeries that may lead to vascular compromise
>
> **Relative**
> - Underlying serious medical condition
> - History of radiation exposure
> - Recent history of isotretinoin intake
> - Pregnancy
> - Photosensitizing medications
> - Fitzpatrick skin type IV–VI
> - History of herpes simplex infection

Also a meticulous inspection for the presence of any inflammatory skin lesions should be noted prior to the start of the peeling session. Inflammatory skin tends to increase the penetration of the peeling agent due to vasodilatation and increased inflammatory mediators in the skin area. The increased absorption of the peeling agent may lead to a deeper wound than intended and thus run a risk of scarring and hyperpigmentation. The presence of psoriasis or lichen planus lesions may lead to Koebner's phenomenon.[7]

Meticulous physical examination is of utmost importance. It is wise to inspect for a previously healed burn or a surgical scar, which may thereby suggest the tendency for keloid formation and other pigmentary abnormalities that the patient may be predisposed to.[8] Box 2 lists the contraindications for chemical peeling.

INFORMED CONSENT

The importance of taking an informed consent cannot be underestimated. Every clinic may have its own consent form. An example of a consent form is given in appendix 1. A detailed discussion with the patient regarding the indication, risks and precautions involved in the procedure is of utmost importance.[9] It also helps in establishing a good doctor-patient relationship. A patient who understands the rationale for which a particular peel is being utilized along with the warning signs and complications that may follow, is the ideal candidate for the peel procedure.

TEST PEEL

Any patient planned for peeling should ideally undergo a test peel. This gives a good opportunity to the physician to assess the likelihood of any postpeel complications/side effects and also instills confidence in the patient to continue with future sessions. The site for the test peel is usually an area that is easily concealed such as the retroauricular area. Test peel gives the physician a chance to look for common complications such as prolonged erythema, hypo or hyperpigmentation and counsel the patient accordingly. Prolonged erythema is often an indicator to the risk of developing a pigmentary complication. For test peel procedures, in our experience a small amount of solution is applied over the retroauricular area for 5 minutes or till burning and stinging occurs.[10] The patch is neutralized and the site is inspected after a week.

It is of prime importance to take baseline and postpeel photographs. Even taking a few photographs during the procedure is ideal, as it can act as a self-educating tool to note the chronology of skin changes after a particular peeling formulation. Both front and side views of the patient at a specified distance with adequate lighting are taken to highlight any textural irregularity, wrinkles and scars over the face. Patients should be shown their respective photographs taken serially in an effort to display the gradual course of improvement and thereby enhance the doctor-patient relationship. Also, at any point of time, if the physician feels that there is a lack of improvement and thus further peeling sessions ought to be discontinued, then such should be clearly discussed with the patient.

WARNING SIGNS

It is important to make the patient aware of some of the important postpeel warning signs. Most common among these is the development of postpeel erythema. Its occurrence is dependent on the depth of the peel. The usual duration for postpeel erythema after a superficial peel is 3-5 days; medium-depth peel is 15-30 days and deeper peel 60-90 days. If the duration of erythema exceeds these periods, it may indicate delayed peeling and risk of scarring.[11,12] Other factors associated with development of prolonged erythema include exacerbation of preexisting skin disease, contact hypersensitivity and sensitive skin. If erythema is associated with induration on palpation, it may herald development of scarring. Such a patient should be started on potent topical steroids immediately and should be kept under observation.

Pruritus may be present as a normal consequence of the healing process. It is more common with medium-depth and deep peels. It is commonly managed with reassurance, topical steroids, oral antihistamines and moisturizers. If pruritus is severe, one should suspect contact sensitization and if it is associated with occurrence of pustules, it may herald an infection.[13]

Pain may commonly accompany medium or deep peel procedures. Pain following a medium-depth peel is transient and does not require analgesic medication. Analgesics and ice can be used to alleviate it. That occurring after a deep peel resolves in 8-12 hours. Persistent severe pain may herald eruption of herpes simplex.

Acne-prone patients should be warned regarding an outbreak of acne following chemical peel. This can be either due to the healing phase of the skin or due to the use of occlusive emollients after the procedure. These eruptions resolve in about a week but can also be managed with the use of oral antibiotics (avoid topical therapy as it may irritate the healing skin).[14] The authors commonly use 20% azelaic acid cream intermittently between peels and have also used salicylic acid peels for the eruptions.[15]

Telangiectasias start becoming visible as the skin starts lightening postpeels. This may occur due to lighter pigmentation following a peel. Patients should be made aware of this possibility beforehand. If the telangiectasias are bothersome to the patient, then they can be managed using vascular lasers.

Edema is a common sequela following medium or deep peels. It usually subsides without causing much alarm to the patient. However, following deeper peels, edema may be severe enough to warrant oral corticosteroids. Severe edema after a peel may also leave behind areas of ecchymosis, especially in the infraorbital area.

Occurrence of milia may be noted in patients 2-3 weeks following re-epithelialization. This may be due to the occlusive emollient use or following healing. Use of retinoic acid in the prepeel period reduces the occurrence of milia formation.[14]

Lines of demarcation may be noticed following medium or deep peels especially at the jaw and neck. These may become a cause of concern for the patient. Feathering the edges of the peel and peeling the earlobes is a good practice to avoid such an occurrence.[16] Box 3 lists the common sequelae following chemical peeling.

BOX 3	Minor sequelae following chemical peel
• Pain	• Acne/milia
• Erythema	• Edema
• Pruritus	

CONCLUSION

Chemical peeling is a safe, simple, and effective procedure done in the dermatology setup. Complications are minimal in well-trained hands. An in-depth knowledge about the nature of the peeling agent, the risks involved and adequate counseling are all important points a physician must consider before commencing the peel procedure.

TAKE HOME POINTS

- Detailed history should be noted to identify patients at risk of developing complications. Patients with history of keloidal scarring and recent facial surgery should be discouraged from undergoing the procedure. Patients with recent radiation exposure, isotretinoin intake, and dark-skinned patients should be counseled about higher risk of developing complications
- Note of the personal habits and skincare regimen is to be made. Patients with the habit of skin picking should be warned about risk of developing pigmentary abnormalities. Use of scrubs, waxing and epilation should be discouraged in the peripeel period
- Stringent use of sunscreen should be stressed upon to the patient. Those predominantly involved in outdoor activities are poor candidates for medium-depth or deep peels
- A thorough physical examination to look for old burn marks and scars may give a clue to the tendency of the patient to develop hyperpigmentation or scarring following a wound
- Informed consent and serial photography in adequate illumination are of paramount importance
- Counseling regarding the nature of the treatment, risks involved in the procedure and the expectant clinical outcome should be done
- Patient should be made aware of certain warning signs such as persistent erythema, edema, pain and itching. Prior knowledge of these signs will reduce patient anxiety
- Always test peel the patient in the retroauricular area prior to commencing a full-face peel. This would help to observe the healing process and identify patients at risk of complications
- Emphasize the importance of postpeel care to the patient. Strict sun protection and use of broad-spectrum sunscreen are a must. Patients should avoid travel outside their respective cities ideally 7 days after a superficial peel and 14 days after a medium or deep peel.

REFERENCES

1. Brody HJ. Complications of chemical resurfacing. Dermatol Clin. 2001;19:427-37.
2. Matarasso SL. Skin characteristics that affect peel penetration. Dermatol Clin. 1997;15(4):569-82.
3. Matarasso SL, Matarasso A. Analysis and treatment of the aging face. Dermatol Clin. 1997;15(4):549.
4. Monheit GD. Fundamentals of cosmetic surgery. Dermatol Clin. 2001;19(3).
5. Rubin M. Manual of Chemical Peels. Philadelphia: JB Lippincott; 1995.
6. Khunger N. Standard guidelines of care for chemical peels. Indian J Dermatol Venereol Leprol. 2008;74:S5-12.
7. Duffy DM. Avoiding complications with chemical peels. In: Rubin MG (Ed.) Procedures in Cosmetic Dermatology Series: Chemical Peels. Amsterdam: Elsevier Inc.; 2006. pp. 137-70.
8. Resnik SS, Resnik BI. Complications of chemical peeling. Dermatol Clin. 1995;13:309-12.
9. Duffy DM. Informed consent for chemical peels and dermabrasion. Dermatol Clin. 1989;7:183-9.

10. Duffy DM. Alpha hydroxy acids/trichloroacetic acids risk/benefit strategies. Dermatologic Surgery 1998;24(2):181-91.
11. Briden ME. Alpha-hydroxyacid chemical peeling agents: Case studies and rationale for safe and effective use. Cutis. 2004;73:18-24.
12. Tung RC, Bergfeld WF, Vidimos AT, et al. Alpha-hydroxy acid based cosmetic procedures. Guidelines for patient management. Am J Clin Dermatol. 2000;1:81-8.
13. Baker TM. Chemical and lasers for skin resurfacing. Aesthetic Surg. 1999;19:325-7.
14. Hevia O, Nemeth AL, Taylor JR. Tretinoin accelerates healing after trichloroacetic acid chemical peel. Arch Dermatol. 1991;127:678-82.
15. Bari AU, Iqbal Z, Rahman SB. Tolerance and safety of superficial chemical peeling with salicylic acid in various facial dermatoses. Indian J Dermatol Venereol Leprol. 2005;71:87-90.
16. Rendon MI, Berson DS, Cohen JL, et al. Evidence and considerations in the application of chemical peels in skin disorders and aesthetic resurfacing. J Clin Aesthet Dermatol. 2010;3:32-43.

CHAPTER 7

Glycolic Acid Peels

Shankila Mittal, Rashmi Sarkar, Sneha Ghunawat

INTRODUCTION

Alpha-hydroxy acids (AHAs) are carboxylic acids derived from various fruits such as glycolic (sugarcane), malic (apples), tartaric (grapes), citric (citrus), mandelic (almonds), lactic (milk), and phytic (rice) acids, thus also called fruit peels.[1]

They are also called lunchtime peels due to quick recovery time and minimum disfigurement.

Alpha-hydroxy acids have been used since ancient times for rejuvenation like sour milk (containing lactic acid) which was applied by Cleopatra and old wine (containing tartaric acid) utilized by French women.[2] However, AHAs used in practice are synthesized chemically.

Glycolic acid (GA) is the most commonly used AHA because it penetrates the skin easily and has the smallest molecular weight. GA acts as very superficial, superficial and medium-depth peels, and can be used for all skin types.

PHARMACOLOGY AND CHEMICAL STRUCTURE

Alpha-hydroxy acids are carboxylic acids with a hydroxyl group on the adjacent (or α) carbon.

Glycolic acid is the smallest AHA with two carbon molecules—one with carboxyl group and other with hydroxyl group.

Properties

- *Structure*:
- *Chemical name*: Hydroxyacetic acid
- *Formula*: $C_2H_4O_3$ (or $HOCH_2CO_2H$)
- Monoprotic metabolic acid (pKa = 3.83)
- *Appearance*: White crystals, colorless, and odorless
- *Solubility*: Water (highly soluble), acetone, alcohol and acetic acid
- *Extracted*: Sugarcane
- Chemically synthesized by passage of carbon monoxide through formaldehyde solution
- pH of pure aqueous solution (at saturated concentration of 80%): 0.5.[3]

According to Henderson–Hasselbalch equation:

$$pH = pK_a + \log([A^-]/[HA])$$

[A^-] = Molar concentration of a conjugate base

[HA] = Molar concentration of an undissociated weak acid (M)

Unbuffered GA has pH 0.5 (which is <pKa) which consists mainly of acid and on gradual

Chemical Peels: A Global Perspective

TABLE 1: Formulations of glycolic acid

Formulation	Properties	Remarks
Free acid	• Aqueous acidic non-neutralized solution • pH range: 0.6 (70% GA) to 1.7 (20% GA)	• Greater reactivity and bioavailability • Greater burning and stinging • Can lead to epidermolysis • More effective
Partially neutralized	• Combines acid with base (e.g., ammonium hydroxide) • pH higher (mean: 3.8)	• Less irritating, safer • Can have longer contact time
Buffered	Resists pH change on addition of acid or alkali	No practical benefit
Esterified	When ester bond forms between carboxyl group of glycolic acid and -OH group of citric acid—glycol citrate solution forms	• Said to be less irritating • Needs further evidence
Gel based	Less free acid which is released slowly, slower penetration	• Less irritating • Less effective • Can be used for sensitive skin or rosacea

GA, glycolic acid.

addition of base, pH of the solution increases such that at half neutralization (i.e., pH = pKa) a solution with 50% GA and salt is obtained. Higher the concentration and lower the pH, more is the peeling effect.

The action of GA is time dependent; it must be terminated by application of water or a neutralizing agent to discontinue its effect. Unneutralized, it may penetrate the dermis and lead to variable healing, crusting and even scarring. Buffered and partially neutralized solutions with a higher pH must be left on the skin longer than pure aqueous 70% GA to achieve the same clinical effects (erythema and peeling).

Various formulations of GA peel are available (Table 1).

CLASSIFICATION OF GLYCOLIC ACID PEELS

Classification of GA peels based on depth is as given in table 2.[4]

TABLE 2: Classification of glycolic acid peel

Depth of peel	Concentration (%)	Time of application (min)
Very superficial	30–50	1–2
Superficial	50–70	2–5
Medium	70	3–15

MECHANISM OF ACTION

Action of GA varies with the pH.[1]
- At higher pH (pH > pKa), it acts as a moisturizer due to presence of salt with moisturizing effect
- At lower pH (pH < pKa), it acts as a keratoregulator. It causes lysis of corneodesmosomes leading to skin exfoliation.

It has a dual mode of action acting at both epidermal and dermal levels.[5-7]

Epidermal Effects

Glycolic acid causes lysis of corneodesomosomes at acidic pH and low concentration.

Topical application of GA leads to:
- Acidification of skin which increases epidermal activity of lipases, phosphatases and transforming growth factor (TGF)-beta
- Decrease in epidermal calcium ion concentration leading to loss of calcium ions from cell junctions and desquamation
- Interference with the working of enzymes responsible for corneocyte adhesion.

Due to the disruption of epidermal barrier, a cascade of secondary events lead to stimulation of the basal layer of the epidermis, which accelerates conversion of keratinocytes into corneocytes leading to regulation of epidermal thickness. Regulation of keratinization leads to smoother skin and decreases dryness.

Also, desquamation of corneocytes from follicular orifices prevents follicular occlusion and leads to improvement in acne. Higher concentrations can reduce melanin synthesis by direct inhibition of tyrosinase.

Dermal Effects

Glycolic acid stimulates fibroblast proliferation and synthesis of collagen, elastin and glycosaminoglycan (GAG) leading to dermal thickening and hydration and reduction in fine lines.

Ultimate effects of GA peel include:
- Thinning of stratum corneum
- Epidermal thickness regularization
- Synthesis of dermal collagen and ground substance
- Decreased pigmentation.

Note: GA does not cause protein coagulation, hence, there would be an absence of frosting. However, grayish discoloration can occur with higher concentrations due to epidermolysis and is a sign of excessive peeling. It has to be neutralized with water or sodium bicarbonate to stop its action. Longer the contact time, deeper is the peel, thus the effect of a GA peel relies heavily on the total time it is left on the skin.

Various advantages and disadvantages of the GA peel are provided in table 3.

TABLE 3: Advantages and disadvantages of glycolic acid peel

Advantages of glycolic acid peel	Disadvantages of glycolic acid peel
- Inexpensive - Appropriate for all Fitzpatrick skin types - Useful in photodamage - Multiple conditions treated simultaneously - Epidermal and dermal improvement - Appropriate for body peel - Mild desquamation - Shorter downtime	- Require multiple treatments to achieve benefits - Cannot remove scars, only lessen their appearance - Neutralization is mandatory

INDICATIONS OF GLYCOLIC PEEL

- *Acne*: Comedonal acne, postacne hyperpigmentation, superficial scarring
- Melasma
- Lentigines, ephelides
- Postinflammatory hyperpigmentation (PIH)
- Dilated pores
- Fine wrinkling
- Superficial scars
- Photoaging
- Seborrhea
- Disorders of keratinization, e.g., keratosis pilaris.

Melasma

Therapeutic options for melasma include photoprotection, topical depigmenting agents, peels and lasers. A combination of modalities is often used to achieve optimum results. Chemical peels benefit in treatment of only epidermal and mixed varieties. There is a risk of complications like hypertrophic scarring, hyperpigmentation, and depigmentation if used in stronger concentration.

Serial glycolic peels at an interval of 2-3 weeks help in improvement of melasma (Figs. 1 and 2). It has been found to be safe for all skin types. The epidermal form responds the best to GA peels thereby giving optimal results; whereas, the dermal variant responds the least. Studies on GA peel and its comparison with other peels have found GA peel to be as effective (Tables 4 and 5). GA peels are the best option considering safety and efficacy and relatively provide for a greater patient satisfaction.[8]

It also shows improvement in ephelides and facial melanosis (Figs. 3 and 4).

Acne

Glycolic acid peels have a role in the management of acne (especially the comedonal variety), PIH and superficial scarring after acne.

Glycolic acid decreases corneocyte cohesion and due to its small size, it can easily penetrate into pilosebaceous units to remove the keratinous plug. It also allows for a better, faster and more efficient penetration of retinoids by decreasing epidermal cell attachment.[22] Tretinoin, when used in conjunction with chemical peels, increases the depth of treatment and exfoliation and thus should be used with due caution. The GA peel is used as adjuvant therapy in acne instead of monotherapy.[5]

Sequential GA peels have also shown improvement in acne (Fig. 5). They also improve PIH and/or coexistent melasma (Figs. 6 and 7).

Various studies have shown benefit of GA in acne, PIH, and superficial scarring (Table 6).

Postinflammatory Hyperpigmentation

Glycolic acid peel decreases PIH by its action on epidermal remodeling and turnover and direct inhibition of tyrosinase activity. GA peel enhances the penetration of other agents like hydroquinone leading to a better therapeutic response. Concentration and contact time of

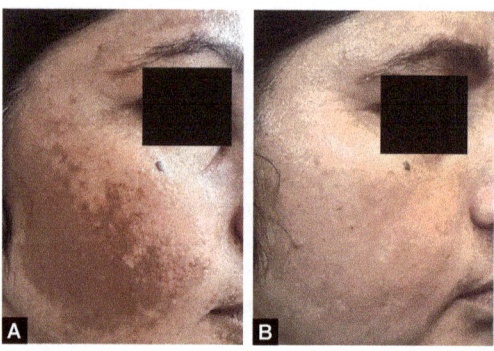

FIG. 1: Improvement in melasma on both sides of face after sequential 35–50% glycolic acid peels.

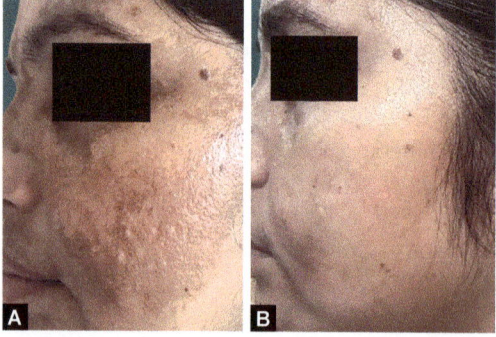

FIG. 2: Improvement in melasma on both sides of face after sequential 35–50% glycolic acid peels.

Glycolic Acid Peels

TABLE 4: Studies on glycolic acid peel in melasma

Study (Study population)	Peel used	Topical therapy, if any	Result
Lim et al.[9] (10 Asian women)	GA peel (20–70%) every 3 weeks on one side of face	Sunscreen, HQ 2% and 10% GA on both sides of face	Significant improvement in combination group
Javaheri et al.[10] (25 Indian patients)	GA 50% once a month for 3 months	Sunscreen, 10% GA	Improvement in 91%. Better improvement in epidermal than mixed group
Grover et al.[11] (15 Indian patients)	Series GA peel	–	Improvement present
Godse et al.[12] (20 Indian patients)	Series GA peel	Sunscreen and triple combination	>50% improvement in half the patients
Hurley et al.[13] (21 Hispanic women)	20–30% GA peels on one side of face	HQ 4% on both sides of face	Improvement on both sides No significant difference
Erbil et al.[14] (28 women)	Serial GA peels Control group: Only topical therapy	Azelaic acid 20% cream twice a day and adapalene 0.1% gel bedtime	Significant difference in improvement in GA peel group
Rendon et al.[15] (20 patients)	Six 2-week cycles of topical cream and 5 GA peels	Triple-combination (fluocinolone acetonide 0.01%, HQ 4%, and tretinoin 0.05%)	>90% showed improvement by 12 week with alternating sequential treatment and was well tolerated

GA, glycolic acid; HQ, hydroquinone.

TABLE 5: Studies comparing glycolic acid peel with other peels for melasma

Study (No. of patients)	Group A	Group B	Result
Sarkar et al.[16] (90 patients)	35% GA	• Group B: SM peel • Group C: Phytic combination peels	• Decrease in MASI in all groups • GA and SM acid peels equally effective and more effective than phytic acid peel
Kalla et al.[17] (100 patients)	55–75% GA	10–15% TCA	Response faster in TCA but relapse and PIH more in this group
Sarkar et al.[18] (40 Indian patients of epidermal melasma)	GA peels with modified Kligman's formula	Modified Kligman's formula	MASI decreased in both but results faster in group A
Khunger et al.[19] (10 Indian patients)	70% GA peel on one side	1% tretinoin peel on other side	Improvement in both, no difference in group A and B
Kumari et al.[20] (40 Indian women)	20–35% GA peel	10–20% TCA peel	• Good response in both groups • GA peel fewer side effects than TCA
Puri et al.[21] (30 women)	35% TCA peel	15% TCA peel	• Both equally effective • Side effects more with TCA peel

GA, glycolic acid; MASI, melasma area and severity index; PIH, postinflammatory hyperpigmentation; SM, salicylic–mandelic acid; TCA, trichloroacetic acid.

Chemical Peels: A Global Perspective

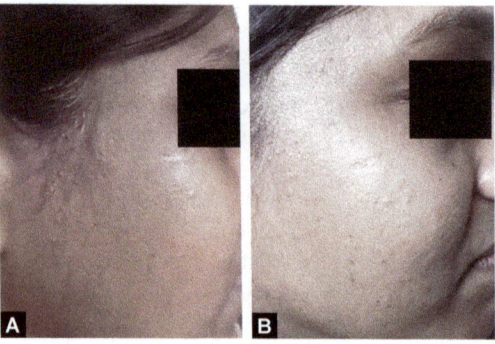

FIG. 3: Improvement in facial pigmentation with 5 sittings of 35–50% glycolic acid peels.

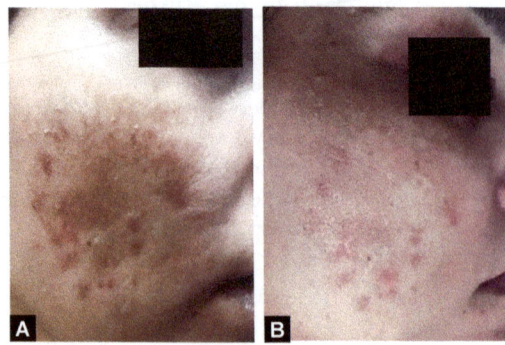

FIG. 6: Dual benefit of 50% glycolic acid peel in acne and pigmentation.

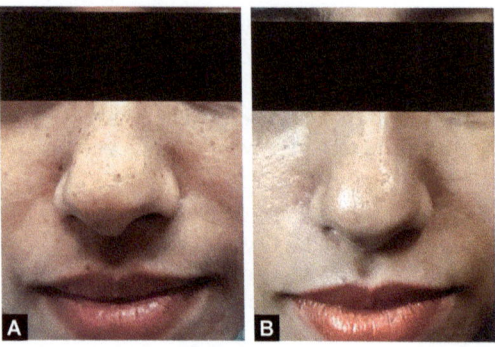

FIG. 4: Improvement in freckles after five sittings of 35–50% glycolic acid peels.

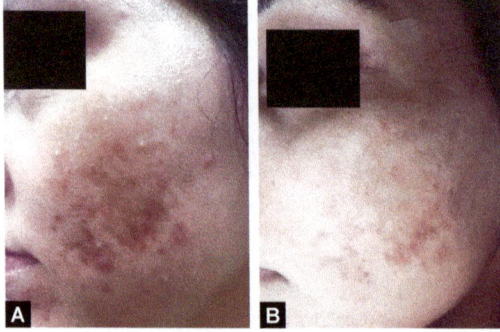

FIG. 7: Dual benefit of 50–70% glycolic acid peel in acne and pigmentation.

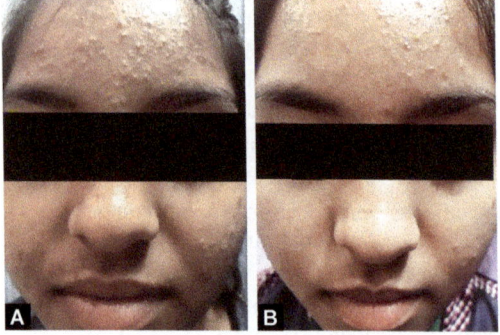

FIG. 5: Improvement in comedones after three sessions of 35% glycolic acid peel.

GA must be increased with caution in darker skin types due to risk of PIH itself. A pilot study conducted in nineteen patients with Fitzpatrick skin type IV-VI with PIH treated with a series of GA peels in addition to topical therapy found rapid and greater improvement in PIH with the peels.[26] Similar results were seen in another study with improvements in skin texture.[11]

Photoaging

Photoaging in the form of dyschromias, actinic keratoses, solar lentigines, fine wrinkling and altered texture show improvement with GA peel alone or in combination with other peels.[29] However, it does not affect deep wrinkles.

Glycolic acid increases the thickness of the viable epidermis and leads to production of glycosaminoglycans in the dermis leading to a reduction of fine lines.

TABLE 6: Studies on role of glycolic acid in acne and acne scars

Study (No. of patients)	Peel used	Results
Wang et al.[23] (40 patients)	• Group 1: 35% GA • Group 2: 50% GA • 15% GA for home care	• Improvement in comedones, papules, and pustules • Improvement of skin texture, acne scars, and cystic lesions • Follicular pores become smaller • Small percentage (5.6%) developed side effects: PIH, skin irritation, and exacerbation of herpes simplex infection
Atzori et al.[24] [80 women (13–40 years)]	70% GA	• Comedonal acne: Most rapid improvement • Papulopustular: Average 6 applications • Nodulo-cystic: Average 8–10 applications • Significant improvement of postacne superficial scarring
Kim et al.[25] (26 patients)	70% GA and Jessner's solution split face 2 weekly	• Improvement after 3 sessions in both groups • More exfoliation in Jessner's solution group • GA peel better tolerated
Grover et al.[11] [41 patients (16 acne)]	10% GA* 1–2 min. Gradually increase time and conc. to 5 min and 30%	• Good response in 75% of patients • Excellent improvement in PIH and scarring • Significant decrease in number of comedones and papulopustules • Nodulocystic acne lesions did not respond well
Kessler et al.[26] (20 patients)	30% GA and 30% SA split face 2 weekly for 6 sittings	• Both peels improved acne • SA peel had better sustained efficacy and fewer side effects than GA (due to better lipophilicity of SA) and was better tolerated than GA peels
Garg et al.[27] [44 patients (post acne scarring and PIH)]	• Group 1: 35% GA • Group 2: SM peel	• Both found to be effective • SM peel had a higher efficacy for active acne and PIH
• Erbagci et al.[28] • Group 1: 23 patients • Group 2: 20 patients • Group 3: 15 patients	• Group 1: Biweekly GA peels increasing conc. 20–70% • Group 2: 15% GA cream twice a day • Group 3: Placebo	• Statistically significant difference in results at week 24 in different groups • Home application of low-strength GA was better tolerated but repeated short-contact 70% GA peels provided superior results • 70% GA peel: Significant improvement in atrophic acne scarring

GA, glycolic acid; PIH, postinflammatory hyperpigmentation; SA, salicylic acid; SM, salicylic/mandelic acid.

The results are more evident with higher concentrations. At lower concentrations, the improvement is much slower being seen only on prolonged use.[22] GA peel can be combined with 5-fluorouracil for treatment of actinic keratosis.

Rosacea

Most physicians avoid using GA in rosacea due to potential irritation and erythema. However, a few studies have found improvement with decrease in the inflammatory process, papules, pustules and erythema.[5] GA may act by preventing attachment of *Demodex* mite in the follicle by decreasing corneocyte adhesion and its acidic pH may deplete bacterial nutrients and its number. GA peels tend to have maximum benefit for the inflammatory lesions and background photodamage but should be used cautiously due to potential for irritation.[22]

Keratosis Pilaris

Glycolic acid peels lead to desquamation of keratotic lesions, but do not improve the associated erythema. Topical GA creams can also be used for maintenance.

CONTRAINDICATIONS[1,3]

- Allergy to chemical peel constituents
- Pregnancy or nursing
- Active infection or open wound in the treatment area (e.g., herpes simplex, impetigo, active bacterial, viral, or fungal infection)
- Inflammatory skin condition at treatment site (seborrheic dermatitis, atopic dermatitis, or contact dermatitis)
- Patient taking photosensitizing drugs
- Deep chemical peel, dermabrasion, or radiation therapy in the treatment area in the preceding 6 months
- Insufficient sun protection (including tanning bed use) pre- or postprocedure
- Unrealistic expectations
- Body dysmorphic disorder.

PATIENT PREPARATION

Steps of patient preparation include:
- Detailed history and examination
- Prepeel counseling
- Priming.

History

Important history points include history of:
- Existing skin condition (atopic dermatitis/eczemas/seborrheic dermatitis, photosensitivity)
- Medication intake [e.g., photosensitizing drugs like tetracyclines, oral contraceptive pills (OCPs)]
- Any medical illness
- Allergy to any drug
- Infections, e.g., herpes labialis, facial warts and molluscum
- Patient's profession (if outdoor worker counsel about strict sun protection).

If history of recurrent herpes infection is present then the patient should be treated prophylactically with oral antiviral agents from the morning of peel as peeling can induce an episode of herpes. If active herpes infection is present on the day of the session, then peeling should be postponed.

Examination

Following points should be noted on examination:
- Fitzpatrick's skin type
- Degree of seborrhea
- Evidence of PIH
- Signs of photoaging
- Presence of infection or inflammatory disease
- Keloid or hypertrophic scarring.

Prepeel Counseling

Before peeling, counsel the patient appropriately explaining the following points:
- Procedure, expected outcome, side effects, and precautions
- Importance of sun protection, avoiding excessive sun exposure, and regular use of sunscreen. If the patient is not motivated

to follow sun protection, then he/she should be excluded from peeling
- Peeling should be avoided if there is a social event that would be taking place within a few days after the peel
- Counsel the patient that improvement can be seen only after a series of sessions with intervals of 2-4 weeks between peels, mostly 6 weeks but can vary from patient to patient and depending on skin condition
- Patient should discontinue following 2-4 days prior to peel
   - Retinoid preparations
   - AHA or beta-hydroxy acid-based products
   - Waxing, bleaching, depilatories, and electrolysis
   - Loofahs, scrubs, and masques
   - Hair dyeing and straightening.
- Avoid shaving and threading 1 day prior to peel
- To avoid makeup on the day of the peel.

Priming

Priming helps to prepare the skin for uniform and better penetration of the peel, enhances healing and reduces the risk of PIH and other complications. Priming should begin about 2-4 weeks before the procedure. When utilizing 4% hydroquinone, it is ideal to prime the skin 4-6 weeks prior to the peel. The priming regimen generally consists of a broad spectrum sunscreen, an AHA (like glycolic acid), hydroquinone and/or a retinoid. A study was conducted on sixty Indian patients with melasma allocated into the following three groups: Serial glycolic acid peel; GA primed with 0.025% tretinoin and GA peel with 2% hydroquinone. The fall in melasma area and severity index (MASI) was highest in those receiving 2% hydroquinone as a priming agent with minimum PIH.[30] Tretinoin should be discontinued 2 days prior to peel.

PEELING TECHNIQUE

Equipment required for peeling (Fig. 8) include:
- Prepeel cleanser, postpeel neutralizer
- Peeling agent
- Petrolatum jelly
- Cold water or spray bottle
- Syringes with normal saline (for irrigation of eyes in case of spillage)
- Glass cup
- Peeling brush or cotton tipped applicator
- Timer
- Gloves
- 2" × 2" cotton gauze pieces
- Fan for cooling.

Steps of Peeling

- Always take pre- and postprocedure photographs of the patient
- Always take informed consent mentioning expected course of events, risk of complications and willingness to adhere to postpeel instructions
- Ask the patient to clean the face with soap and water to remove any dirt or makeup
- Head end should be raised to 45° with eyes closed and a drape placed around the neck

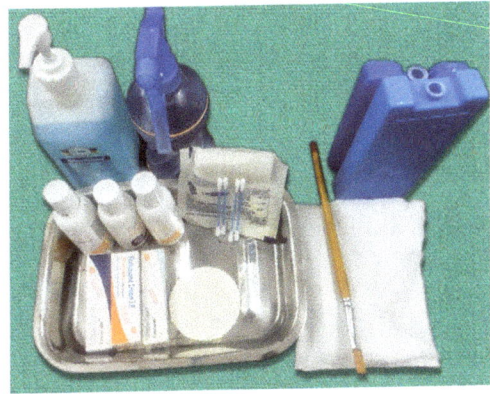

FIG. 8: Materials required for peeling.

- Inspect the face for any abrasions and inflammation
- The face is degreased with prepeel cleanser (usually acetone based). Degreasing removes oil from the skin, thus allowing hydrophilic peel to penetrate better
- Sensitive areas like inner and outer canthi of eyes, nasal alar groove, oral commissures, and lips are protected with petrolatum jelly (to prevent pooling of peel)
- Do a test patch behind the ears to look for any reaction or sensitivity
- Begin peeling by applying GA on the face starting from forehead to cheeks, chin, nose, upper lip with feathering on the neck to prevent any demarcation lines (Fig. 9). Warn the patient that some stinging and burning sensation will be felt
- The peel should be applied quickly in about 30 seconds to 1 minute so that the contact time for entire face is the same
- Timer should start at the beginning of the procedure
- *Endpoint*: Faint erythema (or based on time if no erythema appreciated especially in dark skin types)
- Peel should be neutralized with sodium bicarbonate solution or plain water Neutralization can lead to an exothermic reaction with foaming, thus cool water should be simultaneously sprayed on the face to reduce stinging and heat experienced at the time of neutralization. A handheld fan could be used too
- Apply moisturizer and sunscreen postpeel
- If peel accidentally enters the eye, irrigate the eyes with water or normal saline (do not use sodium bicarbonate in the eye for neutralization)
- Glycolic acid peel can be used for anybody site like chest, back, forearm, hands and legs. However, a lower concentration should be used for the neck
- Always begin with a lower concentration of the peel and a shorter contact time and increase on subsequent visits. Begin with 20–30% GA which if tolerated for 5 minutes can be subsequently increased to higher concentration. But, if erythema develops before 5 min, then on subsequent visit repeat the procedure at the same concentration but longer contact time (up to 5 min).

Common office regimens for GA peel are formulated in table 7.[5]

TABLE 7: Common regimens for glycolic acid (GA) peel*

Regimen A	Regimen B
Month 1: 20% GA for 5 min	Month 1: 20% GA for 4 min
Month 2: 35% GA for 5 min	Month 2: 30% GA for 4 min
Month 3: 50% GA for 5 min	Month 3: 40% GA for 4 min
Month 4: 70% GA for 4 min	Month 4: 50% GA for 4 min
Month 5: 70% GA for 5 min	Month 5: 60% GA for 4 min
Month 6: 70% GA for 7 min	Month 6: 70% GA for 4 min

*Regimens for face and body parts (lower concentrations up to 50% advisable for dark skin)

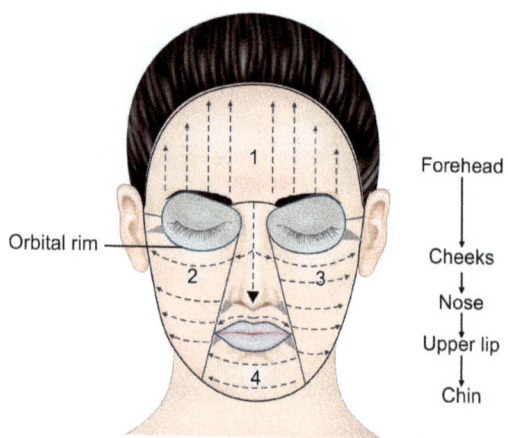

FIG. 9: Direction of application of glycolic acid peel.

Glycolic Acid Peels

POSTPEEL CARE

- It is of utmost importance to counsel the patient that postpeel erythema, exfoliation and/or tightening of the skin may be experienced for a few days. Cold compresses can be done in the event that burning and stinging occur after the peel
- Strict sun protection and use of broad-spectrum sunscreens every 3 hourly should be adhered to
- Use of soap-free cleansers should be advocated
- Moisturizer use about twice a day reduces a certain degree of exfoliation
- Avoid use of irritants, bleaching, facials, and waxing for 1 week postprocedure
- Abstinence from scratching, picking or peeling the skin is important
- Topical maintenance therapy can be started after 2 days of a superficial peel
- Regeneration of epidermis occurs in about 1 week and second sitting can be done after 2–3 weeks.

COMPLICATIONS

Complications with GA peel are minor and rare, if used properly. These include:
- Scabbing
- Persistent erythema
- Frosting or epidermolysis
- Postinflammatory hyper- or hypopigmentation
- Acneiform eruption
- Scarring
- Allergic reaction
- Urticaria.

Epidermolysis

Glycolic acid normally does not lead to frosting as it does not coagulate proteins.

TABLE 8: Skin appearance at different depth of penetration of glycolic acid peel[3]

Skin appearance	Depth of penetration
No erythema	No or minimal peeling
Spotty erythema	Very very superficial
Patchy erythema	Very superficial
Uniform faint erythema	Superficial peel (desired depth)
Frosting	Deep peel (undesirable)

However, presence of frosting indicates deeper penetration than desired leading to epidermolysis (seen as blistering or whitening followed by scabbing).

An idea about depth of penetration can be obtained by observing skin appearance (Table 8).

There is an increased risk of epidermolysis if the patient does not follow a priming regimen, uses loofahs, scrubs or microdermabrasion prior to the peel. This leads to a disruption of the epidermal barrier and promotes a deeper penetration of the peel. Once epidermolysis occurs, moisturization of the affected area with mild potency steroid (hydrocortisone) should be given. If severe edema develops, a short course of oral corticosteroid (e.g., prednisolone 30–40 mg/day) for about 3–5 days can be given.

Hyperpigmentation or Hypopigmentation

Sun exposure after the peel, noncompliance with the postpeel measures, deeper peel penetration and/or scabbing all lead to an increased risk of pigmentary changes on the skin. PIH can be managed with regular use of broad-spectrum sunscreens and topical depigmenting agents like tretinoin and hydroquinone as needed.

COMBINATION TREATMENT

Glycolic acid peel can be combined with:
- Other peels
- Microneedling
- Microdermabrasion
- Lasers
- Botulinum toxin
- Fillers.

Glycolic acid and trichloroacetic acid peels (e.g., Coleman peel) in combination produce deeper and more uniform peeling than either alone and can be performed sequentially for PIH, postacne pigmentation and melasma.[31] Jessner's solution and GA peel can be combined for the treatment of photoaged skin, actinic keratoses and wrinkles but risk of PIH and scarring is higher especially in darker patients.[1]

Microneedling can be combined with GA peel for the treatment of acne scars, PIH and to improve the skin texture. GA peeling can be combined with microdermabrasion for the treatment of acne vulgaris and superficial acne scars. Microdermabrasion leads to exfoliation and may give faster results when combined with GA peel. They can be done at an interval of 2 weeks or in the same session (microdermabrasion followed by peel) but the risk of PIH especially in darker skin types should be kept in mind.[3,32]

Combining GA peels with botulinum toxin and fillers complement each other and thus reduce wrinkles, improve uneven tone and skin laxity. They can be combined in the same sitting or at an interval of 2-4 weeks.[33]

It is important to let the inflammation settle postpeel before undertaking any other resurfacing procedure in an effort to prevent PIH and scarring.

CONCLUSION

Glycolic acid peel is an easy to use, result-oriented, evidence-based and cost-effective peel. It has undergone more studies than any other peel. The treating physician must individualize the concentration, pH concentration/level and application schedule according to the patient's needs.

PRACTICAL TIPS

- Emphasize on regular use of broad-spectrum sunscreen and adequate photoprotection measures
- Start with a lower concentration and gradually advance to higher concentrations or use combination peels which contain lower concentrations of multiple agents having a broad spectrum of activity, yet reducing the chance of overt side effects
- Take consent and pre- and postprocedure photographs
- Give a good home care regimen for better results
- Always follow priming and postpeel protocols and also advise the patient to adhere to instructions to avoid the likelihood of any complication.

TAKE HOME POINTS

- Glycolic acid is the smallest AHA and extensively studied
- It is available in 20-70% concentration
- More the concentration and lower the pH—more is the peeling effect
- Priming must be done before peeling
- Glycolic acid peel must be neutralized—longer the contact time, deeper the peel.

REFERENCES

1. Tung R, Rubin MG. Procedures in Cosmetic Dermatology Series: Chemical Peels, 2nd edition. Philadelphia: Elsevier Health US; 2010. p. 208.
2. Brody H. History of chemical peels. In: Baxter S (Ed.) Chemical peeling and resurfacing, 2nd edition. St Louis: Mosby Year Book Inc; 1997. p. 1-5.
3. Venkataram. ACS(I) Textbook on Cutaneous and Aesthetic Surgery, 1st edition. New Delhi: Jaypee Brothers Medical Publishers Private Limited; 2012. p. 968.

4. Fabbrocini G, De Padova MP, Tosti A. Chemical peels: what's new and what isn't new but still works well. Facial Plast Surg. 2009;25:329-36.
5. Wolverton. Comprehensive Dermatologic Drug Therapy, 3rd edition. Edinburgh: Elsevier Health US; 2012. p. 1024.
6. Okano Y, Abe Y, Masaki H, et al. Biological effects of glycolic acid on dermal matrix metabolism mediated by dermal fibroblasts and epidermal keratinocytes. Exp Dermatol. 2003;12 Suppl 2:57-63.
7. Bernstein EF, Lee J, Brown DB, et al. Glycolic acid treatment increases type I collagen mRNA and hyaluronic acid content of human skin. Dermatol Surg Off Publ Am Soc Dermatol Surg. 2001;27:429-33.
8. Sarkar R, Bansal S, Garg VK. Chemical Peels for Melasma in Dark-Skinned Patients. J Cutan Aesthetic Surg. 2012;5:247-53.
9. Lim JT, Tham SN. Glycolic acid peels in the treatment of melasma among Asian women. Dermatol Surg Off Publ Am Soc Dermatol Surg. 1997;23:177-9.
10. Javaheri SM, Handa S, Kaur I, et al. Safety and efficacy of glycolic acid facial peel in Indian women with melasma. Int J Dermatol. 2001;40:354-7.
11. Grover C, Reddu BS. The therapeutic value of glycolic acid peels in dermatology. Indian J Dermatol Venereol Leprol. 2003;69:148-50.
12. Godse KV, Sakhia J. Triple combination and glycolic acid peels in melasma in Indian patients. J Cosmet Dermatol. 2011;10:68-9.
13. Hurley ME, Guevara IL, Gonzales RM, et al. Efficacy of glycolic acid peels in the treatment of melasma. Arch Dermatol. 2002;138:1578-82.
14. Erbil H, Sezer E, Taştan B, et al. Efficacy and safety of serial glycolic acid peels and a topical regimen in the treatment of recalcitrant melasma. J Dermatol. 2007;34:25-30.
15. Rendon M, Cardona LM, Bussear EW, et al. Successful treatment of moderate to severe melasma with triple-combination cream and glycolic acid peels: a pilot study. Cutis. 2008;82:372-8.
16. Sarkar R, Garg V, Bansal S, et al. Comparative evaluation of efficacy and tolerability of glycolic acid, salicylic mandelic acid, and phytic acid combination peels in melasma. Dermatol Surg Off Publ Am Soc Dermatol Surg. 2016;42:384-91.
17. Kalla G, Garg A, Kachhawa D. Chemical peeling--glycolic acid versus trichloroacetic acid in melasma. Indian J Dermatol Venereol Leprol. 2001;67:82-4.
18. Sarkar R, Kaur C, Bhalla M, et al. The combination of glycolic acid peels with a topical regimen in the treatment of melasma in dark-skinned patients: a comparative study. Dermatol Surg Off Publ Am Soc Dermatol Surg. 2002;28:828-32.
19. Khunger N, Sarkar R, Jain RK. Tretinoin peels versus glycolic acid peels in the treatment of Melasma in dark-skinned patients. Dermatol Surg Off Publ Am Soc Dermatol Surg. 2004;30:756-60.
20. Kumari R, Thappa DM. Comparative study of trichloroacetic acid versus glycolic acid chemical peels in the treatment of melasma. Indian J Dermatol Venereol Leprol. 2010;76:447.
21. Puri N. Comparative study of 15% TCA peel versus 35% glycolic acid peel for the treatment of melasma. Indian Dermatol Online J. 2012;3:109-13.
22. Moy R, Luftman D, Kakita LS. Glycolic Acid Peels. Taylor & Francis; 2002. p. 256.
23. Wang CM, Huang CL, Hu CT, et al. The effect of glycolic acid on the treatment of acne in Asian skin. Dermatol Surg Off Publ Am Soc Dermatol Surg. 1997;23:23-9.
24. Atzori L, Brundu MA, Orru A, et al. Glycolic acid peeling in the treatment of acne. J Eur Acad Dermatol Venereol. 1999;12:119-22.
25. Kim SW, Moon SE, Kim JA, et al. Glycolic acid versus Jessner's solution: which is better for facial acne patients? A randomized prospective clinical trial of split-face model therapy. Dermatol Surg Off Publ Am Soc Dermatol Surg. 1999;25:270-3.
26. Kessler E, Flanagan K, Chia C, et al. Comparison of alpha- and beta-hydroxy acid chemical peels in the treatment of mild to moderately severe facial acne vulgaris. Dermatol Surg Off Publ Am Soc Dermatol Surg. 2008;34:45-50.
27. Garg VK, Sinha S, Sarkar R. Glycolic acid peels versus salicylic-mandelic acid peels in active acne vulgaris and post-acne scarring and hyperpigmentation: a comparative study. Dermatol Surg Off Publ Am Soc Dermatol Surg. 2009;35:59-65.
28. Erbağci Z, Akçali C. Biweekly serial glycolic acid peels vs. long-term daily use of topical low-strength glycolic acid in the treatment of atrophic acne scars. Int J Dermatol. 2000;39:789-94.
29. Sharad J. Glycolic acid peel therapy – a current review. Clin Cosmet Investig Dermatol. 2013;6:281-8.
30. Garg VK, Sarkar R, Agarwal R. Comparative evaluation of beneficiary effects of priming agents (2% hydroquinone and 0.025% retinoic acid) in the treatment of melasma with glycolic acid peels. Dermatol Surg Off Publ Am Soc Dermatol Surg. 2008;34:1032-9.
31. Coleman WP, Futrell JM. The glycolic acid trichloroacetic acid peel. J Dermatol Surg Oncol. 1994;20:76-80.
32. Kempiak SJ, Uebelhoer N. Superficial chemical peels and microdermabrasion for acne vulgaris. Semin Cutan Med Surg. 2008;27:212-20.
33. Rendon MI, Effron C, Edison BL. The use of fillers and botulinum toxin type A in combination with superficial glycolic acid (alpha-hydroxy acid) peels: optimizing injection therapy with the skin-smoothing properties of peels. Cutis. 2007;79:9-12.

CHAPTER 8

Procedure of Glycolic Acid Peel

Sumit Sethi

PREPARING THE PATIENT FOR THE GLYCOLIC ACID PEEL

Aesthetic Skin Consultation: First Visit

At the first visit, assess the patient's Fitzpatrick skin type, Glogau photoaging score—active infections like herpes, wrinkles, acne, scars, oiliness or dryness and presence of any benign vascular or pigmented lesions. Use ultraviolet or Wood's light to determine the extent of pigmentary abnormalities. Discuss routine skin care, sunscreen use and the importance of priming before peel, and offer peel recommendations based on the patient's skin type (Box 1).[1-5]

Preprocedure Skin Care Products

Preparation of the skin prior to chemical peeling using a topical product regimen can enhance peel effects, facilitate postprocedure healing and reduce the risks of complications.

Products used to prepare the skin are typically begun 2-4 weeks preceding the chemical peel and aim at exfoliation, hydration and protection, in particular alpha-hydroxy acids (AHAs) (glycolic acid, lactic acid), sunscreen, tretinoin and tyrosinase inhibitors.[2,5]

BOX 1: Glycolic acid peel preprocedure instructions

- Perform an aesthetic consultation
- Examine the treatment area and document the patient's Fitzpatrick skin type, Glogau photoaging score, acne, wrinkles, scars, oily/dry skin and presence of any benign vascular or pigmented lesions
- Obtain informed consent (Box 2)
- Pretreatment photographs are advised
- Strict sun protection beginning 2–4 weeks prior to the procedure, with a broad-spectrum sunscreen of SPF 30 or greater, containing zinc oxide or titanium dioxide
- 2–3 days prior to treatment, advise patients to discontinue products containing high strength alpha-hydroxy acids (AHAs) and prescription retinoid
- Two days prior to the procedure, start a prophylactic antiviral medication (e.g., acyclovir 400 mg or valacyclovir 500 mg, 1 tablet two times per day) for patients with a history of herpes simplex, and continue for 5 days post-procedure
- Patients are instructed to arrive on the day of the peel with a clean face, free of makeup and moisturizers. Male patients should be asked not to shave on the day of the peel to prevent deeper penetration. Contact lenses and jewelry are to be removed before the procedure

Procedure of Glycolic Acid Peel

BOX 2 Glycolic peel consent

Hospital/Clinic Name... Sr. No.. Date...................................

Patient Name.. Age/Sex.....................................

Address ....

Telephone Number .... Email ID..

Diagnosis..

I, _____, consent to the treatment known as a glycolic acid peel.

I state that I have understood the following information.

- The treatment has been explained to me, and I have had an opportunity to ask questions regarding the procedure, its risks, consequences, alternatives, potential complications, intended benefits and recovery, and received satisfactory answers.
- I am advised that though good results are expected, they cannot and are not guaranteed; nor there is any guarantee against untoward results.
- The procedure may cause my skin to appear somewhat pink and flaky like a mild to moderate sunburn.
- During and after the procedure, the following may be experienced: stinging, itching, burning, mild pain, tightness, peeling, and scabbing of the superficial layer of the skin. These sensations will gradually diminish over the course of the week as the skin returns to its normal appearance. However, some patients may react differently. Although rare, the skin may be uncomfortable and looks like a very bad sunburn. The peeling usually lasts about 3–7 days, although it may last longer. There is a rare incidence of scarring.
- I understand that there is a risk (although small) of developing a temporary or permanent pigment (color) change in the skin. There is a small incidence of the reactivation of "cold sores" (herpes infection) in patients with a prior history of herpes. There is also a rare incidence of a flare of acne-like lesions resulting from the peel.
- I have been given a copy of the post-glycolic acid peel instructions and have reviewed and agreed to follow them as a requisite of the treatment.

I have read and understood the above, and I now authorize _____ to perform a glycolic acid chemical peel.

_____ and any other medical procedure that becomes necessary during the procedure. The consent form has been signed by me and I am not under the influence of any drugs/alcohol. I consent to be photographed before, during and after the treatment and understand that these photographs will be the property of the above doctor(s) and may be published in scientific journal and/or shown for scientific reasons.

I am not known to be allergic to anything except: (list)

_____

_____

Consent

_____
Signature of patient or legal guardian

_____
Signature of staff witness

_____
Signature of physician obtaining consent and witnessing patient's signature

Even Penetration of Acids and Stimulation of Skin Regeneration

Alpha-hydroxy acids (e.g., glycolic acid) break down corneodesmosomes that maintain intercorneocyte cohesion; help in shedding the dead layer of epidermis making the stratum corneum more permeable, so that the acids can penetrate more deeply and evenly. It is best to start with low concentrations (6%) and increase the strength gradually (12%). Cream formulations are preferred for patients with dry skin, lotions for normal skin types, and gels for oily skin. The product should be started nightly for the first 2 weeks, then increased to twice-daily application. This will help develop tolerance to product and determine any unusual sensitivity to glycolic acid prior to peel.

Preprocedure retinoid use especially in thick, oily, or resistant skin for decreasing stratum corneum thickness allows a uniform even peel penetration. Prepeel tretinoin application disperses melanin granules and reduces the overall quantity of melanin in the epidermis, which decreases risk of postinflammatory or postpeel hyperpigmentation. It also helps prepare the skin for chemical peels by activating dermal fibroblasts and stimulating increased collagen deposition. Tretinoin is to be strictly avoided in sensitive-skin patients or if the patient has telangiectasias on face; may lead to irritation.[2,5-10]

Prevention of Pigmentary Changes

Preventive application of tyrosinase inhibitors (hydroquinone, kojic acid, azelaic acid, arbutin, etc.) should begin 3-4 weeks before a glycolic peel when there is a risk of pigmentary change, i.e., in patients with darker Fitzpatrick skin types (IV–VI) who are predisposed to postpeel hyperpigmentation. Hydroquinone is recommended in patients with significant pigmentation, spotty hyperpigmentation, and melasma. It blocks the production of melanin precursors and subsequently epidermal neo-pigmentation during the healing phase by inhibiting the enzyme, tyrosinase.[2,5,10-13]

Prepeel Sun Protection

Effective sun protection should start at least 2 weeks before a superficial peel to inhibit melanocyte activity and avoid excessive stimulation of melanin production before the peel. Physical sunscreen containing zinc oxide or titanium oxide with an SPF of at least 30 should be preferred.[2,5,10,11,13]

Patch Test or Test Peel

A "test patch" may be performed prior to a chemical peel procedure in sensitive-skin individuals to identify potential allergic reaction or intolerance to a specific peel product. Patients with facial dermatitis (rosacea, seborrheic dermatitis, and atopic dermatitis) or a history of multiple allergies and sensitivities to preservatives and/or fragrances have increased risk of adverse reaction to the peel. Test patch should be done in these patients at a site near the treatment area, such as behind the ear, or on the ventral surface of the forearm. The skin is prepared routinely as usual for peeling, and the glycolic test patch applied, timed, and neutralized as indicated. The site is evaluated 48 hours after test peel and the result is noted positive if patient presents with persistent erythema, vesiculation (i.e., epidermolysis) or report of excessive pruritus or pain present at site. Glycolic peel is to be strictly avoided if any adverse effect is noticed at the test site. However, a negative patch test does not ensure that an allergic reaction or adverse response will not occur at the time of treatment with the tested peel.[2,5,10,11,13]

Procedure of Glycolic Acid Peel

FACE PEEL PROCEDURE: EQUIPMENT AND SUPPLIES[2,5,10,11,13]

The equipment needed for a glycolic acid peel is, in general, readily available in a physician's office, with perhaps a few exceptions (Fig. 1 and Box 3).

Steps for Performing a Chemical Peel Procedure (Second Visit)

1. Preparation (position, drape, cleanse and degrease skin, apply eye protection, and apply petrolatum)
2. Chemical peel application
3. Termination
4. Boosting with topical product application.

Immediate Prepeel Preparation

Patient should be made to lie recumbent on the table with head slightly elevated and a drape sheet placed around the patient's neck. Inspect the skin to ensure that there is no existing abrasion, areas of irritation, or inflammation. Patients are instructed to arrive on the day of the peel with a clean face,

| BOX 3 | Equipment for glycolic acid peels |

- Headband or shower cap
- Towel to drape the patient
- Timer/stopwatch
- Battery operated, handheld fan
- Nonsterile gloves
- Eye protection for the patient (goggles or moist gauze)
- Small bowl for water or water spray bottle
- Small ceramic bowl for chemical peel
- 2" × 2" nonwoven gauze sponges
- Cotton-tipped applicators (for petrolatum)
- Petrolatum
- Saline eye wash
- Prepeel facial cleanser (e.g., Cetaphil or episoft cleanser for sensitive skin) or alpha-hydroxy acid facial cleanser for oily, thick skin
- Chemical peel product(s)
- *Topical steroid creams:* Low potency (hydrocortisone), medium potency (fluticasone), and high potency (e.g., halobetasol)
- Postpeel neutralizer
- Postpeel moisturizer that is soothing and nonocclusive
- Broad-spectrum sunscreen of SPF 30 or greater containing zinc oxide or titanium dioxide

free of makeup, and moisturizers. Apply the peel cleansing solution on the clean face to remove any final debris. The cleansing and degreasing allows the hydrophilic peels, which have difficulty in penetrating the oily skin, to penetrate more deeply and evenly. Petrolatum is then applied to the lateral and medial canthi, oral commissures, nasal alar grooves, and lips with a cotton bud. This acts as a protectant against potential pooling sites of the acid after application. A handheld fan should be offered to the patient for personal comfort. Patients should keep their eyes closed during the procedure and protective goggles, or moist gauze applied on them. If the peel solution inadvertently enters the eye, immediately flush it with water.

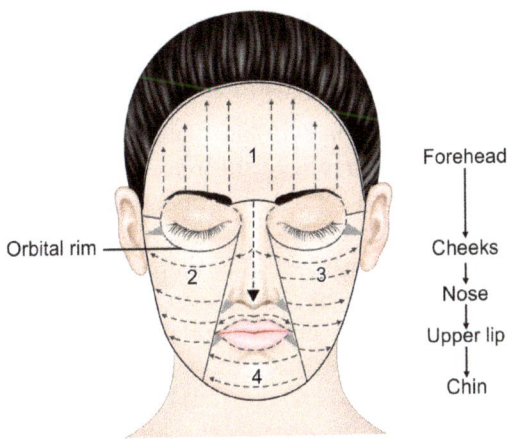

FIG. 1: Application of chemical peel to different areas.

Chemical Peel Application

The chemical peel safety zone is the area within which a chemical peel can most safely be applied to the face. This region includes the full face outside the eye orbits (above the eyebrows and 2–3 mm below the inferior eyelash margin) and excludes the lips. Chemical peels are typically thin liquids that have a tendency to pool in skin folds, which can increase the depth of penetration. Common areas of pooling include oral commissures, marionette lines, nasolabial folds particularly at the ala, and lateral canthal creases. Application of petrolatum to these areas as a barrier to protect them from overtreatment is recommended. Chemical peel is applied to the least-reactive areas first, such as the forehead, then the cheeks followed by application to the medial face starting with the nose, upper lip, and then the chin (Fig. 2).

There are a variety of chemical peel applicators available including non-woven gauze pads (also referred to as cotton squares or gauze sponges), brushes, and cotton-tipped applicators depending on dermatologist's preference and competence. Gauze pads allow easy application whereas more care is needed for the brush technique to prevent drip page. Brushes and cotton-tipped applicators also tend to pick up more products and offer less control. Nonetheless, brushes and cotton-tipped applicators make application for the upper cutaneous lip and lower eyelids technically easier to perform. Consistency is ultimately more important than the type of applicator, which depends on operator's personal choice, as overall results are usually the same.

Dividing the face into four quadrants aids in applying the peel in a systematic manner. The peel procedure is begun by applying the solution to the face, beginning at the forehead and working it down over the cheeks, nose, upper lip, and chin. Use firm even pressure when sweeping the gauze across the skin.

Quadrant 1, forehead: Sweep the gauze from the eyebrow up to hairline. Reapply chemical peel solution to the gauze.

Quadrant 2, right cheek: Sweep the gauze from the temple to the jaw line on one side of the face. The cheek can be covered using either horizontal sweeps from medial to lateral or from superior to inferior. Reapply the chemical peel solution to the gauze.

Quadrant 3, left cheek: Repeat for the contralateral cheek. Do not reapply chemical peel solution to the gauze.

Quadrant 4, medial face: Sweep the gauze down the dorsum of the nose, along each nasal sidewall, above the upper lip, and then across the chin.

Feather the edge of the treatment area with chemical peel by lightly sweeping the peel soaked gauze 1 cm below the jawline. This helps to avoid a possible line of demarcation between treated and untreated skin.

Each patient, even those with type 1 skin, should be treated with the lowest strength peel on the first visit to determine the patient's level of sensitivity. It must be explained to

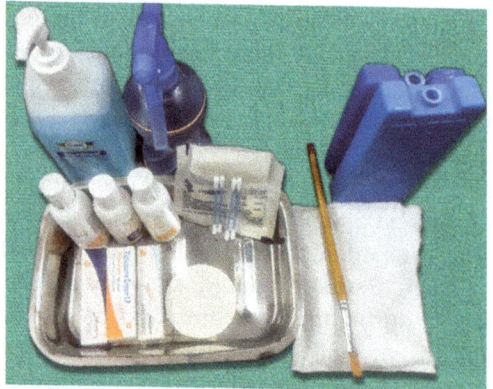

FIG. 2: Equipment for doing chemical peels.

the patients that not much difference will be noticed in their skin after just the first peel because it is a low-strength test peel used to ascertain their ability to tolerate the peel. At each visit, ask if the patient has any forthcoming social obligations to attend, that might be compromised or made embarrassing owing to conspicuous skin flaking or persistent erythema after peel.

The glycolic acid should be left in contact with the skin until the desired endpoint, which is a uniform degree of erythema developing after 2-5 minutes duration. If after a 5-minute contact time, erythema is not visible, it is still recommended that the reaction be terminated. If for any reason, the patient feels discomfort, the reaction can be neutralized before the endpoint of erythema or contact time is reached. Patient's comfort is assessed using a verbal scale from 1 to 10 (with 10 noted as the highest degree of discomfort). Discomfort level up to 5 out of 10 is typically acceptable. Itching, burning, tingling, and stinging sensations are commonly reported peaking within a few minutes after application and then subsiding. Discomfort of level 6 or greater indicates that the peel procedure should be neutralized, with removal of any residual peel product from the face, and the patient's skin cooled. The skin is observed throughout the procedure for desirable and undesirable clinical endpoints.

The chemical peel procedure should be terminated if/when:
- Desired clinical endpoints are achieved. Mild uniform erythema is the desirable clinical endpoint for superficial peels such as glycolic acid
- Desired number of minutes for peeling has been reached (if the peel is a timed procedure)
- Undesired endpoints occur. Undesirable clinical endpoints include excessive patient discomfort with pain greater than 6 out of 10; "frosting" or blanching of the skin which is indicative of epidermolysis.

Neutralization is done with bicarbonate solution (10%) to stop the effect of glycolic acid, designated by a foaming reaction that is readily apparent. At the same time, cool water is sprayed onto the face for the patient's comfort as it helps control the exothermic reaction achieved by the acid–base neutralization procedure. Patient should be apprised prior to neutralization that initial stinging may be experienced that is sometimes more intense than the acid application itself and that swiftly subsides. Neutralization is completed when there is no further foaming reaction on the skin. After the bicarbonate neutralizer and cool water spray, a postpeel moisturizer and a cold mask or frozen 4″ × 4″ gauze sponges are applied for about 5 minutes. This is for furthering patient comfort after the peel.[5,10,11,14-21]

Third Visit and Later

If the glycolic acid 20% or 35% peels solution is tolerated for 4 or 5 minutes, then subsequent glycolic acid peels should be performed at the next higher concentration. If the 5-minute time point has not been achieved, or if erythema occurs earlier than 5 minutes, then the peel should be neutralized. At the next visit, the next peel should resume at the previous concentration but maximized at the 5-minute time point. If the patient complains about flaking skin or erythema, the physician should titrate the peels more slowly. If the patient feels that significant erythema and/or flaking are the sine qua non of an adequate peel, the physician may want to proceed more rapidly. It is best to increase concentrations and contact times gradually with patients whose professional lives will not allow them to spend time locked away recovering (Table 1).

TABLE 1: **Commonly used office glycolic acid peel regimens (personal communications with many cosmetic dermatologists)**

Regimen #1	Regimen #2
Month 1: 20% glycolic acid for 5 min	Month 1: 20% glycolic acid for 5 min
Month 2: 35% glycolic acid for 5 min	Month 2: 30% glycolic acid for 5 min
Month 3: 50% glycolic acid for 5 min	Month 3: 40% glycolic acid for 5 min
Month 4: 70% glycolic acid for 5 min	Month 4: 50% glycolic acid for 5 min
Month 5: 70% glycolic acid for 6 min	Month 5: 60% glycolic acid for 5 min
Month 6: 70% glycolic acid for 7 min	Month 6: 70% glycolic acid for 5 min

Note: Peel in any of these regimen may be neutralized sooner if desired or undesired endpoints are observed.

Nonfacial Treatment Areas

While the face is generally the most coveted site, many patients seek improvement in other areas of the body namely the chest and neck, back, dorsal hands, arms, and legs. The skin on the body differs from facial skin as it has fewer pilosebaceous units, which are the sites of re-epithelialization and sebum production. Therefore, nonfacial skin is relatively drier, repairs more slowly, has less dramatic improvements with treatments, and is more prone to complications compared to the face. Any cosmetic unit can be treated with a glycolic acid peel. In general, chest, back, forearms, dorsal hands, and legs are easily treated with higher concentrations of glycolic acid without fear of overtreatment. However, necks are the more sensitive body area and conservative treatment with lower concentrations first is recommended. Chemical peel application is limited to not more than 25% of the body at any one time. Peeling a large surface area can be associated with excessive discomfort and postprocedure skin care can be challenging. Post-treatment care is the same for peels in nonfacial areas and includes protection with a broad-spectrum sunscreen and hydrating topical products.[2,5,10,11,13]

Aftercare

Erythema, dryness, mild edema, and skin sensitivity are common in the first 3-5 days postprocedure. The skin may also feel tighter, texture, and wrinkles may appear coarser, and patients may report mild pruritus during this time. Desquamation typically starts on day 3-5 postprocedure and ranges from skin flaking to skin sloughing and peeling. If peeling occurs, it usually starts in the mid-face proceeding towards the periphery, and can persist up to 2 weeks. In some cases, flaking or peeling may not occur, particularly in patients whose skin is conditioned (i.e., who regularly exfoliates) and these patients require reassurance that, despite lack of desquamation, the skin has histologic benefits from the peel procedure. For the 1-2 weeks following treatment, soothing and hydrating topical products are used and irritating ingredients such as AHAs or retinoids are avoided until skin becomes normal again. An example of a postpeel regimen would include daily use of a gentle cleanser, broad-spectrum sunscreen of SPF 30 or greater containing zinc oxide or titanium dioxide during the day, and a nonocclusive moisturizer in the evening. If erythema is marked immediately after

Procedure of Glycolic Acid Peel

treatment, hydrocortisone cream may be applied twice daily until erythema resolves. This is particularly important for patients with darker skin types (V–VI) to reduce the risk of PIH. Makeup may be worn 24 hours after the procedure and mineral makeup is preferable. Strict sun (and tanning bed) avoidance for 2 weeks postprocedure is advised as well as the use of other sun protective measures such as a wide-brimmed hat. Patients are instructed to follow-up if they notice prolonged erythema for 5 days or more, severe pruritus, discomfort, pain, crusting, drainage, or other signs or symptoms that deviate from the usual postprocedure course. Regular skin care products may be resumed once the skin is no longer irritated or peeling, usually 1–2 weeks postprocedure (Box 4).[2,5,10,11,13]

> **BOX 4** **Glycolic acid peel or acne wash postprocedure instructions**
>
> - It may take anywhere from 1 to 7 days for the appearance of skin to return to normal depending on the degree of peeling experienced. During the recovery or renewal period, tightening, peeling or desquamation, burning, itching, stinging, mild-to-moderate pain, and peeling along with scabbing of the superficial layer of the skin, may be experienced by the patient. These sensations will gradually diminish over the course of the week as the skin returns to its normal appearance
> - Wash the treated area very gently with cleansers and apply the postpeel glycolic-acid-free moisturizer twice daily for 3–7 days until the skin returns to its normal appearance, and then restart the maintenance regimen
> - Do not use abrasive or exfoliating sponges on the treated area(s)
> - Practice strict photo protection. Continue to apply sunscreen, as tolerated, beginning the day after the peel because postpeel the skin becomes more sensitive to sunlight
> - Avoid peeling, scratching, or picking the skin to prevent scarring

Common Follow-ups and Management

Excessive dryness during the post-treatment period can be managed with reapplication of sunscreen in the daytime and a non-occlusive moisturizer in the evening until dryness resolves.

Lack of peeling or flaking does not indicate that a peel was histologically or clinically ineffective and patients may require reassurance regarding this point.[5,11,13]

PROGRESSIVE PEELING

Progressive peeling refers to increasing the intensity of chemical peels over time. A series of 12 treatments is typically performed where the depth of peeling is progressively increased by gradually increasing the concentration of peels, number of layers applied or the time of their application on skin. This escalation of intensity allows the patient to become acquainted with the experience of peeling gradually, safely gauge the skin's response to particular peels early on in the series and helps ensure patient adherence to postprocedure instructions with use of appropriate home care products. As the series progresses, skin becomes more conditioned as the stratum corneum is thinned and leveled. Towards the end of the treatment series, more intense and effective peels may be safely performed to help achieve maximal results.[3,5,11]

Treatment Intervals

Treatment intervals for peels vary from 2–4 weeks during a series of 12 treatments, and the interval is determined by the treatment intensity and sensitivity of the patient's skin. Low concentration glycolic peels are performed at the beginning of a series and treatment intervals are usually every 2 weeks, as the skin recovers rapidly from these treatments. Higher concentration glycolic peels performed later in the series are associated with a greater degree of exfoliation and require more time for re-epithelialization. Superficial chemical peels are typically performed every 2 weeks.[5,11,13]

REFERENCES

1. Fischer TC, Perosino E, Poli F, et al. Chemical peels in aesthetic dermatology: an update 2009. J Eur Acad Dermatol Venereol. 2010;24(3):281-92.
2. Baumann L, Saghari S. Chemical Peels. In: Baumann L (Ed.). Cosmetic Dermatology, 2nd edition. New York: McGraw-Hill; 2002. pp. 148-60.
3. Zakopoulou N, Kontochristopoulos G. Superficial chemical peels. J Cosmet Dermatol. 2006;5(3):246-53.
4. Khunger N. Standard guidelines for chemical peels. Indian J Dermatol Venereol Leprol. 2008;74:S5-12.
5. Small R, Hoang D, Linder J. Chemical peels. In: Small R, Hoang D, Linder J (Eds). A Practical Guide to Chemical Peels, Microdermabrasion & Topical Products. USA: Lippincott Williams & Wilkins; 2013. pp. 35-110.
6. Matarasso SL, Glogau RG. Chemical face peels. Dermatol Clin. 1991;9(1):131-50.
7. Matarasso ST, Salman SM, Glogau RG, et al. The role of chemical peeling in the treatment of photodamaged skin. J Dermatol Surg Oncol. 1990;16:945-54.
8. Roberts WE. Chemical peeling in ethnic/darker skin. Dermatol Ther. 2004;17:196-205.
9. Murad H, Shamban AT, Premo PS. The use of glycolic acid as a peeling agent. Dermatol Clin. 1995;13:285-307.
10. Deprez P. Textbook of Chemical Peels: Superficial, Medium and Deep Peels in Cosmetic Practice. London: Informa Healthcare; 2007. p. 206.
11. Ditre CM. Alpha-hydroxy acid peels. Chemical Peels. Procedures in cosmetic dermatology. In: Rubin MG (Ed.). Elsevier Inc.; 2011. pp. 27-40.
12. Garg VK, Sinha S, Sarkar R. Glycolic acid peels versus salicylic-mandelic acid peels in active acne vulgaris and post-acne scarring and hyperpigmentation: A comparative study. Dermatol Surg. 2009;35:59-65.
13. Small R, O'Hanlon K. Chemical Peels. In: Usatine R, Pfenninger J, Stulberg D, Small R, (Eds). Dermatologic and Cosmetic Procedures in Office Practice. Philadelphia, PA: Elsevier; 2011. pp. 259-73.
14. Drake LA, Dinehart SM, Goltz RW, et al. Guidelines of care for chemical peeling. Guidelines/Outcomes Committee: American Academy of Dermatology. J Am Acad Dermatol. 1995;33:479-503.
15. Monheit GD, Chastain MA. Chemical peels. Facial Plast Surg Clin North Am. 2001;9(2):239-55.
16. Glogau RG, Matarasso SL. Chemical face peeling: patient and peeling agent selection. Facial Plast Surg. 1995;11(1):1-8.
17. Sharad J. Glycolic acid peel therapy - a current review. Clin Cosmet Investig Dermatol. 2013;6:281-8.
18. Coleman WP 3rd, Brody HJ. Advances in chemical peeling. Dermatol Clin. 1997;15(1):19-26.
19. Landau M. Chemical peels. Clin Dermatol. 2008;26(2):200-8.
20. Slavin JW. Considerations in alpha hydroxy acid peels. Clin Plast Surg. 1998;25(1):45-52.
21. Salam A, Dadzie OE, Galadari H. Chemical peeling in ethnic skin: an update. Br J Dermatol. 2013;169 Suppl 3:82-90.

CHAPTER 9

Salicylic Acid Peels

Surabhi Sinha, Rashmi Sarkar

INTRODUCTION

Unna, a German dermatologist, was the first to describe the properties of salicylic acid (SA). It is a very superficial to superficial chemical peeling agent.

CHEMISTRY

Salicylic acid (ortho-hydroxybenzoic acid) was described as a beta-hydroxy acid by Kligman but Yu and Van Scott later described it as a phenolic aromatic acid.[1,2] It is desmolytic rather than keratolytic in the sense that it removes intercellular lipids that are covalently linked to the cornified envelope, thus disrupting cellular junctions instead of lysing intracellular keratin filaments.[3] It also has anti-inflammatory, antimicrobial and anesthetizing properties. It is also known to enhance the penetration of other topical agents.[4] It is used as a chemical peel in hydroethanolic solutions and, recently, in gel-based formulations, in concentrations ranging from 10–50%.

It is relatively safe in all skin types, and is one of the few peels that have been validated in Asian and dark-skinned patients (Fig. 1).[5-7]

It also has a sebum lowering effect, thus having high utility in the treatment of acne patients. Marczyk et al. compared the effect of 50% pyruvic acid and 30% SA peels on skin lipid films in acne patients and concluded that SA had a greater sebostatic effect.[8]

Of the total, 30% SA peels formulated in polyethylene glycol (PEG) vehicle were found to be efficacious and better tolerated.

INDICATIONS

- Pigmentary disorders:
  ○ Postinflammatory hyperpigmentation (PIH)
  ○ Mild melasma
  ○ Ephelids and lentigines.
- Acne-related conditions:[10]
  ○ Active inflamed acne
  ○ Comedonal acne
  ○ Postacne hyperpigmentation
  ○ Superficial acne scars—mainly boxcar.
- Aesthetic:
  ○ Photoaging (with/without tretinoin or retinol)
  ○ Dilated pores
  ○ Fine superficial wrinkling
  ○ Striae distensae (with yellow peel or microdermabrasion).[11]

Chemical Peels: A Global Perspective

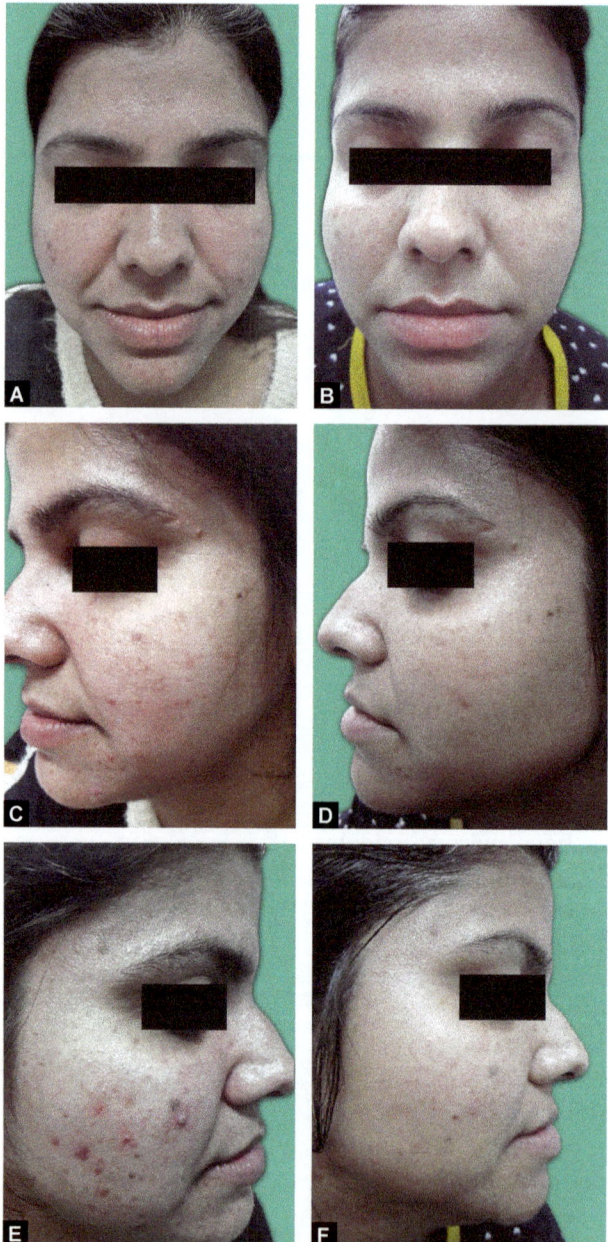

FIG. 1: A,C,E, Photographs of patient at baseline showing acne and post acne hyperpigmentation; **B,D,F,** Photographs show significant reduction in acne and post acne hyperpigmentation and overall improvement in texture at 24 weeks (after 6 fortnightly peels and follow up period of 12 weeks).

CONTRAINDICATIONS

- Known hypersensitivity to aspirin or any component of the peel
- Acute bacterial, viral or fungal infection at the site to be peeled
- Pregnancy and lactation (category C—high dermal penetration present)
- Acute inflammatory dermatoses or open wound over the site to be peeled
- Uncooperative, unreliable patient or patient with unrealistic expectations.

PATIENT PREPARATION

Proper patient selection and assessment of each individual's skin condition is crucial.

Preoperative consultation is important in the following:
- Identifying at-risk patients who are best avoided or necessitate an extra-cautious approach
- Selecting ideal candidates
- Evaluating patients for relative contraindications
- Discuss indications of the procedure
- Assessing and understanding the patient's goals, expectations and anticipated results
- A thorough medical history and physical examination should be done
- The latest American Society for Dermatologic Surgery (ASDS) guidelines task force—consensus recommendations concluded that there is insufficient evidence to justify delaying treatment with superficial chemical peels in patients on/exposed to isotretinoin within the past 6 months. Data on medium and deep chemical peels was insufficient to make recommendations. Many workers have combined oral isotretinoin and SA peels for better and faster results too. Kar et al. compared oral isotretinoin alone versus 20% SA peels and oral isotretinoin in active acne and concluded that both were effective but the combination showed significantly better clearance.[12]

However, in patients with sensitive skin and active inflamed acne, it would be better to stick to the earlier guidelines and avoid even superficial peels while on/within 6 months after isotretinoin intake. Also, while using SA as part of combination or sequential peels, the depth of penetration may be increased and the peel may behave as a medium-depth peel, and thus, it may be a contraindication in patients on oral isotretinoin therapy.

- Patients should be asked about prior resurfacing procedures or cosmetic procedures such as rhytidectomy, coronal brow lift or blepharoplasty, which pose an increased risk of complications
- An interval of 4–12 weeks is recommended between peeling and procedures involving undermining of skin
- Patients with history of recurrent herpes simplex should be given prophylactic acyclovir or valaciclovir beginning 2 days prior to the procedure and continuing for 7–10 days after procedure
- Patients with active inflammation (seborrheic, atopic, irritant or allergic dermatitis, rosacea, psoriasis or vitiligo) may be at an increased risk for complications secondary to alterations in the skin's normal barrier function
- Any history of abnormal scar formation, either hypertrophic scar or keloids
- Patients infected with human immunodeficiency virus (HIV) may experience delayed healing or be at risk for secondary infection after peeling
- A postauricular test peel may be carried out on a 1 cm^2 area. It is useful mostly in patients with sensitive skin, prior history of unexpected reaction to peeling agent applied in the past. Although a favorable test is reassuring, it does not guarantee a positive outcome following full-face resurfacing

- Patient information sheet containing the intended benefits, limitations and risks of treatment should be explained to the patient. An informed written consent should also be taken.

Priming

Priming agents are agents applied to the skin in preparation for peeling. They have the following benefits:
- They help to achieve a more uniform penetration of peeling agents by reducing sebum and thinning stratum corneum
- Accelerate re-epithelialization; reduce wound healing time
- Have a lightening effect by enhancing dispersion of melanin granules.

Some of the mild priming agents include the following:
- 0.025% tretinoin
- Adapalene
- Alpha-hydroxy acids (6% glycolic acid, lactic acid and mandelic acid)
- Kojic acid
- Azelaic acid 10–20%
- Broad-spectrum sunscreens.

Pretreatment with 2–4% hydroquinone twice daily and topical tretinoin (0.05% and 0.1%) or retinoic acid nightly 2–4 weeks prior to peeling reduces chances of PIH and promotes faster healing in the immediate postpeel period. Hydroquinone, when applied for a period of 4 weeks prior to the peel, attains better results than that applied for a shorter duration.

PEEL TECHNIQUE

- Prior to peel application, the skin is cleaned with spirit and degreased with acetone-soaked sponges. A superficial peel like lactic acid has little or no effect if the skin is poorly prepared. The cleansed skin should be checked for presence of residual oil; if required, cleansing can be repeated
- Salicylic acid peel, like all others, is applied quickly within 1 minute according to cosmetic units. Perioral, infraorbital and medial parts of cheeks are treated in the end. Feathering should be done at the edges to blend with the surrounding areas
- Approximately 1 mL is needed to cover the face
- Patients experience a stinging sensation for 3–5 minutes, following which it ceases and SA crystallizes to form a pseudo-frost—this is more frequently and clearly seen in solution-based peels as it indicates the deposition of SA after its hydroethanolic vehicle has volatilized. This is an advantageous property as the endpoint is easily visualized and there is no need to neutralize
- If pseudofrost is not visible, then the cessation of stinging sensation usually after 3–5 minutes is considered as the endpoint
- A cooling fan can be used to reduce the stinging sensation. Wiping or neutralizing with ice cold water can also help
- Salicylic acid alone is a very superficial or superficial depth peel, can be done two weekly
- Salicylic acid can be used as part of a combination formulation or as sequential therapy 2 to 4 weekly.

PRECAUTIONS

- Always check the label on the bottle of the chemical to be applied
- Never pass an open container of acid or applicator wet with acid over patient's face
- Always elevate patient's head by 45° during procedure
- Keep water-filled syringes ready.

POSTPEEL CARE

- Strict sun avoidance and sun-protective measures during postoperative period
- Erythema, edema and tightness can persist for 1–3 days post superficial peels and 5–10 days in case of deeper peels. A moisturizing cream should be applied frequently throughout the day especially in the first 2–3 days postpeeling
- Mild non-soap based cleansers should be used starting from the day after peeling
- Patients should be counseled not to smoke, as it impairs healing
- Resume prepeel regimen only after complete re-epithelialization which may take a few days
- To avoid scratching
- To avoid epilation on treated areas
- To avoid using makeup within the first 24 hours
- To avoid cleansing aggressively.

COMPLICATIONS[3]

- Prolonged erythema—harbinger of PIH or scarring
- Intense exfoliation
- Crusting
- Excessive dryness and tightness
- Contact sensitization
- Pigmentary dyschromias
- Salicylism (rare)
- Hypoglycemia (rare).

PRACTICAL TIPS

Salicylic acid can be used in a diverse number of ways as a very superficial to a superficial or sometimes even medium-depth peel. It is a user-friendly peel with visible endpoints and is compatible with many peels for combination or sequential use too. It has excellent comedolytic properties and is very good for acne and its sequelae. Additionally it has a whitening effect and it improves the overall texture of the skin too.

TAKE HOME POINTS

- Salicylic acid peels are user friendly and have a wide range of use. They can be used as very superficial to even medium-depth peels
- Salicylic acid has excellent effects in acne and acne-related sequelae and it has an overall whitening effect. Plus, it also improves the overall skin texture, leading to greater patient satisfaction.

REFERENCES

1. Kligman AM. Salicylic acid: an alternative to alpha-hydroxy acids. J Geriatr Dermatol. 1997;5:128-31.
2. Yu RJ, Van Scott EJ. Salicylic acid: not a beta-hydroxy acid. Cosmet Derm. 1997;10:27.
3. Arif T. Salicylic acid as a peeling agent: a comprehensive review. Clin Cosmet Invest Dermatol. 2015;8:455-61.
4. Grimes PE. Salicylic acid. In: Tosti A, Grimes PE, Padova MP (Eds). Color Atlas of Chemical Peeling, 2nd edition. New York, USA: Springer-Verlag; 2006.
5. Garg VK, Sinha S, Sarkar R. Glycolic acid peels versus salicylic-mandelic peels in active acne vulgaris and post-acne scarring and hyperpigmentation: a comparative study. Dermatol Surg. 2009;35:59-65.
6. Grimes PE. The safety and efficacy of salicylic acid chemical peels in darker racial – ethnic groups. Dermatol Surg. 1999;25:18-22.
7. Ahn HH, Kim I. Whitening effect of salicylic acid peels in Asian patients. Dermatol Surg. 2006;32:372-5.
8. Marczyk B, Mucha P, Budzisz E, et al. Comparative study of the effect of 50% pyruvic and 30% salicylic acid peels on the skin lipid film in patients with acne vulgaris. J Cosmet Dermatol. 2014;13:15-21.
9. Dainichi T, Ueda S, Imayama S, et al. Excellent clinical results with a new preparation for chemical peeling in acne: 30% Salicylic acid in PEG vehicle. Dermatol Surg. 2008;34:891-99.
10. Kessler E, Flanagan K, Chia C, et al. Comparison of alpha and beta hydroxy acid chemical peels in the treatment of mild to moderately severe facial acne vulgaris. Dermatol Surg. 2008;34:45-51.
11. Karia UK, Padhiar BB, Shah BJ. Evaluation of various therapeutic measures in striae rubra. J Cutan Aesthet Surg. 2016;9:101-5.
12. Kar BR, Tripathy S, Panda M. Comparative study of oral isotretinoin versus oral isotretinoin plus 20% Salicylic acid peels in the treatment of active acne. J Cutan Aesthet Surg. 2013;6:204-8.

Trichloroacetic Acid Peels

Jaishree Sharad

INTRODUCTION

Trichloroacetic acid (TCA) peel is a cost effective, simple office procedure used for a plethora of indications like acne, postinflammatory hyperpigmentation, melasma, xanthelasma, solar lentigines, actinic keratosis, etc. It has enhanced therapeutic and cosmetic effect when combined with other peels like glycolic acid and modalities like solid CO_2.

TRICHLOROACETIC ACID AS A CHEMICAL AGENT[1]

Trichloroacetic acid (also known as trichloroethanoic acid) is an acetic acid analog in which the three hydrogen atoms of the methyl group have been replaced by chlorine. It is an anhydrous, colorless crystalline solid with a sharp pungent odor. It is soluble in water, ethanol and diethyl ether. The pKa value is 0.26. TCA has a protein dissociation constant (pKa) of 0.52, making it an inherently stronger acid than alpha-hydroxy acids (pKa of glycolic acid: 3.83). The hygroscopic nature of TCA makes it absorb moisture from air.

MECHANISM OF ACTION

Trichloroacetic acid causes structural cell death by protein denaturation and coagulative necrosis of the cells. The coagulation of proteins is clinically seen as frosting. Intensity of frosting correlates with depth of penetration. Further, higher the concentration of the peel, deeper is the penetration. Frosting is followed by inflammation and re-epithelialization leading to even skin tone and enhanced texture. Medium-depth peels cause collagen remodeling and eliminate fine lines and wrinkles. TCA peels are self-neutralizing and hence do not get absorbed into the systemic circulation.[2,3]

Different TCA concentrations and its level of penetration into the skin:
- 10–20%: Till stratum granulosum
- 25–30%: Full thickness of the epidermis
- 40–50%: Till the papillary dermis
- 50% and more: Till the reticular dermis.

Frosting is considered as the endpoint of peeling. The following table explains the various levels of frosting (Table 1).[4]

FORMULATIONS

PG Unna first used TCA in 1882 as a peeling agent.[5] It can be used as superficial, medium-depth and/or deep peel, depending on the concentration of the peel.

Different concentrations can be formulated by adding distilled water or normal saline to the crystals. Tremendous variations

TABLE 1: Various levels of frosting

Level of frosting	Clinical features
Level 0	No frost. Little or no erythema
Level I	Erythema with a stringy or blotchy frosting, seen with light chemical peels
Level II	White-coated frosting with erythema showing through
Level III	• A solid white enamel frosting with little or no erythema • The peel penetrates through the papillary dermis • A deeper level III frosting must be limited only to areas of heavy actinic damage and thicker skin

were found in the relative concentrations of TCA in solutions. To avoid mishaps and complications, the weight to volume (wt/vol) method should be used. For example, to make 15% TCA solution, 15 g TCA crystals should be added in distilled water to make 100 mL. Another method is to dilute the product by mixing purified water with the 100% TCA. For a 50% mixture, combine one part 100% TCA and one part water. For a 25% solution, combine one part 50% TCA and one part water. For a 12% solution, combine one part 25% TCA with one part water.

Once formulated, it has to be stored in airtight bottles and also prolonged air contact should be avoided during the procedure because of its hygroscopic nature. Old crystals should not be used to formulate the peel and every 6 months, new solution should be prepared. The solution is not light sensitive and can be stored at room temperature.

If methyl salicylate is added, activation of TCA is achieved. Methyl salicylate works as a carrier. It increases the degree of penetration and allows for a faster and more intense whitening effect.[6]

Trichloroacetic acid peel penetrates to various depths depending on the concentration.[7]

- 10–15% TCA: very superficial peeling
- 15–25% TCA: superficial peeling
- 35–50% TCA: medium-depth peeling.

Concentration above 40% is not recommended as it causes scarring and dyschromias.

INDICATIONS[8-12]

Superficial-depth Peels

- Acne
- Postinflammatory hyperpigmentation
- Epidermal melasma
- Photoaging
- Dilated pores
- Freckles and lentigines
- Rough skin texture
- Dyschromias
- Periorbital melanosis.

Medium-depth Peels

- Postinflammatory hyperpigmentation
- Superficial acne scars
- Keratosis pilaris
- Dermal melasma
- Warts
- Lentigines
- Xanthelasma palpebrarum
- Actinic keratosis
- Seborrheic keratosis.

CONTRAINDICATIONS

- Active viral (e.g., Herpes or warts), fungal or bacterial infection
- History of keloidal tendency or hypertrophic scarring (medium-depth peel)
- History of taking photosensitive drugs
- History of recent radiation treatment
- Insufficient sun protection
- Patients with unrealistic expectations

- Atrophic skin or recent facial surgical procedures within last 6 months
- Medium-depth peels should be used cautiously in dark-skinned patients to avoid postinflammatory hyperpigmentation and dyschromias.

COMBINATION TREATMENTS

- *Coleman's peel*: 70% glycolic acid and 35% TCA[13]
- *Brody's peel*: Solid CO_2 and 35% TCA[14]
- *Monheit's peel*: Jessner's solution and 35% TCA and 15–25% TCA[15]
- CO_2 laser and 3% TCA[16]
- Sand abrasion.[17]

A study done by Coleman et al. showed significant improvement in pigmentary dyschromias and actinic damage. 70% GA application for 2 minutes followed by 35% TCA application resulted in medium-depth peel.[13]

Another variation of TCA peeling is the Obagi Blue Peel®, a compound of fixed concentration of TCA, added to a nonionic blue base containing glycerin and saponins.[18]

METHOD OF APPLICATION

Preprocedure Care

Priming of the skin for at least 2–4 weeks before any peel is very important because not only does it increase the peel efficacy, it also reduces the risk of postinflammatory hyperpigmentation.

- Hydroquinone (2–5%) and retinoic acid, kojic acid (1–2%) are commonly used as priming agents and priming cream should be discontinued 2 days before the peel treatment[19]
- Sun protection is essential which can be done using broad-spectrum sunscreen along with physical protection
- Patients with a history of herpes simplex must undergo prophylactic antiviral therapy (acyclovir 200 mg five times a day or Valacyclovir 500 mg twice a day for 5 days)[6]
- All other treatments like waxing, threading, bleaching, microdermabrasion and other lasers should be avoided for at least 1 week before peel
- A test peel may be done in the postauricular area for patients with a sensitive skin a week or two prior to the procedure.

Peel Procedure

Written informed consent and photographic documentation should be taken before commencement of the procedure.

- A hair band is used to ensure that hair does not fall on the face while conducting the procedure
- The skin is cleaned with alcohol and chlorhexidine gluconate. Acetone is used to degrease the skin. This ensures even penetration of the peeling agent
- Contact lenses must be removed before performing the peel
- Petroleum jelly is applied on the sensitive areas like corners of the mouth, nasolabial fold and outer canthus of the eyes
- Performing the peel at an angle of 45° is found to be most ergonomic. A uniform coat of the TCA solution is applied quickly, using cotton tipped swab or a 2" × 2" gauze piece on different cosmetic units of the face starting from the forehead. The perioral and periorbital areas are treated last. Feathering strokes are applied to prevent demarcation lines. A cooling fan is advisable to reduce any burning sensation
- Use a lower concentration of peel (10–15%) when peeling for the first time, depending on skin type

Trichloroacetic Acid Peels

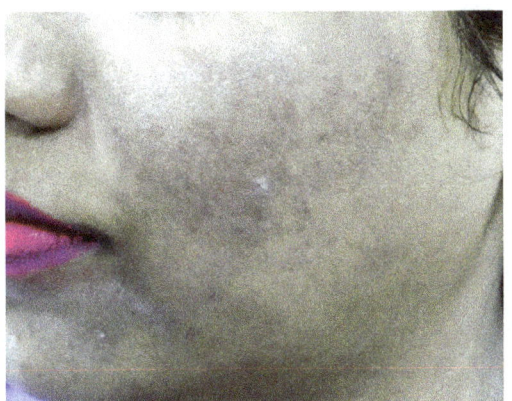

FIG. 1: Frosting is the endpoint.

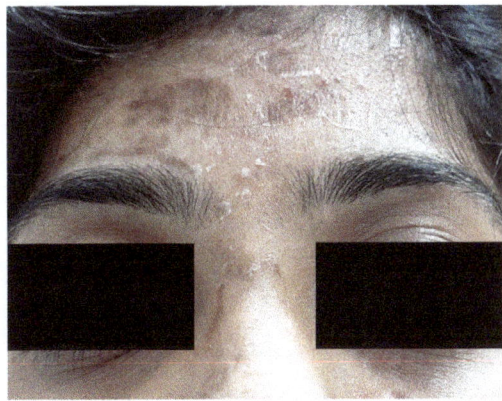

FIG. 2: Peeling in 3–4 days with 20 % trichloroacetic acid peel.

- When adequate frosting is achieved, the area is immediately neutralized with cold distilled water.[20] The patient is asked to wash the face with plain water to remove any traces of remaining peel (if any) (Fig. 1)
- This is followed by ice application till the burning completely stops
- Thick layer of sunscreen is applied before stepping out.

POSTPEEL CARE

A postpeel instruction form should be given to all patients undergoing the peel having the following instructions:[21]

- Strict use of sunscreen is a must which includes adequate quantity and repeated application every 3 hours
- Mild soap or non-soap cleanser may be used
- A bland moisturizer should be used till desquamation subsides or in case of dryness. Flaking or dryness may be seen in superficial peels. In case of a stronger peel if there is crusting, the patient should be counseled that skin spots may look darker and usually returns to normal in 2–5 days.

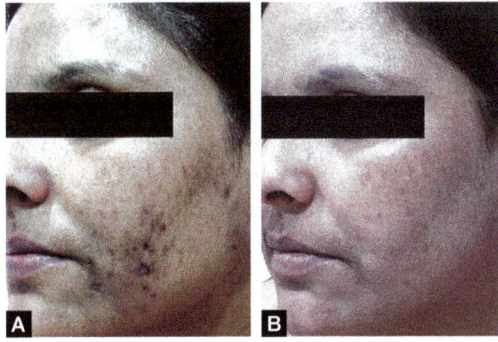

FIG. 3: **A,** Before and **B,** after 15% trichloroacetic acid peel (4 sessions at intervals of 2 weeks).

In cases of TCA peels above 20%, the patient is asked to apply a combination of mid potent steroid and antibacterial cream for a few days along with a moisturizer (Fig. 2)
- Topical antiacne creams and topical skin lightening creams should be started a week after the peel
- The peels can be repeated every 15 days till satisfactory results are achieved. Maintenance peels can be done once a month or once in 2 months (Figs. 3 and 4).

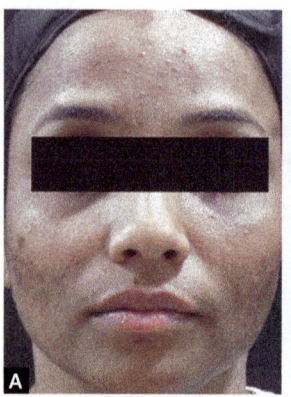 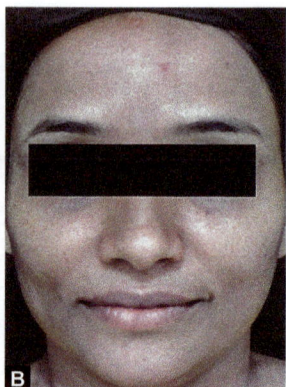

FIG. 4: **A,** Before and **B,** after 20% trichloroacetic acid peel (4 sessions at an interval of 2 weeks).

TCA CROSS (CHEMICAL RECONSTRUCTION OF SKIN SCARS)[22]

As the name suggests, it is a focal application of a high concentration of TCA peel (50–100%) for the treatment of ice pick scars. The peel causes inflammation and necrosis of the tissue. Increased collagen production with glycosaminoglycan and elastin fragmentation and reorganization helps to fill up the atrophic scar. After preparing the skin, a sterile wooden toothpick is used to apply the peel in the depth of the scar. This is done with due caution without spilling it on to the surrounding skin. Within 10–15 seconds, a dense focal pin-point area of frosting could be denoted post-application. The healing is faster and it is associated with fewer complications because of the sparing of adjacent normal tissue.

TRICHLOROACETIC ACID PEEL FOR NONFACIAL SKIN

Trichloroacetic acid 15–35% can be effectively used on nonfacial skin, namely the chest, back, hands and legs to primarily treat pigmentary disorders. A study done by William R et al. combined the use of 70% glycolic acid gel with 40% TCA on nonfacial skin. This combination provided consistently good results on the skin of the neck, chest, arms, hands and back thereby facilitating for a smoother skin texture, decreased wrinkling and striae, fading of lentigines and other pigmentary abnormalities.[23]

SIDE EFFECTS[7,24-29]

Immediate Effects

- Erythema, irritation and pruritus: Avoid excessive peel concentration and sun exposure. Topical bland emollients and steroid can be used
- Pain
- Edema
- *Allergic reaction*: Always perform a postauricular patch test in patients with a sensitive skin. In case of a reaction, give oral antibiotics and topical antibacterial cream with emollient
- Photosensitivity.

Delayed Effects

- *Acneiform eruptions*: Topical and oral antibiotics and topical azelaic acid can used. Low dose isotretinoin can be started after antibiotic course

- *Infection*: Avoid itching, rubbing and peeling of the skin
  - *Bacterial infection*: This is mostly seen in medium-depth peels due to delayed healing and premature peeling of the skin. Topical and oral antibiotics should be started immediately
  - *Herpetic infection*: Topical and oral antiviral drugs should be used. If the patient is already on prophylactic antiviral and herpes still occurs, then it is advisable to double the dose
  - *Fungal infection:* It is seen in the form of oral thrush or angular cheilitis. Oral fluconazole or itraconazole with topical antifungal preparations should be used.
- *Demarcation lines*: These are seen at the junction of peeled and unpeeled areas. Seen commonly in medium-depth peels. This problem can be prevented by feathering the peeling agent at the border of the area of peeling
- *Postinflammatory hyperpigmentation or hypopigmentation*: Ethnic or Fitzpatrick photo type III–VI skin is particularly vulnerable to dyschomia. The use of estrogen containing medication, photosynthesizing drugs and early exposure to sunlight increase the risk of hyperpigmentation. Priming the skin and strict photo protection play a very important role in preventing this side effect. Triple combination cream or modified Kligman's regimen can be started after the completion of desquamation of the skin (Fig. 5)
- *Persistent erythema*: Persistent erythema is erythema lasting for a longer period than expected. It is a predictor of scarring
- *Scarring:* It is seen if a concentration of more than 50% is used. The scars can be flat or depressed. Hypertrophic scars can be treated with topical steroids and pulsed dye laser

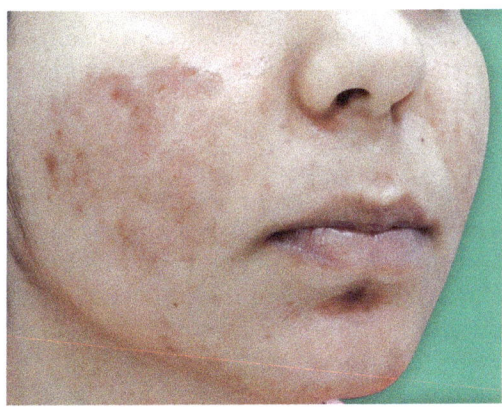

FIG. 5: Postinflammatory hyperpigmentation.

- Milia
- Delayed healing
- Textural changes
- *Ectropion and ocular complications*: This can be prevented by applying petrolatum around the eyes. In case of accidental spillage, immediate saline irrigation of eyes and ophthalmology reference is advised.

Patient education is important to prevent the side effects.

DISCUSSION

Trichloroacetic acid peels can be safely used in Indian skin in concentrations ranging from 10–35%. Medium-depth peels should be used very cautiously to prevent hyperpigmentation and scarring. There should be a minimum interval of 2 weeks between two peels. The level of frosting determines the penetration of the peel. It is advisable to avoid waxing, threading, scrubbing, steaming, laser hair reduction and similar procedures for a week after the peel. This will not only prevent hyperpigmentation but will also help in faster healing of skin. This self-neutralizing peel is not absorbed systemically and can be used on larger areas of the body as well. TCA peels can be readily combined with other resurfacing and rejuvenation procedures, often providing synergistic treatment for patient specific needs.

CONCLUSION

Trichloroacetic acid peels are easy, cheap and an effective modality of treatment. However, due caution must be taken when performing the peel especially in skin of color, due to an increased possibility of postinflammatory hyperpigmentation. It is technique dependent and the results vary with the physician and the concentration of the peel used. Clinicians must be aware of the strengths and limitations of the peel in order to prevent untoward side effects. Skin type, area of skin to be treated, pre- and postpeel care, healing time and patient compliance, should also be taken into account for best overall results.

REFERENCES

1. National Center for Biotechnology Information. PubChem Compound Database CID=6421. Trichloroacetic Acid. [online] Available from https://pubchem.ncbi.nlm.nih.gov/compound/6421 [Accessed March 2018].
2. Ragunath A, Venkataram M, Khunger N. Non-glycolic acid peels—salicylic acid and trichloroacetic acid peel. In: Venkataram M (Ed.). ACSI Textbook of Cutaneous and Aesthetic Surgery, 2nd Edition. New Delhi: Jaypee Medical Publishers; 2017. pp. 745-7.
3. Dewandre L. The Chemistry of Peels and a Hypothesis of action mechanisms. In: Rubin MG (Ed.). Chemical Peels. Procedures in Cosmetic Dermatology. St Louis, MO: Elsevier Inc.; 2006. pp. 1-12.
4. Antonella T, Grimes PE, Padova M (Eds). Color Atlas of Chemical Peels. Berlin: Springer; 2012.
5. Brody H. History of chemical peels. In: Baxter S (Ed.). Chemical Peeling and Resurfacing, 2nd edition. St. Louis: Mosby Year Book Inc; 1997. pp. 1-5.
6. Yokomizo VMF, Benemond TMH, Chisaki C, et al. Chemical peels: review and practical applications. Surg Cosmet Dermatol. 2013;5(1):5868.
7. Khunger N. Trichloroacetic acid peels. In: Khunger N (Ed.). Step by Step Chemical Peels, 2nd edition. Jaypee Medical Publishers; 2014. pp. 79-108.
8. Chun EY, Lee JB, Lee KH. Focal trichloroacetic acid peel method for benign pigmented lesions in dark skinned patients. Dermatol Surg. 2004;30:512-6.
9. Kontochristopoulos G, Kouris A, Platsidaki E, et al. Combination of microneedling and 10% trichloroacetic acid peels in the management of infraorbital dark circles. J Cosmet Laser Ther. 2016;18(5):289-92.
10. Kumari R, Thappa DM. Comparative study of trichloroacetic acid versus glycolic acid chemical peels in the treatment of melasma. Indian J Dermatol Venereol Leprol. 2010;76(4):447.
11. Savant SS. Superficial and medium depth chemical peeling. In: Savant SS (Ed.). Textbook of Dermatosurgery and Cosmetology, 2nd Edition. Mumbai: ASCAD; 2005. pp. 177-95.
12. Al-Waiz MM, Al-Sharqie AI. Medium- depth chemical peels in the treatment of acne scars in dark- skinned individuals. Dermatol Surg. 2002;28(5):383-7.
13. Coleman WP III, Futrell JM. The glycolic, trichloroaceticacid peel. J Dermatol Surg Oncol. 1994;20:76-80.
14. Brody HJ, Hailey CW. Medium depth chemical peeling of the skin: A variation of superficial chemosurgery. J Derm Surg Oncol. 1986;12:1268.
15. Monheit GD. The Jessner's + TCA peel: A medium depth chemical peel. J Dermatol Surg Oncol. 1989;15: 953-63.
16. Fulton JE, Rahimi D, Helton P, et al. Neck rejuvenation by combining Jessner/TCA peel, dermasanding, and CO2 laser resurfacing. Dermatol Surg. 1999;25:745-50.
17. Harris DR, Noodleman FR. Combining manual dermasanding with low strength trichloroacetic acid to improve actinically injured skin. J Dermatol Surg Oncol. 1994;20:436-42.
18. Obagi ZE, Obagi S, Alaiti S, et al. TCA-based blue peel: a standardised procedure with depth control. Dermatol Surg. 1999;25(10):773-80.
19. Garg VK, Sarkar R, Agarwal R. Comparative evaluation of beneficiary effects of priming agents (2% hydroquinone and 0.025% retinoic acid) in the treatment of melasma with glycolic acid peels. Dermatol Surg. 2008;34(8):1032-9.
20. Roberts WE. Chemical peeling in ethnic/dark skin. Dermatol Ther. 2004;17:196-205.
21. Sharad J. Glycolic acid peel therapy – a current review. Clin Cosmet Investig Dermatol. 2013;6:281-8.
22. Bhardwaj D, Khunger N. An Assessment of the Efficacy and Safety of CROSS Technique with 100% TCA in the Management of Ice Pick Acne Scars. J Cutan Aesthet Surg. 2010;3(2):93-6.
23. Cook KK, Cook WR Jr. Chemical peel of nonfacial skin using glycolic acid gel augmented with TCA and neutralized based on visual staging. Dermatol Surg. 2000;26(11): 994-9.

24. Khunger N. Standard guidelines of care for chemical peels. Indian J Dermatol Venereol Leprol. 2008;74 (Suppl.): S5-12.
25. Resnik SS, Resnik Bl. Complications of chemical peeling. Dermatol Clin. 1995;13:309-12.
26. Liu H, Khachemoune A, Rashid RM. Chemical burn following 50% trichloroacetic acid for acne: Presentation of a case and a focused review. J Dermatol Dermatologic Surg. 2015;20:71-4.
27. Rubin MG. Manual of Chemical Peels. Philadelphia, PA: Lippincott; 1995.
28. Nikalji N, Godse K, Sakhiya J, et al. Complications of medium depth and deep chemical peels. J Cutan Aesthet Surg. 2012;5(4):254-60.
29. Salam A, Dadzie OE, Galadari H. Chemical peeling in ethnic skin: an update. Br J Dermatol. 2013;169 (Suppl. 3):82-90.

Lactic Acid Peels

Surabhi Sinha, Gunjan Verma

INTRODUCTION

The use of chemical peels in treating various skin disorders is well established and poses minimal risk when performed by educated practitioners. In this chapter, we will discuss about lactic acid peels in dermatology. Lactic acid is derived from sour milk and is an alpha-hydroxy acid (AHA). AHAs are naturally occurring compounds that contain a hydroxyl group in the alpha position. The use of AHAs in skin care products dates back to ancient Egypt, chiefly Cleopatra, who was said to have applied sour milk to her face to enhance its youthfulness. Lactic acid is a popular AHA that is found in many at-home products and prescription moisturizers. It is one of the mildest AHAs, much milder than the more commonly used glycolic acid (GA) peels. It is an ideal primary peel especially in sensitive skin.

CHEMISTRY

Lactic peel is an AHA and is classified as a superficial peel according to the depth of peel used. Chemically it is 2-hydroxypropanoic acid. It occurs naturally in sour milk, bilberries, pickled vegetables, cheese, wine and beer. It is a natural by-product of glycolysis, having an essential role in carbohydrate metabolism in the body. It is also an important component of the natural moisturizing factor (NMF) in the skin.[1] Several studies on the activity of buffered 12% ammonium lactate lotion have documented its moisturizing ability.[2] It has been shown to increase skin firmness and thickness and improvement in skin texture and moisture content using 5% and 12% lactic acid. These effects were limited to the epidermis as no effect on dermal firmness or thickness was seen.[3]

Alpha-hydroxy acids exert a profound influence on epidermal keratinization.[4] They affect corneocyte cohesiveness at the lower level of stratum corneum, where they alter its pH.[5] When they are applied at a high concentration on the skin, there is a resultant detachment of keratinocytes and epidermolysis; application of a lower concentration reduces intercorneocyte cohesion directly above the granular layer, advancing desquamation and thinning of stratum corneum.[5] This has two major effects—quickening of the cell cycle (which is slowed in aged skin) and increased desquamation, which results in improvement of hyperpigmentation and a smoother skin surface. Without causing deep injury, they have a stimulatory effect on collagen production in fibroblasts. Lactic acid also has a moisturizing and humectant action, increases flexibility and gives a shiny appearance to the skin.

Chemical Formulations

The formulation of lactic acid as a peel or as a moisturizing agent, depends on its pH. Lactic acid above a pH of 3.5 is used as moisturizer. At a pH lesser than 3.5, it is utilised as a peeling agent. In concentrations above 30%, it works as a chemical peel.

PROPERTIES OF LACTIC ACID

- *Keratolytic*: Exfoliation of stratum corneum and stimulation of proliferation in stratum basale
- *Hydrating*: This is unlike the drying effect other AHAs have. Lactic acid is one of the components of NMF and hence improves skin turgor, smoothens skin texture and decreases fine lines and wrinkles
- *Sebostatic and comedolytic:* Lactic acid decreases sebum secretion and unclogs clogged follicular openings
- *Whitening effect due to exfoliation*: It facilitates uniform distribution of melanin in the epidermis. It is also an inhibitor of tyrosinase
- *Bacteriostatic*: Due to the acidifying effect of ionized lactic acid
- *Antioxidant*: As it decreases free radical production.

Its advantages over other AHAs include its significant hydrating effect and its lack of photosensitizing potential, qualities which would make it safer to use in sensitive and darker skin types. Its drawback is that unlike other AHAs, it has no effect on dermal firmness and thickness.

Different pharmaceutical companies provide lactic peel in various formulations and base used. It is also available in gel form which improves the tolerability of the peel. Few brands provide pure lactic acid peel without any added agent. It is also used in combination with many peels. It is a component of Jessner's solution with salicylic acid and resorcinol. Various whitening and depigmenting peels also have lactic acid peel in varying concentrations.

Singh et al. used lactic acid peels in melasma and concluded that 82% lactic acid peel is well tolerated and effective in melasma.[6]

Marked improvement of texture, pigmentation and appearance of superficial acne scars was reported by Sachdeva with full strength (92%) (pure) lactic acid peel.[7]

A study conducted to see clinical efficacy of superficial peeling with 85% lactic acid versus 70% GA in periorbital wrinkling found that both agents were effective in reducing fine wrinkles of the outer lateral eye area after three applications.[8] Vavouli et al. observed that the combination of trichloroacetic acid 3.75% and lactic acid 15% showed encouraging results in improving periorbital hyperpigmentation (POH).[9] Dayal et al. compared GA and lactic acid peels in POH and concluded that both the peels were effective, though GA peels were better from the 12th week onwards but also had more side effects.[10]

INDICATIONS

The role of lactic acid peels is basically to reduce fine lines and wrinkles, reduce uneven pigmentation and to improve texture of photoaged skin.
- *Acne*:[5]
    - Post-acne hyperpigmentation
    - Mild active acne
    - Superficial scarring
    - Acne excoriée.

- *Epidermal dyschromias*:
  - Melasma[5]
  - Postinflammatory hyperpigmentation
  - Periorbital melanosis
  - Frictional dermal melanosis.
- *Rejuvenation*:
  - Photodamaged skin
  - Aging skin
  - Hand rejuvenation.

CONTRAINDICATIONS

- Known hypersensitivity to any component of the peel
- Acute herpes simplex virus infection
- Pregnancy and lactation
- Acute inflammation over the site to be peeled.

PATIENT PREPARATION

Proper patient selection and assessment of each individual's skin condition is crucial. Preoperative consultation is important in:
- Identifying at-risk patients who are best avoided or necessitate an extra-cautious approach
- Selecting ideal candidates
- Evaluating patients for relative contraindications
- Discuss indications of the procedure
- Assessing and understanding the patient's goals, expectations and anticipated results
- A thorough medical history and physical examination should be done
- Past (within last 6 months) or present use of systemic isotretinoin must be ascertained, since retinoids are known to be associated with a greater risk of scarring. This is, however, less relevant in lactic acid peels since it is a superficial peel
- Patients should be asked about prior resurfacing procedures or cosmetic procedures such as rhytidectomy, coronal brow lift or blepharoplasty—increased risk of complications
- An interval of 4–12 weeks is recommended between peeling and procedures involving undermining of skin
- Patients with history of recurrent herpes simplex should be given prophylactic acyclovir beginning the day of the procedure and continuing for 3–5 days after procedure
- Patients with active inflammation (seborrheic, atopic, irritant or allergic dermatitis, rosacea, psoriasis or vitiligo) may be at an increased risk of complications secondary to alterations in the skin's normal barrier function
- Any history of abnormal scar formation, either hypertrophic scar or keloids
- Patients infected with human immunodeficiency virus may experience delayed healing or be at risk for secondary infection after peeling
- A postauricular test peel may be carried out on a 1 cm^2 area. It is useful mostly in patients with sensitive skin, prior history of unexpected reaction to peeling agent applied in the past. Although a favorable test is reassuring, it does not guarantee a positive outcome following full-face resurfacing
- Patient information sheet containing the intended benefits, limitations and risks of treatment should be explained to the patient and an informed written consent should be taken.

Priming

Priming agents are agents applied to the skin in preparation for peeling. They have the following benefits:
- They help to achieve a more uniform penetration of peeling agents by reducing sebum and thinning the stratum corneum
- Accelerate re-epithelialization; reduce wound healing time

- Have a lightening effect by enhancing dispersion of melanin granules.

Multiple combinations exist with a few key players such as topical tretinoin, hydroquinone, AHAs, kojic acid and low-potency steroids.

Pretreatment with 2–4% hydroquinone twice daily and topical tretinoin (0.05% and 0.1%) or retinoic acid nightly 1 month prior to peeling reduces dyschromias and promotes faster healing in the immediate postpeel period.

PEEL TECHNIQUE

Prior to application of peel, the skin is cleaned with spirit and degreased with acetone-soaked sponges. A superficial peel like lactic acid has little or no effect if the skin is poorly prepared. The cleansed skin should be checked for presence of residual oil, if needed, cleansing can be repeated.

- The area is then rinsed with water and dried
- Lactic peel is applied with a brush or Q-tipped applicator on the whole face in a sequential manner within 30 seconds to 1 minute. Feathering is done on the edges to avoid lines of demarcation (Fig. 1)
- Endpoint is pink erythema. But, this may not always be visible in darker skins. This is why time limits are usually set for termination of peeling

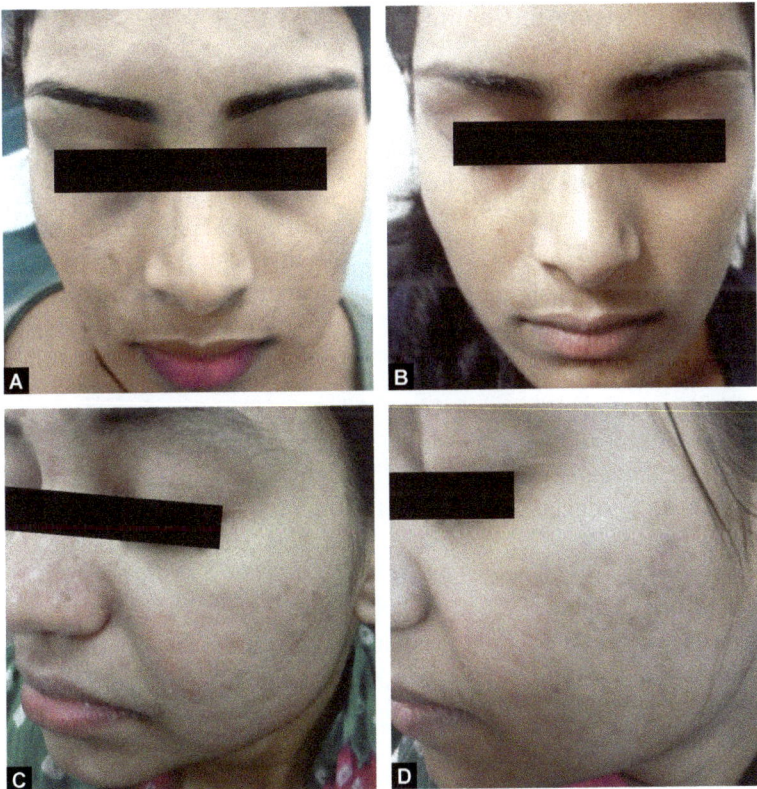

FIG. 1: A, Postacne hyperpigmentation on bilateral malar areas; **B,** Reduction in postacne hyperpigmentation after six sittings of fortnightly lactic acid peels; **C,** Postacne scarring and persistent erythema and textural abnormalities; **D,** Reduction in postacne scars and erythema and improvement in skin texture after six sittings of fortnightly lactic acid peels.

- First sitting is usually done with half-strength (HS—46%) lactic acid peel (1-2 coats) for a maximum of 2-3 minutes depending upon the patient's tolerance. Time and number of coats are increased gradually with further sittings. Contact time can be increased up to 10-15 minutes according to patient tolerance
- During this time, patients may experience mild stinging and burning with minimal discomfort
- Neutralization is done with water or ice-cold sponges
- Peeling is done at an interval of 2 weeks for 4-8 sessions.

PRECAUTIONS

- Always check label on the bottle of chemical to be applied
- Never pass an open container of acid or applicator wet with acid over patient's face
- Always elevate patient's head by 45° during procedure
- Keep water-filled syringes ready.

POSTPEEL CARE

- Strict sun avoidance and sun-protective measures during postoperative period
- Redness and tightness can persist for 2 days. Moisturizing cream should be applied frequently, especially in the first 2-3 days
- Patients should be counseled not to smoke, as it impairs healing
- Resume prepeel regimen only after complete re-epithelialization—may take a few days
- To avoid scratching
- To avoid epilation on treated areas
- To avoid using makeup within the first 24 hours
- To avoid cleansing aggressively.

COMPLICATIONS

- Mild peeling agent; burning and irritation is rare
- Less therapeutic indication
- Sometimes, as a single peeling agent, it is not effective
- Can act as adjuvant to other peels or medical treatment.

PRACTICAL TIPS

Lactic acid is a mild AHA peel. It would be preferable for first-timers to be cautious, start with low strengths (HS) and then move onto full-strength peels and longer contact times. Epidermolysis is always a potential adverse effect especially on periorbital and sensitive skins.

TAKE HOME POINTS

- Lactic acid is one of the largest AHAs; so penetration into the skin is much slower thus leading to less irritation potential
- Lactic acid peels can be used by starters as a first peel, albeit carefully
- Lactic acid is a natural humectant, thus it does not lead to the sensation of dryness and tightness associated with other AHAs.

REFERENCES

1. Middleton JD. Sodium lactate as a moisturizer. Cosmet Toiletries. 1978;93;85.
2. Wehr R, Krochmal L, Bagatell F, et al. A controlled two-center study of lactate 12 percent lotion and a petrolatum-based creme in patients with xerosis. Cutis. 1986;37(3):205-7, 209.
3. Smith WP. Epidermal and dermal effects of topical lactic acid. J Am Acad Dermatol. 1996;35(3 Pt 1):388-91.
4. Van Scott EJ, Yu RJ. Control of keratinization with alpha-hydroxy acids and related compounds. I. Topical treatment of ichthyotic disorders. Arch Dermatol. 1974;110(4):586-90.
5. Berardesca E, Distante F, Vignoli GP, et al. Alpha hydroxy acids modulate stratum corneum barrier function. Br J Dermatol. 1997;137(6):934-8.

6. Singh R, Goyal S, Ahmed QR, et al. Effect of 82% lactic acid in treatment of melasma. Int Sch Res Notices. 2014;14:407142.
7. Sachdeva S. Lactic acid peeling in superficial acne scarring in Indian skin. J Cosmet Dermatol. 2010;9(3):246-8.
8. Prestes PS, Oliveira MM, Leonardi GR. Randomized clinical efficacy of superficial peeling with 85% lactic acid versus 70% glycolic acid. An Bras Dermatol. 2013;88:900-5.
9. Vavouli G, Katambas A, Gregoriou S, et al. Chemical peeling with trichloroacetic acid and lactic acid for infraorbital dark circles. J Cosmet Dermatol. 2013;12:204-9.
10. Dayal S, Sahu P, Jain VK, et al. Clinical efficacy and safety of 20% glycoloc peel, 15% lactic peel, and topical 20% vitamin C in constitutional type of periorbital melanosis: a comparative study. J Cosmet Dermatol. 2016;15:367-73.

CHAPTER 12

Mandelic Acid Peels

Seemal R Desai, Jacob R Stewart

INTRODUCTION

Mandelic acid is a large alpha-hydroxy acid often utilized in dermatology as a superficial chemical peel. Other superficial chemical peels include other alpha-hydroxy acids such as glycolic acid, beta-hydroxy acids and lipohydroxy acids.[1] Mandelic acid is used alone or in conjunction with salicylic acid as a treatment for several common skin conditions such as wrinkles, irregular pigmentation and acne. Although mandelic acid is not as widely used as some other chemical peels, its efficacy for the treatment of multiple dermatological conditions combined with its favorable side-effect profile in multiple skin types (Fitzpatrick I–VI) make it a favorable treatment option.

CHEMISTRY AND CHEMICAL FORMULATIONS USED

Mandelic acid (2S)-2-hydroxy-2-phenylacetic acid) is a chiral, 8-carbon alpha-hydroxy acid.[2] Other alpha-hydroxy acids include glycolic acid, citric acid and lactic acid, which are effective agents in organic synthesis of pharmaceuticals. Mandelic acid's chemical formula is $HOCH(C_6H_5)COOH$ and its chemical properties include a pKa of 3.41 and a high melting point of 119°C.[2,3] The relatively large size and amphiphilic (soluble in water and lipids) nature of the compound also contribute to mandelic acid's ability to slowly and uniformly penetrate the epidermis.[4]

Some of the chemical formulations used include 2–10% mandelic acid concentration washes, gels or lotions, as well as solutions containing vitamins or sunscreen formulations. Chemical peels may contain 30–50% mandelic acid.[3] Beta-hydroxy acids may also be used in combination, such as salicylic-mandelic acid formulations, often 20% salicylic acid and 10% mandelic acid.[5]

INDICATIONS

Pigmentary Disorders

The efficacy of chemical peels in treating a variety of skin conditions is well known, but individuals with ethnic skin have an increased risk of adverse events such as pigmentary disorders, hypertrophic scars and keloid scarring.[6] In patients with darkly pigmented skin types (Fitzpatrick IV to VI), mandelic acid combined with salicylic acid was shown to be well-tolerated compared to glycolic or phytic acid peels.[4,5] This formulation of salicylic–mandelic acid (20% and 10%, respectively) is also more effective for treating postinflammatory hyperpigmentation and melasma than phytic acid peels.[4,5] Dermal melasma and faintly-pigmented lentigines, however, may not respond as quickly or as robustly as superficial melasma, sometimes taking months for lesions to gradually fade.[3]

Skin Rejuvenation

Mandelic acid is an effective chemical peel to decrease fine lines and wrinkles. The rejuvenation of the skin may occur quickly, within days to weeks, and this effect may be sustained as the treatments are continued.[3] The mechanism of action of chemical peels to achieve this result is postulated to be through both the removal of old epidermal cell structures and inducing the production of matrix metalloproteinases and thus collagen remodeling.[7] Mandelic acid was also shown to increase sebum production in the skin of aging women, possibly contributing to the reduction of fine wrinkles in patients following treatment.[7]

Acne and Post-acne Complications

Significant improvement of active acne vulgaris, especially grade III or less with inflammatory lesions, may occur with mandelic acid treatment.[3,4] The antibiotic properties of mandelic acid may contribute to its efficacy in treating active acne lesions, with some patients being able to treat their acne with this chemical peel instead of traditional acne treatment methods.[3] Post-acne scarring and inflammatory hyperpigmentation may also be treated with mandelic acid. One study by Garg et al showed an increased efficacy of mandelic acid combined with salicylic acid compared to glycolic acid in patients with active acne and postinflammatory hyperpigmentation. Antibiotic resistant acne, rosacea and folliculitis are additional conditions which may be treated with mandelic acid.[3]

Antibiotic Properties

Another intriguing aspect of mandelic acid is its properties as an antibiotic. This characteristic of mandelic acid has been used in medicine for many years, particularly for its utility as a urinary antiseptic, inhibiting multiple pathogens including E*scherichia coli, Staphylococcus aureus, Bacillus proteus* and *Enterobacter aerogenes*.[3] In this manner, mandelic acid may be utilized in conjunction with other treatments by acting synergistically to treat skin pathology and prevent potentially devastating gram-negative bacterial infections.[8] When combined with laser resurfacing, one study with over 100 patients resulted in no gram-negative infections.[3]

PATIENT PREPARATION

Patient preparation is one of the most crucial steps in performing any type of chemical peel. Pretreatment screening for any possible contraindications, eliciting a thorough medical history, and discussing the risks and benefits of the procedure is of paramount importance. Once these steps have been completed, the next step is to ensure patient preparation is complete for an efficacious and safe treatment outcome. The patient should undergo a thorough history taking, physical examination, and assessment to understand the the diagnoses, establish expectations, and provide proper education. The basic principles of pretreatment 2–4 weeks before the chemical peel are generally similar for patients being treated with mandelic acid, including photoprotection (sun avoidance and broad-spectrum sunscreen application), gentle facial cleansing, tretinoin and hydroquinone for darker skin types.[9,10] Treatment with antiviral medications is not necessary but must be individualized at times for patient's needs, as mandelic acid is a superficial chemical peel. Within 1 week of the treatment, patients should not do any bleaching, waxing, massaging or scrubbing of the skin and hydroquinone or tretinoin pretreatment should be discontinued a few days before the peel to prevent irritation.[11]

Immediately before the application of mandelic acid, the patient's skin should be made free of debris and facial oil. This may be done by cleansing the face with spirit and degreasing the face with acetone and water, drying the skin gently afterward.[1] Hair should be removed from the face and sensitive areas of the face may be protected by applying a thin layer of petrolatum.

PEEL TECHNIQUE

Mandelic acid may be applied using any classic applicator such as a brush or gauze applicator. The volume of mandelic acid may be approximately 1 mL, taking 30–45 seconds to apply.[4] Patients should be positioned comfortably and be warned about possible discomfort such as a stinging or burning sensation. An endpoint of peeling should be observed, such as mild erythema, stinging or burning sensation described by the patient, or a white frost-like crust developing.[4]

POSTPEEL CARE

The total duration of each peeling session may last from 1–5 minutes, after which patients should wash their face with cold water, being careful to avoid rubbing their skin and rather should pat or air dry the same. Each session should finish with the application of a moisturizer, sunscreen and instructions to avoid sunshine.[1] Patients should continue these precautions and avoid applying other chemicals such as retinoids or salicylic acid in the immediate period following the mandelic acid peel.

Patients may resume hydroquinone or tretinoin after 2 days to 1 week postpeel, allowing for 2–4 weeks between chemical peels.[10]

COMPLICATIONS

Many studies have examined the favorable side-effect profile of mandelic acid. Mandelic acid is much larger than the traditional alpha-hydroxy acid used in chemical peels, namely glycolic acid. As a large chemical peel, mandelic acid penetrates the epidermis slowly, uniformly and may remain in the skin for a longer period.[5] These characteristics make it useful for patients with sensitive skin, as it is associated with fewer complications compared to other peels.[7] A majority (76%) of patients treated with salicylic–mandelic acid do not experience any side effects after treatment, but the most common side effects are a burning sensation (17-25%), dryness (14%) and some photosensitivity or acne flairs.[4,5] It has been observed that erythema and desquamation occurred in 15-20% of patients treated with glycolic acid, while very few patients treated with salicylic–mandelic acid exhibit these adverse events. Patients treated with mandelic acid, however, are more likely than patients treated with glycolic acid to experience a burning sensation (25% to nil, respectively). Further studies are warranted to elucidate the effectiveness and safety profile of this chemical peel compared to similar compounds, as well as in combination with salicylic acid.

PRACTICAL TIPS

Mandelic acid follows much of the same treatment algorithm of other superficial chemical peels. In addition, careful attention should be taken when applying mandelic acid to attain a proper endpoint of treatment. Mandelic acid is a large alpha-hydroxy acid, and slowly penetrates the stratum corneum compared to similar agents. Specific planning and documentation may help the clinician to chart the patient specific endpoint (usually mild erythema, stinging or burning sensation, or white pseudofrost). This will allow effective and careful titration of treatment for subsequent applications and maximize likely therapeutic benefit while minimizing deleterious side effects. We must emphasize, however, that the stringent compliance of the patient to pretreatment and post-treatment skin care is paramount.

TAKE HOME POINTS

- Mandelic acid is effective in treating pigmentary disorders, acne and fine lines or wrinkles
- This chemical peel is a favorable option for patients with ethnic skin (Fitzpatrick IV–VI)
- Mandelic acid has fewer side effects compared to other superficial chemical peels and should be considered for patients with sensitive skin
- Mandelic acid may be used as an adjunct with other therapies such as laser resurfacing, due to its antibiotic properties and safety profile.

REFERENCES

1. Fischer TC, Perosino E, Poli F, et al. Chemical peels in aesthetic dermatology: an update 2009. J Eur Acad Dermatol Venereol. 2010;24(3):281-92.
2. Drugbank. (2005). (S)-Mandelic acid. [online] Available from: https://www.drugbank.ca/drugs/DB03357. [Accessed March 2018]
3. Taylor MB. Summary of mandelic acid for the improvement of skin conditions. Cosmet Dermatol. 1999;12:26-8.
4. Garg VK, Sinha S, Sarkar R.Glycolic acid peels versus salicylic–mandelic acid peels in active acne vulgaris and post-acne scarring and hyperpigmentation: A comparative study.
5. Sarkar R, Garg V, Bansal S, et al. Comparative evaluation of efficacy and tolerability of glycolic acid, salicylic mandelic acid, and phytic acid combination peels in melasma.
6. Jackson A. Chemical peels. Facial Plast Surg. 2014;30(01):26-34.
7. Wójcik A, Kubiak M, Rotsztejn H. Influence of azelaic and mandelic acid peels on sebum secretion in ageing women. Postepy Dermatol Alergol. 2013;30(3):140-5.
8. Brody HJ. Complications of chemical peeling. J Dermatol Surg Oncol. 1989;15(9):1010-9.
9. Monheit GD, Chastain MA. Chemical peels. Facial Plast Surg Clin North Am. 2001;9(2):239-55.
10. Salam A, Dadzie OE, Galadari H. Chemical peeling in ethnic skin: An update. Brit J Dermatol. 2013;169:82-90.
11. Anitha B. Prevention of Complications in Chemical Peeling J Cutan Aesthet Surg. 2010;3(3):186-8.

13 CHAPTER

Pyruvic Acid Peel

Ishad Aggarwal

INTRODUCTION

Pyruvic acid is an alpha-keto acid.[1] It was first shown to be an effective agent for chemical peeling by Griffin in the late 1980s and early 1990s.[2] Since its earliest demonstration as a treatment for actinic keratosis, pyruvic acid is now used for a variety of dermatological indications.

PROPERTIES

- Pyruvic acid is an alpha-keto acid (CH_3-CO-COOH). The C=O group in alpha-keto acids makes them less hydrophilic compared to the O-H group of the alpha-hydroxy acids. Thus, pyruvic acid is a good peeling agent for oily skin
- Because of its low pKa and its small dimension, it penetrates rapidly and deeply through the skin
- It is soluble in both water and ethanol
- At the epidermal level, pyruvic acid induces detachment of keratinocytes, epidermolysis and thinning of the upper epidermal layer
- At dermal levels, pyruvic acid causes an increase in dermal collagen, elastin and other glycoproteins
- It is also known to have antimicrobial properties
- Effect of pyruvic acid depends upon the concentration used, the duration and number of applications and also upon the solvent being used
- Converts physiologically into lactic acid.

FORMULATIONS

The commercially available formulations of pyruvic peels in concentrations of 40–70% are well-balanced solutions of water and ethanol. Pyruvic peels are generally available in combination solutions with lactic acid and salicylic acid.

INDICATIONS

- Greasy, oily skin
- *Acne*: Inflammatory acne especially the microcystic variant
- Moderate acne scars
- Actinic keratosis
- *Photoaging*: Diffuse dyschromias, mottled yellowish pigmentation, fine wrinkles and mild alterations of skin texture
- Melasma
- Warts.

CONTRAINDICATIONS

- History of recent herpes simplex infections

- Pregnancy
- Continuous or daily sun exposure.

PEELING TECHNIQUE

- Degrease the skin with alcohol or acetone
- The peel can be applied either by the brush or cotton tip applicator for 1–3 minutes until erythema appears
- Pyruvic acid can decompose over time, forming carbon dioxide gas and acetaldehyde; these vapors, if inhaled, may be caustic and irritating to the upper respiratory tract. Prevention is achieved with the use of a fan during application
- Neutralization is achieved by sodium bicarbonate solution. Water can also be used to remove the peeling agent from the surface of the skin
- Skin should be adequately hydrated with moisturizer after the peels and adequate sun protection should be given with a sunscreen
- Four to six sessions are needed with a gap of 4 weeks between individual peel sessions.

POSTPEEL CARE

- Adequate sun protection
- Liberal use of moisturizers
- Cessation of irritating products like retinoids.

SIDE EFFECTS

Pyruvic acid application usually induces intense burning and the postpeeling period is characterized by erythema, desquamation and sometimes, crusting. Frosting may happen which can last for a few days.

ADVANTAGES

- Exfoliation and desquamation with pyruvic peels is mild and superficial and generally does not cause discomfort in day-to-day activity of patients after the procedure
- Erythema that may happen after the peel is short lived
- There are little chances of postinflammatory hyperpigmentation, hence its safe to use in type IV–V skin.

DISADVANTAGES

- Intense burning sensation during the procedure
- Since vapors are produced by pyruvic acid, irritation to upper respiratory tract may happen.

RESULTS

- *Acne*: Pyruvic acid peels tend to improve moderate acne of both the inflammatory and noninflammatory variety. Pyruvic acid is strongly lipophilic, thus easily penetrates the pilosebaceous units causing a reduction in sebum and comedolysis. It also has antimicrobial effects. All these properties make pyruvic acid a useful peel for treatment of acne. Cotellessa et al. have reported reduction in lesions of acne in 90% of the cases with pyruvic acid peels.[1] Pyruvic acid has demonstrated comparable efficacy to salicylic acid in treatment of mild to moderate acne in some studies.[3] In 2006, a study by Tosson et al. took place in Egypt.[4] In response to pyruvic acid 40–50%, among 30 patients with acne, 33.3% had very good response (complete healing), 20% had a good response (more than 75% healing), and 36.7% had a moderate response (50–75% improvement). In their study, a clear relation was observed between acne severity and the response to pyruvic acid. The patients with mild acne had revealed much better response to the treatment

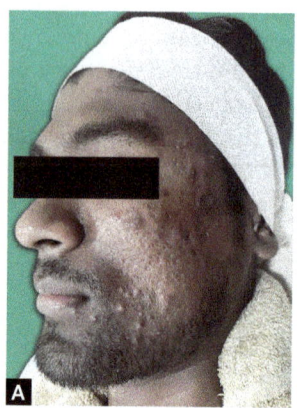 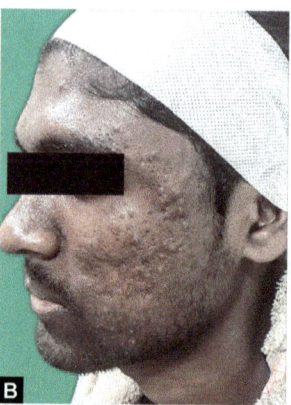

FIG. 1: **A,** A patient of acne before treatment and **B,** after 6 sessions of pyruvic peel. We can also appreciate the difference in texture and pigmentation of the skin.
Courtesy: Manmit K Hora, Consultant Dermatologist, Kolkata.

than other patients. Peeling with pyruvic acid leads to significant reduction in the Global Acne Grading System (GAGS) and Acne Severity Index. In comparison to the 30% salicylic acid peel, there is no significant difference between both the peels in terms of patient tolerability, redness and itching. Only one study reported higher amount of exfoliation with pyruvic peels in the fourth session. Pyruvic peels have shown reduction in both the severity and number of lesions of acne in the author's experience (Fig. 1)

- *Photoaging*: Since pyruvic peel is known to induce collagen and elastin production, it is well suited for treatment of photoaged skin. A study was conducted by Berardesca et al. to evaluate the effects of pyruvic peels.[5] Four peeling sessions were performed once every 2 weeks. The patients were evaluated clinically and by means of several noninvasive methods in order to monitor the following parameters: hydration, color (erythema and pigmentation), elasticity, skin smoothness, skin roughness, scaliness and wrinkles. Instrumental evaluations showed a significant increase in skin elasticity and an improvement of the degree of wrinkling in all the patients. The patients did not report any discomfort neither during the peeling session nor during the postpeeling period, without any impact on their social life. Ghersetich et al. have reported that clinical evaluation of the patients after the peeling sessions with 50% pyruvic acid demonstrated a smoother texture and less evident fine wrinkles[6]
- *Warts*: 70% pyruvic acid is caustic in nature and cause keratolysis. It has been used successfully in treatment of viral warts.[4,7] Tosson et al. in Egypt reported that 70% pyruvic acid used topically twice daily for a period of 2–3 weeks on warts is a safe, effective and painless treatment and can also be used in children.[4] Their results are in agreement with Halasz who reported clearance of warts on using 70% pyruvic acid with and without 5-fluorouracil[7]
- *Hyperpigmentation*: Pyruvic peel has been shown to reduce hyperpigmentary conditions and induce skin lightening.[4-6] A reduction of 3.5 in the mean Melasma

Area and Severity Index (MASI) score was observed in patients of melasma by Tosson et al.[4] Similar findings were reported by Berardesca et al. Pyruvic peels have also shown to reduce other hyperpigmentary conditions like freckles and lentigines.[5]

CONCLUSION

Pyruvic acid is a versatile agent of chemical peeling because of its unique properties. It can be used for a variety of indications like acne, photoaging, melasma and even viral warts. It is well suited for darker skin types because of lesser chances of postinflammatory hyperpigmentation and offers the advantage of lesser downtime and better patient tolerability.

TAKE HOME POINTS

- Pyruvic acid is an alpha keto acid
- It has unique properties
- Well suited for dark skin types
- Common indications are acne, warts, actinic keratosis and melasma.

REFERENCES

1. Cotellessa C, Manunta T, Ghersetich I, et al. The use of pyruvic acid in the treatment of acne. J Eur Acad Dermatol Venereol. 2004;18(3):275-8.
2. Griffin TD, Van Scott EJ, Maddin S. The use of pyruvic acid as a chemical peeling agent. J Dermatol Surg Oncol. 1989;15:1316.
3. Jaffary F, Faghihi G, Saraeian S, et al. Comparison the effectiveness of pyruvic acid 50% and salicylic acid 30% in the treatment of acne. J Res Med Sci. 2016;21:31.
4. Tosson Z, Attwa E, Al-Mokadem S. Pyruvic acid as a new therapeutic peeling agent in acne, melasma and warts. Egypt Dermatol Online J. 2006;2(2):7.
5. Berardesca E, Cameli N, Primavera G, et al. Clinical and instrumental evaluation of skin improvement after treatment with a new 50% pyruvic acid peel. Dermatol Surg. 2006;32:526-31.
6. Ghersetich I, Brazzini B, Peris K, et al. Pyruvic acid peels for the treatment of photoaging. Dermatol Surg. 2004;30(1):32-6.
7. Halasz CL. Treatment of warts with topical pyruvic acid: with and without added 5-fluoruracil. Cutis. 1998; 62(6):283-5.

14
CHAPTER

Jessner's and Resorcinol Peels

Sonali Langar

INTRODUCTION

First formulated by Dr Max Jessner, a German dermatologist in 1950s, and extensively worked on by Dr FC Combes in 1960s, Jessner's solution or Combes formula has since earned its name as a safe and effective superficial peel for skin rejuvenation. It is a superficial peel and induces wounding up to the level of the papillary dermis. It is classified as a blended peel because it combines multiple acids each at a lower concentration to maximize the therapeutic outcome and minimize the potential side effects of any one ingredient when used at a higher concentration. Jessner's peel is self-neutralizing as it spontaneously terminates in a short while after being applied by the water and other skin components. No neutralization by application of a base such as 10–15% sodium bicarbonate solution or water is needed.[1] It can be safely used in all skin types including dark-skinned patients.

However, caution during peeling and judicious application of number of coats should be done when being used in Fitzpatrick skin type IV–VI so as to minimize the possible risk of complications.[2] As with other self-neutralizing peels, increased depth of peel penetration can be achieved by pressure applied during application, number of coats applied and effective skin preparation prior to the peel.

CHEMISTRY AND CHEMICAL FORMULATION

Standard Jessner's solution contains 14 g salicylic acid, 14 g resorcinol, 14 g 85% lactic acid with 95% ethanol added to create a total volume of 100 ml. It is to be kept in a glass, light-protected bottle. It has a shelf life of more than 2 years when kept in the refrigerator and may develop yellow hue after exposure to air and light.

Modified Jessner's solution contains 17 g lactic acid, 17 g salicylic acid and 8 g citric acid with 95% ethanol added to create a total volume of 100 ml. This combination is formulated so as to replace resorcinol and avoid possible allergic reactions and hyperpigmentation problems attributed to it, especially in Fitzpatrick skin types V and VI.

Enhanced Jessner's solution contains, in addition, hydroquinone or kojic acid to target hyperpigmentation.

Jessner's peel exerts its action not only by pH of its solution but also through metabolic effects of lactic acid and toxic effects of resorcinol and salicylic acid. Cell structure and synthesis is interfered with modification or stimulation without causing their destruction.[3]

Salicylic Acid

The properties and the use of salicylic acid (ortho-hydroxybenzoic acid), a beta-hydroxy acid occurring naturally in bark of the willow tree, were first described by Dr Unna, a German dermatologist. It is a lipophilic agent and removes intercellular lipids that are covalently linked to the cornified envelope surrounding cornified epithelioid cells.[4] Due to its comedolytic, keratolytic, anti-inflammatory and antimicrobial properties, it is widely used in the treatment of acne.[5] It has an antihyperplastic effect on the epidermis improving the texture and roughness.[6] It has a mild anesthetic effect and causes less discomfort when applied.[7]

Lactic Acid

Lactic acid (2-hydroxypropanoic acid, gamma-hydroxypropionic acid) is an alpha-hydroxy acid (AHA) occurring naturally in sour milk. It is a weak acid and acts by either metabolic or caustic effect. At low concentration (<30%), it reduces sulfate and phosphate groups from the surface of corneocytes, breaks the intercellular desmosomal bonds thereby inducing exfoliation of the epidermis.[8] At higher concentration, its effect is mainly destructive.[9] It also appears to have dermal effects and has been shown to increase the production of mucopolysaccharides and collagen in the dermis resulting in increased skin thickness and improved skin hydration and suppleness.[10]

Resorcinol

Resorcinol (meta-dihydroxybenzene), a phenol derivative with antibacterial properties, was used in the treatment of minor wounds before the advent of antibiotics. Dr Unna described the use of resorcinol as a peeling agent in 10, 20 and 30% concentrations which was later modified to get a 50% concentration of resorcinol. The paste was prepared using benzoinated axungia as a vehicle, and zinc oxide and ceyssatite as drying agents to obtain a uniform consistency.[11]

Resorcinol is used as a peeling agent at 5-15% concentrations.[12] It is seen that its peeling action starts only at 10% concentration.[13] Resorcinol has proteolytic properties and breaks the weak hydrogen links of keratin causing epidermal exfoliation. It also increases mitosis and accelerates turnover in the basal cell layer resulting in increased thickness of the epidermis. It stimulates fibroblasts in the papillary dermis to synthesize new collagen and glycosaminoglycans.[14]

When used at higher concentrations, resorcinol causes precipitation of skin proteins and protein coagulation. It has been used in many antipruritic formulations mainly in the form of paste known as Unna's paste.[15] Resorcinol has also been shown to control inflammation by stimulating prostaglandin E2 formation.[16]

Traditionally, resorcinol has been used as a peel in a compact paste formulation. The paste which should be freshly prepared (<2 weeks) is softened by putting it in a hot water bath for 5-10 minutes before using it. It is empirical to keep the patient hydrated to encourage diuresis and facilitate elimination of resorcinol metabolites. After covering the eyes, a thick coat of peel is applied uniformly on the face and 2 cm below the jawline using a tongue depressor avoiding the eyebrows and the hair margins. The paste is rubbed gently on the skin to make it more homogenous. The paste can be kept on the face for an average of 30 minutes, and on the trunk for 1 hour. The peel is terminated by removing the paste by tongue depressor and dry gauze and cleaning the skin with tincture of benzoin. Short contact second and third sessions can be done at intervals of a few hours to 2 days.

Peeling of larger surface areas should be avoided in a single session as resorcinol when used alone in higher concentrations has a propensity to cause side effects as myxedema and methemoglobinemia.[11]

INDICATIONS

- Melasma (Fig. 1)
- Postinflammatory hyperpigmentation (Fig. 2)
- Acanthosis nigricans (Figs. 3 and 4)
- Acne vulgaris (Figs. 5 and 6)
- Fine superficial wrinkling
- Lentigines and ephelids
- Photoaging
- Seborrheic keratosis.

PATIENT PREPARATION

Preparing the patient's skin 2–4 weeks prior to the actual peel is the key to get better therapeutic results and overall efficacy of

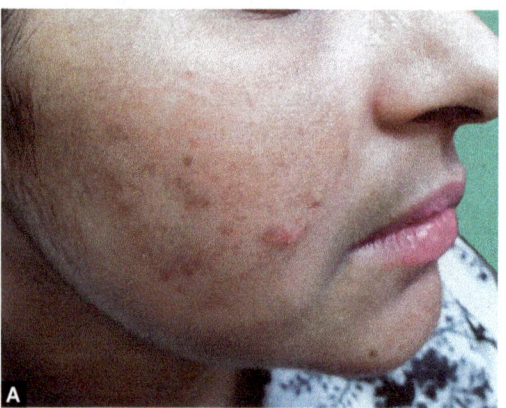 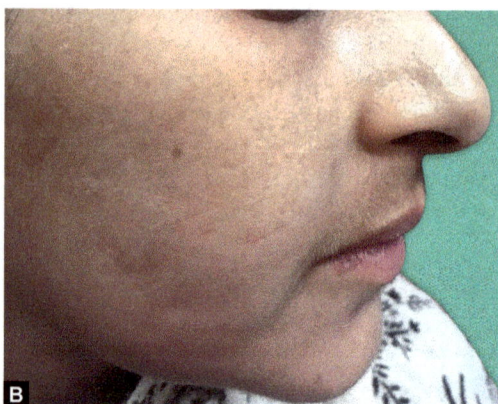

FIG. 1: Significant improvement in melasma and acne seen after 6 sessions of 2-weekly Jessner's peel.

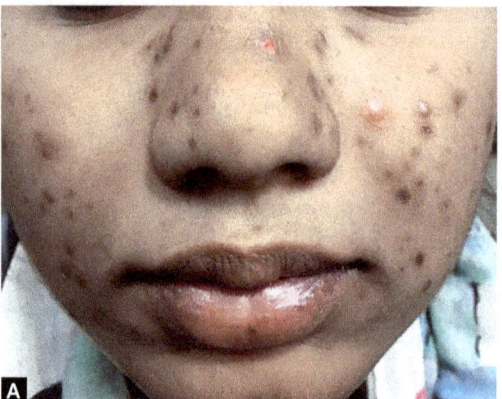 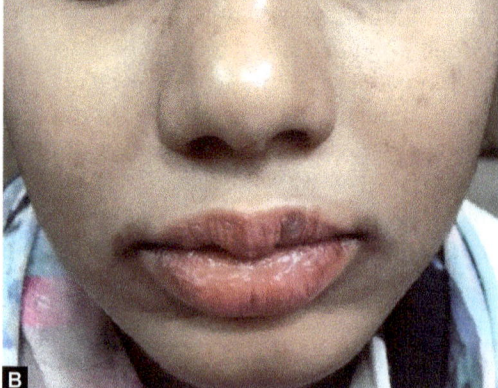

FIG. 2: Marked improvement in postacne pigmentation and scarring seen in the patient after 6 sessions of 2-weekly Jessner's peel.

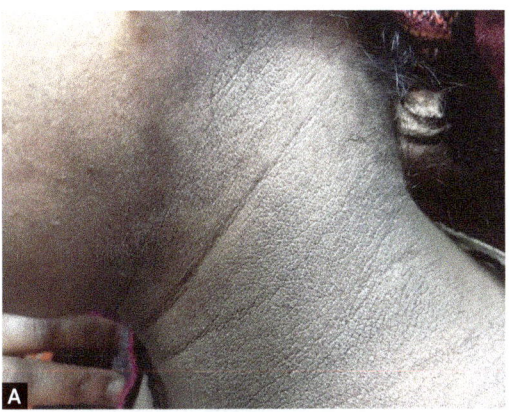 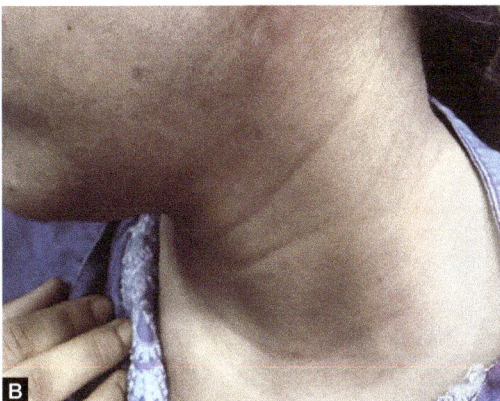

FIG. 3: Marked improvement in acanthosis nigricans seen after 6 sessions of Jessner's–35% trichloroacetic acid peel done at 3 weekly intervals.

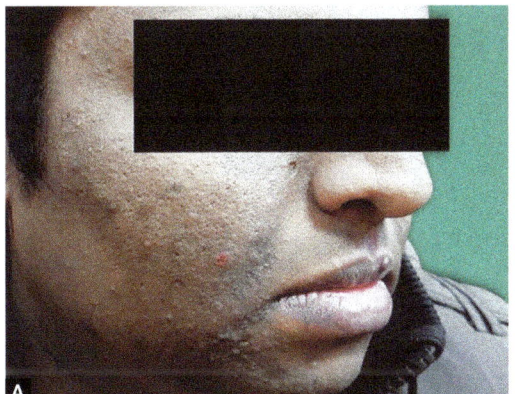 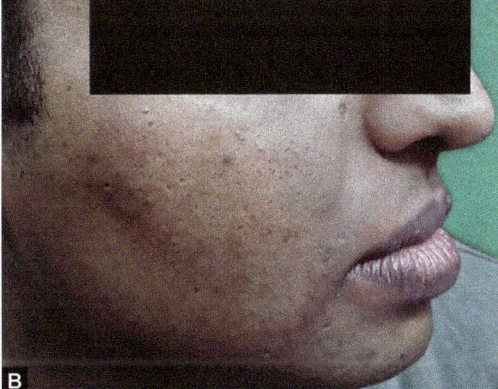

FIG. 4: Marked improvement of skin with regard to thickness, texture and pigmentation seen in the patient after 6 sessions of 3 weekly Jessner's 15% trichloroacetic acid peel.

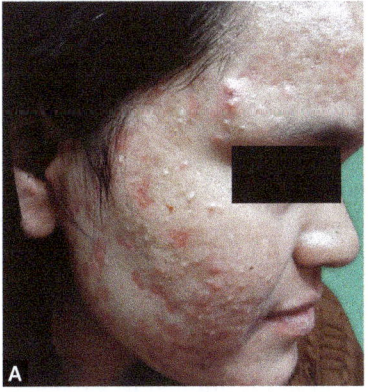 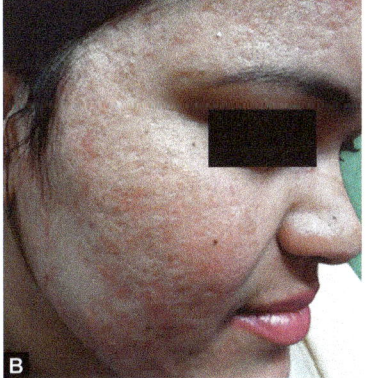

FIG. 5: Complete subsidence of acne and marked improvement in scarring and postinflammatory hyperpigmentation seen after 8 sessions of Jessner's peel in the patient with concomitant oral isotretinoin intake.

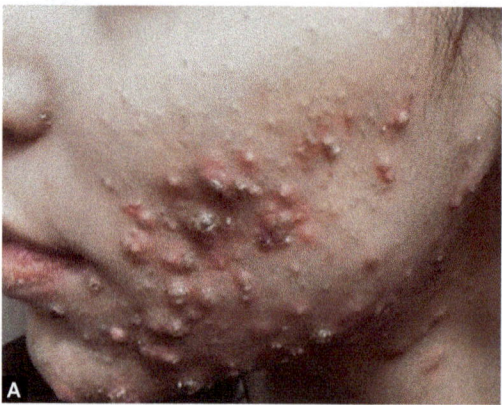 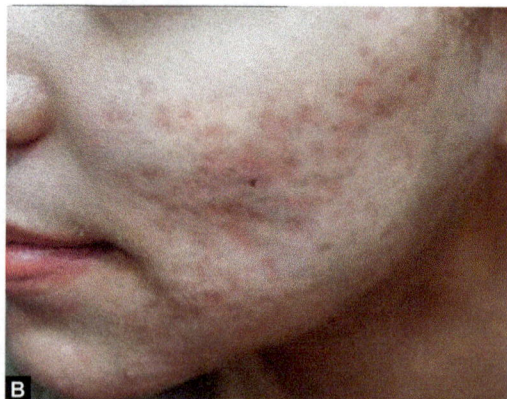

FIG. 6: Marked improvement in acne and postacne pigmentation seen after 8 sessions of 2-weekly Jessner's peel.

the peel. Pretreatment enhances even and increased peel penetration and minimizes chances of potential post peel complications. The regular use of topical pretreatment medications psychologically prepares the patient for the procedure and also enforces compliance for the use of topical medications post peel.

Agents which can be used to prepare the skin include topical retinoids, bleaching agents such as azelaic acid, kojic acid, arbutin, licorice and AHAs as glycolic acid and lactic acid.[17] A broad-spectrum ultraviolet (UV) A or UVB sunscreen with a minimum of SPF 30 should accompany any regimen. Use of topical retinoids (tretinoin cream 0.025-0.05%) for 2-4 weeks prior to peeling thins the stratum corneum, enhancing the penetration of the peeling agent. These agents increase epidermal turnover, reduce the content of epidermal melanin and facilitate epidermal wound healing. The use of topical retinoids should be stopped at least 2-3 days prior to the peeling procedure to avoid postpeel complications such as excessive erythema, desquamation and postinflammatory hyperpigmentation.[18] When treating for dyschromias, the skin should usually be prepared for 2-4 weeks with either a formulation of hydroquinone 2-4% or with any of the bleaching agents to reduce epidermal melanin.[19,20] The AHAs in low percentages decrease keratinocyte adhesion causing desquamation and thinning of epidermis enhancing the overall uniform penetration of peel.[14]

Informed consent should be obtained from each patient. The consent form should list details of the procedure, its limitations and possible complications. It should specifically state the possibility of inclusion of more procedures for attaining desired results. It is worthwhile to mention that providing apt information of the procedure and advising the patient to have realistic expectations is also an important step of patient's preparation.

An allergy test is essential, especially because of the possibility of contact dermatitis due to resorcinol in the formula. Skin sensitivity test should be done behind the patient's ear about a week before the peel. As contact with resorcinol can sensitize the patient to it, the sensitivity test must be repeated before each peel session. A small quantity of resorcinol paste or Jessner's solution is applied to a patch of skin 2 cm × 2 cm behind the ear and left for 15 minutes. The test is read immediately and then at

48 hours and 4-5 days later.[21] A localized skin reaction in the form of erythema and scaling is normal and should not be confused with allergy to the peel. Increased erythema, vesiculation and oozing should arouse suspicion and peel should not be done. The author, however, has not encountered contact sensitivity to Jessner's peel and routinely performs the procedure without allergy testing.

As mentioned earlier, Jessner's peel is safe and well tolerated. General contraindications include infection, dermatitis and active inflammation in the area to be treated, any history of abnormal or delayed wound healing and pregnancy. History of allergies to resorcinol, salicylic acid or lactic acid is an absolute contraindication. Patients with overenthusiastic and unrealistic expectations should not be enrolled. After taking informed consent for photographs, full-face frontal and lateral photos at baseline and each subsequent visit with consistent lighting and positioning should be taken to document improvement.

PEEL TECHNIQUE

The patient is to be laid in a supine position and a headband can be used to secure hair away from the face. A towel is draped across the neck and chest to avoid any spillage of peel on the clothes. The patient shoud be instructed to keep the eyes closed throughout the procedure to avoid accidental eye contact with the peeling agent. Cleansing and degreasing of the skin is carried out with gauze pad or cotton ball soaked with alcohol and acetone. Care should be taken not to abrade the skin manually while degreasing. Application of peel should be done evenly with constant pressure either with a cotton-tip applicator, brush, cotton balls or 2 × 2 gauze sponges.

Apply on the forehead right to left or eyebrows to hairline. Resaturate the applicator each time applying on either cheeks following medial to lateral or horizontal sweep directions. Resaturate and apply down the dorsum of nose, each nasal sidewall, upper lip and across the chin. Apply peel to 1 cm below the jawline so as to avoid the possibility of demarcation line between the treated and untreated areas. If deep wrinkles are present on the skin, stretching of skin is required to avoid pooling of the solution. Prior communication regarding the discomfort that the peel might give in the form of burning, tingling or itching will keep the patient at ease.

Erythema and sporadic pinpoint frosting can be seen after application of the first coat. Pseudofrosting due to precipitation of salicylic acid on the skin can be seen after the ethanol has evaporated. Pseudofrost can be wiped off easily with a gauze unlike true frosting which occurs due to protein coagulation. An additional 2-3 coats can be applied similarly. It is important that each coat be left to dry for 4-5 minutes before applying the next one. As the depth of penetration of the peel depends on the number of coats applied, careless application of one coat immediately over the other would take the peel beyond the desired effect and increase the risk of complications. Also, as the depth of peel depends on the pressure of application, patients with thin skin should be treated with comparative lighter hand pressure.

Undesirable clinical endpoints as increased erythema and frosting can be dealt with by removing the excess peel from the skin using water-saturated gauze. As Jessner's peel is self-neutralizing, application of base is not needed to terminate the acid. It is imperative not to overpeel in the initial session. The first treatment should ideally consist of only one coat and this can be gradually increased to

3-4 coats with successive sessions, assessing the tolerability and safety of the peel on the patient's skin.

Jessner's with 35% Trichloroacetic Acid—Monheit Technique

This technique was developed by Dr Gary Monheit to improve the efficacy, and facilitate more rapid and uniform penetration of trichloroacetic acid (TCA) peel.[22] After the coat of Jessner's solution dries, 35% TCA peel is applied on the skin. This facilitates quick and more even penetration of TCA in the skin because of the breakdown of the epidermal barrier. This technique could be used on patients with thick and oily skin when better TCA penetration is needed. The TCA concentration can be adjusted between 15 and 35% depending upon the patient's thickness of skin and Fitzpatrick type (Fig. 4).

Jessner's with Alpha-hydroxy Acid—Moy Technique

After the coat of Jessner's solution dries, glycolic acid is applied on the skin till erythema spreads and is then neutralized. Jessner's peel improves the depth and even penetration of AHA through the skin. As some degree of erythema is already caused by Jessner's solution, it is difficult to appreciate the progress of the AHA peel which may penetrate too deeply causing unexpected frosting and potential risk of complications. Thus, this technique should be reserved for patients with very thick and oily skin.[23]

Using Retinoid Boost

This is recommended for Fitzpatrick skin types I-III. Additional retinoid peel application is done after application of the last layer of Jessner's peel to expedite the desquamation process. It is noteworthy to mention that the patient's skin type can act as a guide for the treatment to be aggressive or not and can also predict the treatment response. Patients with lighter skin types (Fitzpatrick I-III) typically tolerate more aggressive treatments while patients with darker skin types (Fitzpatick IV-VI) have greater risks of developing post-procedure pigmentary changes and thus should be dealt with a little more meticulously.

POSTPEEL CARE

A single coat application of Jessner's peel only causes little dryness of the skin. Peel sessions consisting of 2-3 coats trigger pronounced erythema and cloudy white frosting making the patient's skin feel dry and tight postpeel. The dry top layers of the epidermis appear transparent and eventually shed by flaking within 5-7 days. Some areas may turn brownish where Jessner's solution had penetrated more deeply and heal in a week's time. Sessions consisting of three coats or more cause more pronounced flaking; the skin becomes brownish and is shed in a strip-like manner. The skin takes 10-14 days to heal. Prior information about the time taken for recovery of skin postpeel should be given as it minimizes anxiety in the patient.

Postpeel care includes regular use of bland moisturizers and a broad-spectrum sunscreen of SPF 30 or higher. Low to mid potency steroid cream can be used for 2-3 days in case of pronounced erythema. Topical antibacterial ointment should be used to prevent bacterial infection in case of crusting. Analgesics though routinely not needed may be advised in case of persistent burning. The flaking should not be picked or scrubbed as fiddling can lead to scarring and pigmentary changes. Waxing and laser hair reduction should be avoided at least 2 weeks postpeel. Avoid any strenuous activity that causes excessive perspiration and avoid the use of steam rooms, saunas and excessively hot showers during the first few days following the peel as this can increase the risk of complications. Use of general skin care products, topical retinoids and bleaching agents can be resumed after peeling subsides. Makeup can be worn to camouflage peeling.[24]

COMPLICATIONS

General Complications

Jessner's peel is a well-tolerated and safe despite concerns regarding resorcinol and salicylate toxicity. Complications usually occur due to improper patient preparation, aggressive peeling (especially in dark skin type), wrong patient selection, inadequate sun protection and picking on the flakes and crust postpeel. Prolonged erythema can occur which is usually mild and transient and can last from 2–3 days to a week postpeel. It usually responds to application of a mild to mid-potent topical steroid cream. Localized or pan facial postinflammatory hyperpigmentation can occur which can be managed by skin lightening creams, vitamin C and adequate sun protection. Reactivation of herpes should be anticipated in susceptive individuals particularly when Jessner's solution is combined with TCA making it a medium-depth peel. Prophylaxis with oral antivirals should be given. Secondary bacterial infections can occur post picking of flakes and crust and should be treated to prevent scarring.

Specific Complications

Contact Dermatitis

Higher concentrations of resorcinol (10–50%) used in peel preparations in the early part of the 20th century were associated with increased incidence of side effects such as allergic contact dermatitis, irritant contact dermatitis and skin discoloration. Subsequent formulation of Jessner's solution using a lower concentration of resorcinol (14%) has rarely been associatied with any allergic reactions. The incidence of allergy to resorcinol is documented to be less than 0.1%. A skin sensitivity test behind the patient's ear a week before a resorcinol peel can be done.[25]

Resorcinol Toxicity

Antithyroid effects of resorcinol have been documented in the past where large amounts of resorcinol-containing ointments were applied to barrier compromised skin for a long time.[26] There has also been a case report of induction of exogenous ochronosis after application of resorcinol for a long time.[27] Cases of methemoglobinemia have been described after application of resorcinol on leg ulcers but not after a peel on normal skin.[28]

Salicylate Toxicity

Application of higher concentrations of salicylic acid particularly on nonintact skin has been documented to cause salicylism manifesting as nausea, tinnitus and disorientation. However, no such case report has been published with the localized use of salicylic acid in concentrations of 14% in Jessner's peel. Cases of salicylism have been described after application of Jessner's solution to the face, chest, arms and legs in a single session. It is, therefore, advisable to avoid large peeling sessions involving more than 25% of the body surface area to reduce the risk of toxicity.[29]

CONCLUSION

Jessner's solution is a versatile and safe peel with minimal downtime useful in all skin types; however, caution should be exercised when using it in darker skin. As previously mentioned, it is critical to wisely choose the appropriate number of peel coats in the patient in order to achieve maximum therapeutic results with minimal risk of complications. Starting with one peel coat and increasing the number of coats with each successive session not going beyond three coats in the colored skin, is imperative to avoid undue complications. Due to its diverse indications, Jessner's peel is surely here to stay for long.

TAKE HOME POINTS

- Jessner's solution is a safe, efficacious peel useful in all skin types; however, overenthusiastic peeling sessions should be avoided when dealing with dark skin types
- Effective prepeel preparation of the skin and religious adaptation of sun protective measures is an important determinant of peel results
- It is critical to wisely choose the appropriate number of peel coats in the patient in order to achieve maximum therapeutic results with minimal risk of complications
- Single peeling sessions involving more than 25% body surface areas should be avoided
- Jessner's peel can be used to prepare the skin for subsequent TCA or alpha-hydroxy acid peels.

REFERENCES

1. Small R. Chemical peel introduction and foundation concepts. In: Small R, Hoang D, Linder J, editors. A practical guide to chemical peels, microdermabrasion and topical products. 1st ed. Philadelphia: Lippincott Williams & Wilkins; 2013. pp. 40-4.
2. Kadhim KA, Al-Waiz M. Treatment of periorbital wrinkles by repeated medium depth chemical peels in dark skinned individuals. J Cosmet Dermatol. 2005;4(1):18-22.
3. Dewandre L, Tenenbaum A. The chemistry of peels: a hypothesis of action mechanisms and a proposal of a new classification of chemical peelings. In: Tung R, Rubin MG (Ed.) Chemical Peels. Philadelphia: Saunders/Elsevier; 2010. pp. 1-16.
4. Lazo ND, Meine JG, Downing DT. Lipids are covalently attached to rigid corneocyte protein envelope existing predominantly as beta-sheets: A solid state nuclear magnetic resonance study. J Invest Dermatol. 1995;105:296-300.
5. Lee HS, Kim IH. Salicylic acid peels for the treatment of acne vulgaris in Asian patients. Dermatol Surg. 2003;29:1196-9.
6. Kligman D, Kligman AM. Salicylic acid peels for the treatment of photoaging. Dermatol Surg. 1998;24:325-8.
7. Grimes PE. The safety and efficacy of salicylic acid chemical peels in darker racial ethnic groups. Dermatol Surg. 1999;25:18-22.
8. Rawlings AV, Davies A, Carlomusto M. Effect of lactic acid isomers on keratinocyte ceramide synthesis, stratum corneum lipid levels and stratum corneum barrier function. Arch Dermatol. 1996;228:383-90.
9. Van Scott EJ, Yu RJ. Alpha-hydroxy-acids: Procedures for use in clinical practice. Cutis. 1989;43:222-8.
10. Deprez P. Alpha hydroxy acids. In: Deprez P, editor. Textbook of Chemical Peels—Superficial, Medium and Deep Peels in Cosmetic Practice. Boca Raton: Taylor & Francis; 2017. pp. 45-6.
11. Karam PG. 50% resorcinol peel. Int J Dermatol. 1993;32(8):569-74.
12. De Groot AC. Dermatological drugs, topical agents and cosmetics. In: Dukes MN, Aronson JK, editors. Meyler's side effects of drugs. Amsterdam: Elsevier; 2000. p. 473.
13. Mills OH, Kligman AM. Drugs that are ineffective in the treatment of acne vulgaris. Br J Dermatol. 1983;108:371-4.
14. Lettessier S. Chemical peel with resorcin. In: Roenigk RK, Roenigk HH, editors. Dermatologic Surgery, Principles and Practice. Oxford: Marcel Dekker; 1999. pp. 1115-9.
15. Alanko J, Riutta A, Holm P, et al. Modulation of arachidonic acid metabolism by phenols: Relation to positions of hydroxyl groups and peroxyl radical scavenging properties. Free Radic Biol Med. 1993;14:19-25.
16. Levy BD, Clish CB, Schmidt B, et al. Lipid mediator class switching during acute inflammation: signals in resolution. Nat Immunol. 2001;2:612-9.
17. Matarasso SL, Glogau RG. Chemical face peels. Dermatol Clin. 1991;9:131-50.
18. Hevia O, Nemeth AJ, Taylor JR. Tretinoin accelerates healing after trichloroacetic acid chemical peel. Arch Dermatol. 1991;127(5):678-82.
19. Garg VK, Sarkar R, Agarwal R. Comparative evaluation of beneficiary effects of priming agents (2% hydroquinone and 0.025% retinoic acid) in the treatment of melasma with glycolic acid peels. Dermatol Surg. 2008;34(8):1032-40.

20. Resnik Bl. The role of priming the skin for peels. In: Tung R, Rubin MG, editors. Chemical Peels. Philadelphia: Saunders/Elsevier; 2010. pp. 23-6.
21. Monheit GD. The Jessner's-trichloroacetic acid peel. An enhanced medium-depth chemical peel. Dermatol Clin. 1995;13:277-83.
22. Moy LS. Superficial chemical peels with alpha-hydroxy acids. In: Robinson JK, Arndt KA, Le Boit PE, Wintroub BU, editors. Atlas of Cutaneous Surgery. Philadelphia: WB Saunders Co.; 1996. pp. 345-50.
23. Fulton JE Jr. The Progressive Peel: The Combined Jessner, TCA, Retinoid Peel. In: Tung R, Rubin MG, editors. Chemical Peels. Philadelphia: Saunders/Elsevier; 2010. pp. 49-60.
24. Barbaud A, Modiano P, Cocciale M, et al. The topical application of resorcinol can provoke a systemic allergic reaction. Br J Dermatol.1996;135:1014-5.
25. Lynch BS, Delzell ES, Bechtel DH. Toxicology review and risk assessment of resorcinol: thyroid effects. Regul Toxicol Pharmacol. 2002;36:198-210.
26. Thomas AE, Gisburn MA. Exogenous ochronosis and myxoedema from resorcinol. Br J Dermatol. 1961;73:378-81.
27. Manquat A. Traité Élementaire de Thérapeutique de Matière Médicale et de Pharmacologie. 5th ed. Paris: JB Librairie J. Baillière et Fil; 1903. pp. 240-60.
28. Grimes P E. Salicylic acid peel. In: Tung R, Rubin MG, editors. Chemical peels. Philadelphia: Saunders/Elsevier; 2010. pp. 41-8.
29. Ekmekçy P, Bostanci S, Gurgey E. The efficacy of chemical peeling performed with Jessner's solution and 35% TCA in the treatment of melasma. Klin J Dermatol. 2001;11:211-6.

Tretinoin and Retinol Peels

Latika Arya

INTRODUCTION

Tretinoin and retinol peels have become popular peeling agents because of the favorable results shown by their use in a few of the recent studies.[1,2] The other reasons for their popularity are ease of application, lack of burning sensation and patient satisfaction. They offer predictable depth control and produce superficial exfoliation. They are considered safe, with a low incidence of side effects. Clinical and histological evidence confirms the favorable results.[1] Effectiveness of topical tretinoin (retinoid acid) in the treatment of photoaging was first suggested by Kligman et al. in 1980.[3] Tretinoin was first used as a peel by Cuce et al. for melasma. They observed a thicker epidermis with a better organization histologically and an improvement in the texture and appearance of the skin clinically.[4]

CHEMISTRY AND CHEMICAL FORMULATIONS USED

The retinoid family comprises vitamin A (retinol) and its natural derivatives such as retinaldehyde, retinoic acid and retinyl esters, as well as a large number of synthetic derivatives.[5] Retinol is a 20-carbon molecule that consists of a cyclohexenyl ring, a side chain with four double bonds (all in transconfiguration) and an alcohol end group, hence the name all-trans retinol. The oxidation of the alcohol end group in retinol results in the formation of an aldehyde (all-trans retinaldehyde or retinal), which can be further oxidized to a carboxylic acid (all-trans retinoic acid or tretinoin).

Mode of Action

Tretinoin activates three nuclear retinoic acid receptors (RAR-alpha, RAR-beta and RAR-gamma), which bind to regulatory regions in DNA and activate many gene transcriptions. This is responsible for the various epidermal and dermal changes seen with retinoids (Table 1).[6,7] Tretinoin lead to mainly epidermal changes, dispersion of melanin and collagen stimulation in the dermis.[8] Tretinoin affect cellular differentiation by exfoliation and compaction of the stratum corneum, stimulating epidermal hyperplasia. It also stimulate the formation of new collagen and blood vessels in the papillary dermis and induces biosynthesis and deposition of glycosaminoglycans. Clinically, there is an improvement in the texture, pigmentation and overall appearance of the treated skin.

Tretinoin and Retinol Peels

TABLE 1: Epidermal and dermal changes seen with retinoids[6,7]

Mechanism of action	Clinical effects
• Epidermal changes 　○ Cellular differentiation 　○ Compaction of stratum corneum 　○ Epidermal hyperplasia	• Improvement in texture ○ Increased smoothness and reduced roughness
Melanin dispersion	Improvement in pigmentation
Collagen stimulation	• Reduction in fine wrinkles • Improvement in atrophy

Also, there is reduction in fine wrinkles and improvement of atrophy.[1,9,10] The mechanism of action of retinoid peels is similar to that of topical retinoids with the advantage of producing faster results.[4,11]

Tretinoin, retinol and retinal are useful in higher concentrations as peeling agents.[12] They penetrate the stratum corneum and the upper layers of the stratum spinosum in the epidermis, thus producing a very superficial peel. Tretinoin is usually employed in the concentration of 1–10%.[2,13] Tretinoin can also be used as a peeling mask in a concentration of 10%.[14] Retinol, however, is the more commonly used agent among the retinoid peels, typically used in concentrations of 10–15%.

INDICATIONS

Retinoid peels can be used in all skin types to treat a variety of conditions.[1,2,15] These chemical peels can be applied to the face and the body.[1]

The usual indications are:
- Photoaging: Solar lentigines, dullness and rough skin texture
- Fine lines
- Enlarged pores
- Melasma
- Ephelides
- Postinflammatory hyperpigmentation
- Comedonal acne and papulopustular acne
- Acne-induced pigmentation (Fig. 1)
- Atrophic acne scars
- Actinic keratosis
- Keratosis pilaris
- Stretch marks.

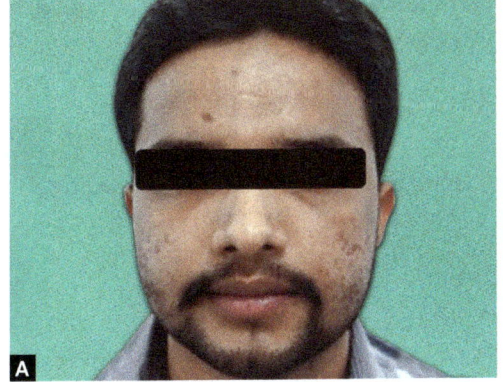 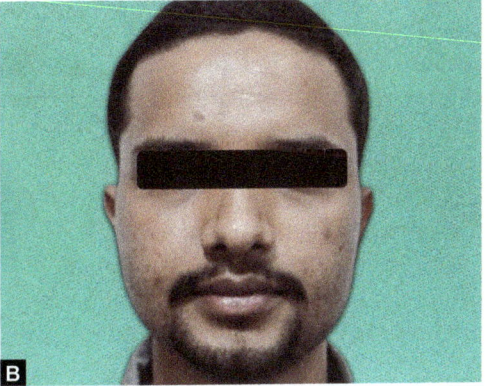

FIG. 1: A, Before treatment; **B,** After treatment. Lightening of postacne hyperpigmentation with 4 sessions of monthly retinol peel. Significant lightening of normal skin also noted.

PATIENT PREPARATION

Prepeel Preparation

The patient's medical history is reviewed and the cutaneous examination is performed. The indications for the peel like pigmentation, acne, scars and wrinkles are noted. The patient's skin type, oiliness/dryness and the current skin condition are noted as well. Pretreatment photographs are taken.

Preparation of the skin for the peel, called priming, is done at least 2–4 weeks prior. It consists of a skin care regimen including a broad-spectrum sunscreen of SPF 30 or greater during the daytime and a retinoid, or alpha-hydroxy acids (AHAs) containing product with or without a skin lightening agent like hydroquinone (2–4%) at night. This helps to prepare the skin by decreasing stratum corneum thickness, thereby allowing even peel penetration. It also helps to enhance peel effects, facilitate postprocedure healing and reduce the risk of complications such as postinflammatory hyperpigmentation. Patients are advised to avoid sun exposure before and during the duration of treatments. Patients are advised to discontinue products containing AHAs and retinoids 4–5 days prior to the peel to ensure that skin is intact at the time of the peel, so as to prevent unintended deeper penetration of the peel. Patch testing is recommended for all chemical peels, wherein the agent is applied on a small area behind the ear and later observed for any undue adverse effects.

If there is a history of herpes, prophylactic antiviral medication (e.g., acyclovir 400 mg or valacyclovir 500 mg, twice daily) should be started 2 days prior to the procedure and continued for 3 days after the procedure.

PEEL TECHNIQUE

Prepeel

Informed consent should be taken. On the day of the procedure, the treatment area is washed and any jewelry or contact lenses are removed. The patient is made to lie in a comfortable semireclining position and is draped. The skin is cleansed to remove topical products or makeup by an hydroxy acid cleanser and an astringent toner or alcohol to degrease the skin (Fig. 2). This preparation helps ensure even application and enhance peel penetration. Petrolatum is applied at the medial and lateral canthi, alar crease, and mentolabial angle to prevent pooling of peel solution in these creases and causing inadvertent deeper peel penetration.

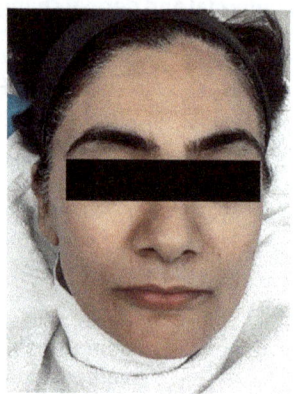

FIG. 2: Prepeel skin preparation. Patient made to lie in a comfortable position and draped; skin cleansed and degreased by hydroxy acid cleanser and an astringent toner or alcohol.

Chemical Peel Application

Retinoid peels range from solutions to cream formulations. Application techniques vary according to the consistency of the product.[16]

Solutions

The peel solution is applied to the least reactive areas first, such as the forehead, then the periphery of the cheeks, followed by nose, upper lip, chin and then to the more sensitive areas such as the medial face. Open bottles or soaked applicators should never be passed over the patient's eyes. If peel solution enters the patient's eyes, flush the eye immediately with normal saline solution or water.

Creams

The cream formulation is applied using gloved hands in a single layer. A coin-sized amount of retinol cream is dispensed onto a gloved hand. An equal-sized amount is placed in 4 quadrants of the face, namely, forehead, bilateral cheeks and medial face (nose, upper lip and chin) (Box 1).[17]

The cream is spread and lightly massaged using fingertips in small circular motions. A small amount is applied along the jawline to feather the edges of the treatment area. The patient is asked to communicate any sensation of discomfort they may be feeling on a pain scale of 1–10, according to the author. Discomfort up to 3 or 4 out of 10 is acceptable. However, usually there is no or minimal discomfort associated with the retinol peel, except for a mild tingling or warm sensation and fanning is rarely required. The cream is continued to be massaged until it is absorbed and almost dried. The skin feels slightly tacky and shows a yellow discoloration due to the yellow color of retinoid peels (Fig. 3).

The skin is observed throughout treatment for any signs of irritation such as excessive burning, pain greater than 5 out of 10, erythema and/or vesiculation. However mild erythema is a desirable endpoint.[17]

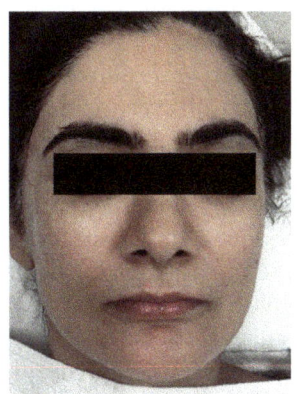

FIG. 3: The yellow appearance of the face after application of a 4% retinol cream peel.

Termination

Retinoid peels are self-neutralizing and therefore do not require application of a neutralizing agent. The peel is left on the skin and patient is instructed to wash the face at home after 4–8 hours with a gentle cleanser.

However, if excessive irritation occurs such as excessive burning, vesiculation or whitening of the skin, then the peel is terminated by removing the peel product using a dry gauze. The face is then wiped briskly from the center to the periphery using gauze moistened with water and repeated 2–3 times until the entire peel is removed. Cold packs or cold wet gauze may be applied to the face for a few minutes and fanning may be done if needed, to reduce discomfort.

POSTPEEL CARE

After the peel has been removed by washing, a soothing bland moisturizer is applied. However, if there is moderate to severe erythema, a low-to-mid-potency steroid cream is applied (e.g., hydrocortisone 1.0%, or fluticasone propionate 0.05%). To protect the skin from ultraviolet exposure, a broad-spectrum sunscreen of SPF 30 or higher containing zinc oxide or titanium dioxide is applied at the end.

BOX 1 | **Application technique for cream-based retinoid peel**

Distribution of cream-based retinoid peel on face
- Coin-sized peel amount distributed in 4 quadrants
    - Quadrant 1, forehead
    - Quadrant 2, cheek
    - Quadrant 3, cheek
    - Quadrant 4, medial face (nose, upper lip and chin)
- Massaged until absorbed

The patient experiences mild erythema, dryness, pruritus and skin sensitivity in the first 3-5 days after procedure. The skin may also feel tighter with accentuation of wrinkles. Desquamation usually starts on day 3-5 after procedure and is visible as mild flaking, scaling, or peeling. It usually starts in the mid face proceeding peripherally and persists for 1 week. In some cases, flaking or peeling may not be visible, particularly in patients whose skin is regularly exfoliated. These patients need to be counseled that despite lack of visible peeling, the skin does receive the benefit of the peel procedure.

During the exfoliating phase after the peel, the patient is instructed to apply soothing and hydrating topical products and avoid irritating ingredients such as AHAs or retinoids. A gentle cleanser and a broad-spectrum sunscreen of SPF 30 or greater containing zinc oxide or titanium dioxide during the day are also recommended. Strict sun avoidance for 1 week postprocedure is advised as well.

If there is marked erythema after peel, a low potency steroid cream (hydrocortisone 1.0%) can be prescribed for a few days to avoid postpeel hyperpigmentation, especially in patients with darker skin types (IV–VI). Makeup may be used 24 hours after the procedure. Regular skin care products may be resumed once the desquamation phase has subsided, usually 7-10 days postprocedure.

The patient is asked to follow up if there is occurrence of any prolonged erythema, severe irritation, pruritus, or crusting.

COMPLICATIONS

Retinoid peels are generally predictable with very low risk of untoward complications. They are considered safe even in darker phototypes, due to their inhibitory effect on melanin synthesis.[14] Usually, they are well tolerated and do not cause burning, stinging, pain, or irritation.

However, occasionally one may see the following complications:
- Burning sensation
- Transient hyperpigmentation
- Prolonged erythema[18]
- Excessive scaling in localized areas, such as the cheeks, eyelids and the perioral region
- Contact dermatitis
- Vesiculation[19]
- Infection
- Acne exacerbation
- Herpes simplex activation.

PRACTICAL TIPS AND AUTHOR'S SUGGESTIONS

- The patient's preprocedure product regimen can alter the skin and its response to chemical peel treatment
- The patient should be counseled regarding variability of desquamation intensity. Excessive desquamation during the post-treatment period can be managed by application of a moisturizer twice or thrice daily, along with a sunscreen in the daytime. On the other hand, lack of peeling or flaking does not indicate that a peel was ineffective and patients may require reassurance regarding this
- Retinoid peels can be used alone, or sequentially over other superficial peels, such as AHAs, beta-hydroxy acids, Jessner's peel and AHA combination peels to intensify the effect and enhance results
- Treatment intensity of a retinoid peel treatment may be increased at a subsequent visit if a patient has demonstrated tolerability to a given peel procedure. The intensity can be increased by either increasing the peel concentration, using a stronger retinoid, or instructing the patient to leave the retinoid peel on for a longer duration. Modify one treatment parameter at a time (e.g., concentration

or duration of application) to increase treatment intensity in a predictable and safe manner.

CONCLUSION

Retinoid peels are effective in the treatment of a wide variety of conditions including photoaging, fine wrinkles, dyschromia, acne, acne scars, actinic keratosis, striae and superficial scarring. They can be used as a stand-alone peel, combination peel, or a sequential peel. They are also of reasonable cost, easy to execute, well tolerated and have a low side effect profile.

TAKE HOME POINTS

- Retinoids—tretinoin, retinol and retinal are useful in strong concentrations as superficial peels
- They are effective in treating a wide variety of indications including photoaging, fine wrinkles, dyschromia, superficial scars, acne, acne scars, actinic keratosis and striae
- They offer ease of application, predictable depth control, safety and efficacy
- They are available as solution and creams and are self-neutralizing leave on peels
- Retinoid peels can be used alone, or as sequential or rotational peels.

REFERENCES

1. Hexsel D, Mazzuco R, Dal'Forno T, et al. Microdermabrasion followed by a 5% retinoid acid chemical peel vs. a 5% retinoid acid chemical peel for the treatment of photoaging–a pilot study. J Cosmet Dermatol. 2005;4(2):111-6.
2. Khunger N, Sarkar R, Jain RK. Tretinoin peels versus glycolic acid peels in the treatment of Melasma in dark skinned patients. Dermatol Surg. 2004;30(5):756-60.
3. Kligman AM, Grove GL, Hirose R, et al. Topical tretinoin for photoaged skin. J Am Acad Dermatol. 1986;15:836-59.
4. Cucé LC, Bertino MC, Scattone L, et al. Tretinoin peeling. Dermatol Surg. 2001;27:12-4.
5. Antille C, Tran C, Sorg O, et al. Penetration and metabolism of topical retinoids in ex vivo organ-cultured full-thickness human skin explants. Skin Pharmacol Physiol. 2004;17:124-8.
6. Darlenski R, Surber C, Fluhr JW. Topical retinoids in the management of photodamaged skin: from theory to evidence-based practical approach. Br J Dermatol. 2010;163(6):1157-65.
7. Baldwin HE, Nighland M, Kendall C, et al. 40 years of topical tretinoin use in review. J Drugs Dermatol. 2013;12:638-42.
8. Sarkar R, Bansal S, Garg VK. Chemical peels for melasma in dark-skinned patients. J Cutan Aesthet Surg. 2012;5(4):247-53.
9. Ramos-e-Silva M, Hexsel D, Rutowitsch MS, et al. Alpha-hydroxy acids and retinoids in cosmetics. Clin Dermat. 2001;19(4):460-6.
10. Griffiths CE, Finkel IJ, Tranfaglia MG, et al. An in vivo experimental model for topical retinoid effects on human skin. Br J Dermatol. 1993;29:389-99.
11. Kligman DE, Draelos ZD. High-strength tretinoin for rapid retinization of photoaged facial skin. Dermatol Surg. 2004;30(6):864-6.
12. Mukherjee S, Date A, Patravale V, et al. Retinoids in the treatment of skin aging: an overview of clinical efficacy and safety. Clin Interv Aging. 2006;1(4):327-48.
13. Magalhães GM, Borges MF, Queiroz AR, et al. Double-blind randomized study of 5% and 10% retinoic acid peels in the treatment of melasma: Clinical evaluation and impact on the quality of life. Surg Cosmet Dermatol. 2011;3:17-22.
14. Ghersetich I, Troiano M, Brazzini B, et al. Melasma: Treatment with 10% tretinoin peeling mask. J Cosmet Dermatol. 2010;9:117-21.
15. Sumita JM, Leonardi GR, Bagatin E. Tretinoin peel: A critical view. An Bras Dermatol. 2017;92(3):363-6.
16. Rubin ME. Manual of Chemical Peels: Superficial and Medium Depth. Philadelphia: Lippincott; 1995.
17. Small R. A Practical Guide to Chemical Peels, Microdermabrasion & Topical Products. Philadelphia:Lippincott Williams & Wilkins, 2013.
18. Faghihi G, Fatemi-Tabaei S, Abtahi-Naeini B, et al. The Effectiveness of a 5% Retinoic Acid Peel Combined with Microdermabrasion for Facial Photoaging: A Randomized, Double-Blind, Placebo-Controlled Clinical Trial. Dermatol Res Pract. 2017;2017:8516527.
19. Magalhães GM, Rodrigues DF, Oliveira ER Jr, et al. Tretinoin peeling: when a reaction is greater than expected. An Bras Dermatol. 2017;92(2):291-2.

16 CHAPTER

Phytic Acid Peel

Rashmi Sarkar, Sneha Ghunawat

INTRODUCTION

The alpha-hydroxy acids also called as fruit acids have been widely used as peeling agents since the 1980s. Although they are commonly found in fruits, the ones used in dermatology practice are synthetically derived.[1] The most commonly used alpha-hydroxy acid is glycolic acid (2 carbon), while others include lactic acid (3 carbon), citric acid (6 carbon), malic and tartaric acid (4 carbon). They are nontoxic substances and have a wide number of indications. The excellent safety profile has made these peeling agents popular even in dark skinned patients. Glycolic acid is the smallest alpha-hydroxy acid that penetrates the stratum corneum with relative ease.[2]

Unlike trichloroacetic acid (TCA) which combines with epidermal and dermal proteins and undergoes neutralization, alpha-hydroxy acids have to be neutralized externally. TCA when applied on the skin causes ultrastructural changes in the skin, visible as frosting. Frosting is an indication that the peel has made its effect and has neutralized. Alpha-hydroxy acids have to be neutralized with a basic solution at the appropriate time to produce the desired peeling effect. Too quick neutralization causes under peeling, while too late neutralization leads to over peeling and undesired effects. Thus, the correct time of neutralization is subjective (appearance of erythema) and dependent on the physician's expertise. The proprietary, phytic acid peel is thus an alpha-hydroxy acid peel which has a low pH and does not require neutralization.[3] It overcomes the shortcomings of the other classical alpha-hydroxy acid peels. Since no external neutralization is required, the action of the peel will continue till self-neutralization occurs. This also implies that the problems linked with too late and too early neutralization are not faced with this peel. It is thus a slowly progressive peel with sequential actuation of the acid. Easy phytic acid peel has a pH of 0–1, which implies that it contains free acid as the active agent. Due to its slow controlled release, the usual side effects such as burning sensation experienced with glycolic acid peel are not noticed.

Commercially used brands like phytic peel (a proprietary peel) contain a mixture of glycolic, lactic, mandelic and phytic acid. All the acids penetrate the skin at different rates (glycolic acid being the fastest and mandelic acid being the slowest). As the acids penetrate from the topmost layer of the skin to the dermis, they progressively lose their effect and undergo self-neutralization. Phytic acid is not an alpha-hydroxy acid; it is a large molecule with an antioxidant effect. Skin undergoing chemical peel treatment generates free radicals as a result of inflammation and vasodilation. These free radicals damage the surrounding structures and have been cited as the major cause for the aging process. The phytic acid present in the Easy phytic acid peel penetrates the skin after the alpha-hydroxy acids have caused inflammation and vasodilation. It then scavenges the free radicals thus generated, decreasing the damage to the surrounding tissues.[3,4]

Phytic acid combination peels is a formulation that does not require neutralization even at low pH when the amount of free acid is high. It has an added advantage of combined antioxidant and anti-tyrosinase activity of phytic acid.

EFFECTS OF PHYTIC ACID ON SKIN

Skin Lightening Effect

Phytic acid inhibits the activity of tyrosinase and helps in reducing melanin content of the skin. Optimal concentration of phytic acid in skin lotion for the lightening effect is 0.5 wt%.

Improvement in Skin Elasticity

The dermis is composed of cellular components (fibroblasts, stellate cells) along with intercellular matrix composed of elastin and collagen. With age, the ability of skin to form new cells decreases, along with weakening of the connective tissue network. It accounts for decrease in skin elasticity. Phytic acid has been shown to increase the moisture content of the dermis and thus, improves skin elasticity.

Effect on Skin Moisturization and Sebum

Skin moisture is maintained by sebum secretion from the sebaceous glands. The absorption of phytic acid into the sebaceous glands help to regularize moisture content of the skin.

Effect on Skin Deodorization

Phytic acid inhibits the growth of gram-negative bacteria and helps to improve body odor.

Effect on Acne and Melasma

In the study by Al-Mokadem et al.[4] to study the effect of phytic acid combination peel on acne and melasma, significant improvement in the degree of papulopustular acne and response to treatment was noted ($p < 0.05$). Global acne grading system was used to assess the response to treatment. Very good response was noted in 20%, good response in 30%, moderate in 25% and mild in the rest 25%. In the melasma group, the difference in Melasma Area Severity Index (MASI) scores before and after the treatment was statistically significant ($p < 0.001$). The clinical improvement among the patients was noted as early as after the first session. Only mild tingling sensation was reported by the patients, without any other noteworthy adverse events. In a split face study by Faghihi et al.[5] comparing the effect of combination of azelaic acid (20%), resorcinol (10%) and phytic acid (6%) versus glycolic acid (50%) in the treatment of melasma, it was found that both the treatment modalities were equally effective in melasma treatment. The difference in decreased MASI score compared to baseline and at each session was not statistically different between the two groups. Similarly, the difference in response to treatment between the two groups was not statistically significant. On comparing the safety between the two groups, the group receiving glycolic acid reported more incidence of burning and dyspigmentation, than the group receiving combination treatment. The authors thus concluded that the two treatments were equally effective, but the combination had a much safer adverse event profile as reported by the patients.

In another study by Sarkar et al.[6] comparing the efficacy of glycolic acid, salicylic acid and phytic acid peel in melasma, peeling sessions were done at two weekly intervals till 12 weeks. Follow-up was done till 20 weeks. Good response was noted in 18.2% patients receiving phytic acid peel, followed by fair in 77.2% and poor in 4.2%. Statistically significant decrease in MASI score was noted at the end of the study compared to the baseline, although the gratification noted by the patients was less than the glycolic acid and salicylic mandelic acid group. The lower response rate compared to the other two groups was attributed to more number of mixed melasma in the phytic acid group. Persistent erythema was noted in 31.8% patients. The number of dropouts were maximum in this group; the postulated explanation by the authors was that the overnight application of the peel might have led to patient inconvenience.

CHEMISTRY

Phytic acid (myoinositol hexaphosphate) is the six phosphate ester of inositol (Fig. 1). It is an intermediate in inositol metabolism. It is found in grains, fibers and plants in the form of insoluble calcium and magnesium salts

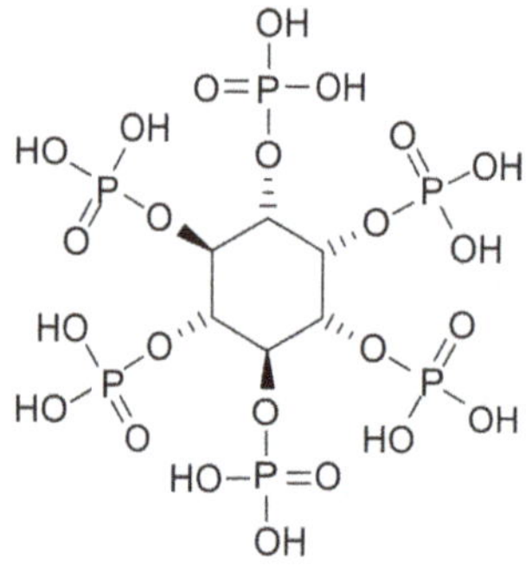

FIG. 1: Structure of phytic acid.

(phytin). Phytic acid was discovered in 1903, as a saturated cyclic acid, being a principal storage form of phosphorus in many plant tissues.[7] It is considered a phytonutrient with an antioxidant property. It protects the seed from oxidative damage during storage. It has been shown to inhibit oxidation of vitamin C, stabilize sorbic acid, prevents preoxidation and hydrolysis of fats and oils. Phytic acid along with vitamin E has shown synergistic effects in preventing lipid oxidation. Other suggested functions of phytic acid include storage of cations and high energy phosphoryl groups. It is a strong chelator of copper, iron, zinc and magnesium. Dietary chelators have been shown to prevent over mineralization of bones and blood vessels.[8] Easy phytic acid is a commercial product composed of glycolic, lactic, mandelic and phytic acid. It does not require neutralization and is a slow release formulation.

Phytic acid has many important functions in the body. It has an antioxidant effect. It has a role as an anticancer agent, reduces blood clots, reduces cholesterol and triglyceride levels as well as prevents heart diseases.[9] It also has a wide range of applications in the industries, where it is used as an additive to metal coating, for the treatment of hard water, as an antioxidant, preservative and stabilizer.

Its action on skin is multimodal. It works by its exfoliant action, inhibition of tyrosinase (action in hyperpigmentary conditions), antioxidant, skin whitening, anti-inflammatory, rejuvenating and lifting effect. It blocks the entrance of iron and copper and prevents formation of melanin. Because of the strong antioxidant effect, it chelates the pro-oxidative ions that lead to postinflammatory hyperpigmentation. Oral administration has been shown to improve blood circulation and fingernail growth. It also finds use in preparation of antidandruff lotions and rinses. Phytic acid molecule has a large molecular size and thus does not penetrate the skin deeply. Even at high concentration of the acid and low pH, it does not cause damage to the skin. Phytic acid precipitates most proteins at low pH, in the absence of cations by binding to the basic residues. At higher pH and in presence of cations it forms ternary-metal-phytate-complex.[10,11]

HIGHLIGHTS OF THE EFFECTS OF PHYTIC ACID ON SKIN

- Improves the texture and smoothens the skin (makes skin smooth and radiant)
- Decreases pigmentation
- Lifting effect
- Reduces pore size
- Improves function of sebaceous and sweat glands
- Antioxidant and anti-inflammatory effect
- Improves metabolic effect and regeneration of damaged tissue
- Improves fine lines and wrinkle depth
- Induction of collagen and elastin
- Improves skin quality and removes dead cells
- Improvement in acne and acne scars
- Improves skin moisturization
- Improves skin elasticity.

INDICATIONS

- Hyperpigmentation
- Acne (Fig. 2)
- Aging skin
- Stretch marks
- Photoaging
- Fine lines
- Enlarged pores
- Keratomas.

PEEL TECHNIQUE

- Skin is cleansed using commercial cleansing foam. No acetone or alcohol is used to clean the face. Skin is pat dried after washing
- Cotton balls are the best applicator. Cotton balls are moistened with the Easy phytic acid solution and even coat is applied on the face. Two coats applied without rubbing are sufficient. Care should be taken while applying to avoid contact with the eyes. If the solution accidently gets into the eyes, wash with copious amount of saline
- Patient may experience stinging sensation, which may persist for 30 minutes or more. Do not neutralize at this stage.

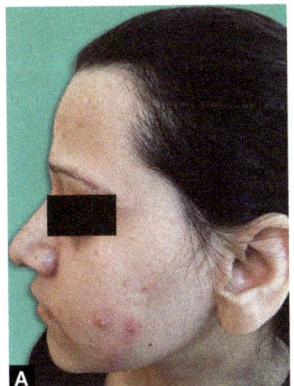 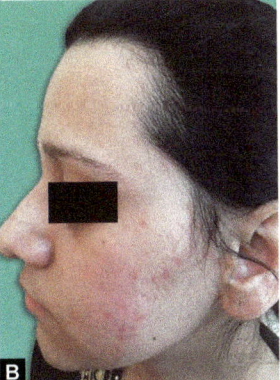

FIG. 2: Before and after pictures of two sessions of phytic acid peel (2 weeks apart) in pustular acne.

- Mild massaging is done to aid in the even penetration of the peel
- No frosting is expected to be seen with this peel. If it occurs, it indicates deep penetration and should be immediately neutralized with basic neutralizer
- The peel is left on the skin until the next morning.

FREQUENCY OF PEELING

Phytic acid combination peels is applied once weekly, but can be repeated twice weekly if a more stimulative effect is wanted. Maintenance peeling can be repeated at two weekly or monthly intervals.

POSTPEEL CARE

- Strict sun protection is advised in the immediate postpeel period to prevent the development of postinflammatory hyperpigmentation
- Mild peeling may be noticed by some patients in the immediate postpeel period. Liberal use of moisturizers is effective to prevent development of dryness
- In case of postpeel reactions involving peeling and dryness, mild topical steroid can be prescribed
- In case of persistent postpeel hyperpigmentation, topical hydroquinone is an effective agent.

CONTRAINDICATIONS

- Pregnancy/lactation
- Active infection over skin
- Hypersensitivity to any of the peel components
- Underlying systemic illness (renal/hepatic insufficiency)
- Active skin disease such as psoriasis, eczema.

DRAWBACKS OF PHYTIC ACID PEEL

- High cost
- Lack of studies on the clinical efficacy of this molecule
- Slight tingling sensation during the procedure.

COMPLICATIONS

- Skin dryness
- Transient patchy erythema
- Transient red itchy nodules that disappear in 2–3 days
- Activation of herpes
- Allergic reaction to the peel components
- Transient swelling due to the anti-inflammatory mediators.

CONCLUSION

Phytic acid is an alpha-hydroxy acid peel with certain advantages over the conventional peels. Due to its large molecular size, it penetrates slowly into the skin and thus is suitable for sensitive skin types. It is gentler on the skin causing less dryness and irritation. Its large molecular size and ability of self neutralization does not allow it to penetrate deep, making it a safe peeling option. It has free radical scavenging effect decreasing oxidative damage to surrounding tissue along with skin lightening and rejuvenating effects. However, studies supporting the efficacy of phytic acid peel are limited and further studies are thus warranted.

TAKE HOME POINTS

- Phytic acid has multiple actions such as antityrosinase, exfoliant and antioxidant effects
- Due to the slow release formulation of the peel, it causes lesser side effects such as burning and stinging

- Due to the ability of phytic acid to scavenge free radicals, the oxidative damage on the skin postpeel is reduced, further decreasing the risk of hyperpigmentation. This makes it a good peeling option among dark skinned patients
- Does not require external neutralization, free from the risks of over/under peeling
- Studies have shown beneficial effects of phytic acid in acne and melasma.

REFERENCES

1. Ramos-e-Silva M, Hexsel DM, Rutowitsch MS, et al. Hydroxy acids and retinoids in cosmetics. Clin Dermatol. 2001;19:460-6.
2. Ditre CM, Griffin TD, Murphy GF, et al. Effects of α-hydroxy acids on photoaged skin: A pilot clinical, histologic, and ultrastructural study. J Am Acad Dermatol. 1996; 2(pt 1):187-95.
3. Deprez P. Easy phytic solution: A new alpha-hydroxy acid peel with slow release and without neutralization. Int J Cosmet Surg Aesthetic Dermatol 2003;5:45-51.
4. Al-Mokadem S, Al-Aasser O, Nassar A, et al. Easy phytic peel as a therapeutic agent in acne vulgaris and melasma. The Egyptian Journal Dermatology and Venereology. 2013;33:6-11.
5. Faghihi G, Taheri A, Shahmoradi Z, et al. Solution of azelaic acid (20%), resorcinol (10%) and phytic acid (6%) versus glycolic acid (50%) peeling agent in the treatment of female patients with facial melasma. Adv Biomed Res. 2017;6:9.
6. Sarkar R, Garg V, Bansal S, et al. Comparative evaluation of efficacy and tolerability of glycolic acid, salicylic mandelic acid, and phytic acid combination peels in melasma. Dermatol Surg. 2016;42(3):384-91.
7. Ngozi OOP, Nkiru OA. Evaluation of tannin, phytate and mineral composition of different indigenous dishes based on pumpkin (Cucurbita pepo). International Journal of Nutrition and Food Sciences. 2014; 3(6): 493-6.
8. Ohlrogge JB, Kernan TP. Oxygen-dependent aging of seeds. Plant Physiology. 1982;70(3):791-4.
9. Jariwalla RJ, Sabin R, Lawson S, et al. Lowering of serum cholesterol and triglycerides and modulations by dietary phytate. J Appl Nutr. 1990;42:18-28.
10. Graf E. Phytic Acid: Chemistry and Applications. Journal of the American Oil Chemists' Society, 1983;60(11): 1861-7.
11. Mene R. Will phytic acid replace hydroquinone? 3º Congresso Nazionale Di Medicina Estetica: Milano, Italy; 2011.

CHAPTER 17

Medium-depth Peeling with Special Consideration to Ethnic Skin

Sidharth Sonthalia

INTRODUCTION AND HISTORICAL PERSPECTIVE

The use of caustic chemicals for skin peeling procedures finds mention in Papyrus Ebers, one of the most ancient medical documents of the world, from ancient Egypt traced to about 1550 BC.[1] After the initial description of the actions of salicylic acid, resorcinol, trichloroacetic acid (TCA) and phenol on the skin by Unna in 1882, the use of phenol was further developed in France after World War I.[1,2] It was in 1940s, when the first systematic description on the use of phenol, resorcinol, salicylic acid and CO_2 for scar treatment was described by Eller and Wolff of the United States.[3] Mackee of England published his results on the use of phenol for scars in 1952.[4] Finally, in the 1960s, the development of modified phenol solutions (addition of croton oil, septisol and water) by Baker and Gordon,[5] and histological assessment of peeling results of phenol and TCA peels[6] marked the commencement of the modern era of peeling.

The classification of chemical peels based upon their depth of penetration and wounding in the skin is well known and has been dealt with in detail in a previous chapter of this book. While the superficial peels halt at the epidermal basal layer, medium-depth peels reach the upper layers of the dermis down to the papillary dermis, and deep peels remove the papillary dermis and reach the reticular dermis.[7] A medium-depth peel penetrates the skin up to a depth of 200 µm.

It is important to know that a particular chemical or substance cannot be simply labelled as an effector of superficial, medium or deep peeling. Apart from the substance, several factors determine the depth of peeling, including its concentration, the pH of the solution, number of coats applied and the time of application. A chemical like TCA or glycolic acid (GA) can provide the desired depth of peeling depending on their concentration. Use of combination of different peeling agents in different concentrations can also provide a deeper peeling effect. This chapter is focused on medium-depth peels.

COMMONLY USED AGENTS FOR MEDIUM-DEPTH PEELING (BOX 1)

- *Trichloroacetic acid and its combinations*: The classic agent to achieve medium depth peeling is TCA. As a single agent, 35% TCA produces superficial peeling and for it to achieve stable penetration

Medium-depth Peeling with Special Consideration to Ethnic Skin

> **BOX 1** **Medium-depth chemical peeling agents and combinations**
>
> - Glycolic acid 70%, applied for a variable time (3–15 min)
> - Pyruvic acid 60%, applied for a variable time (3–5 min)
> - Trichloroacetic acid (TCA): 35–50%
> - Augmented TCA
> - Monheit's combination: Jessner's solution plus TCA 35%
> - Coleman's combination: Glycolic acid 70% plus TCA 35%
> - Brody' combination: Solid carbon dioxide plus TCA 35%
> - Jessner's solution: Multiple coats
> - Phenol 88%
> - Modified phenol-based combination peels

to the level of the upper reticular dermis, an initial epidermal injury is essential. While in the past, this was achieved by application of refrigerant solid CO_2 block,[8] later on the use of GA 70%[9] and Jessner's solution (JS)[10] was introduced for pre-TCA (35%) application; which are commonly referred to as *augmented TCA peels*—GA-TCA and JS-TCA peels, respectively.[11] Proprietary TCA-based agents are now available to provide medium-depth peeling effect. Although, a higher concentration of TCA, e.g., 40% or 60% as a single agent can provide medium-depth peeling but the dermal penetration also becomes deeper and the outcome is unreliable and unpredictable.[12] Thus, this approach is best avoided in skin of color (SOC), owing to a significant possibility of postinflammatory hyperpigmentation (PIH) as well as scarring

- *Jessner's solution*: Traditional JS combines salicylic acid, resorcinol and lactic acid 85% mixed in ethanol (95%). Apart from its use as a coat preceding TCA 35% (JS-TCA peel), multiple coats of JS *per se* can also provide medium-depth peeling. Jessner's solution provides the synergistic effect of three keratolytic agents, as well as the additional benefit of resorcinol, a phenolic skin-lightening agent.[13] Jessner's solution must be stored in a dark bottle to prevent photo-oxidation.[14] In the author's experience of using multiple coats of JS to provide medium-depth peeling in SOC, gratifying results are obtained in acne scars, melasma and PIH. Although there is a possibility of pigmentary complications with JS in skin types V–VI, the same can be minimized by proper priming, patch peel testing and restricting the multiple coats to the affected areas, after the first uniform coat on the entire face
- *Glycolic acid*: Apart from its role in combination with TCA 35% (GA-TCA), unbuffered solution of 70% GA (time-dependent) can itself result in medium-depth peeling. The pH of the solution should preferably be more than 2.0 to avoid excessive tissue necrosis. Other measures to increase safety of 70% GA solution in SOC include use of a buffered or partially neutralized acid, and timely neutralization with water or 1% bicarbonate solution[14]
- *Pyruvic acid*: Pyruvic acid 60% applied for 3–5 minutes can provide medium-depth peeling. Details of pyruvic acid peel may be found in another chapter in the book
- *Phenol*: Unoccluded full-strength phenol (88%) has been successfully used as single agent medium-depth chemical peel, especially for medical conditions, but has distinct disadvantages compared with TCA-based combination approach for cosmetic indications.[13,14] Modified phenol-based peels are now popular as safe and effective medium-depth peeling agents. Readers are advised to refer to the chapter on phenol peels in this book for details.

MECHANISM OF ACTION AND HISTOLOGIC EFFECTS OF MEDIUM-DEPTH PEELS

Medium-depth peeling agents, such as TCA, induce epidermal destruction, dermal inflammation and edema with coagulation of membrane proteins. The depth of skin necrosis correlates closely with the potency of the medium-depth peel. Eventually, abnormal keratinocytes are replaced by healthier cells and the dermis is stimulated to produce new collagen.[13,14] By wounding the skin to the upper reticular dermis, the medium-depth peel yields a more significant sloughing of the upper layers of skin. Complete re-epithelialization that develops from nests in the adnexal structures occurs within 7 days.[11] Neocollagenesis occurs in the papillary and upper reticular dermis; grenz zone, i.e., normal-appearing zone of expanded papillary dermis is usually visible 90 days after the peel.[15] Although both JS-TCA and GA-TCA peels can cause neoelastogenesis, experimentally, the GA-TCA peel generated more new elastic fibers than the JS-TCA peel.[11]

INDICATIONS OF MEDIUM-DEPTH PEELS[13,14,16,17]

Indications of medium-depth peels are given in table 1.

BEFORE YOU PEEL: PREPEEL PROTOCOLS

- Confirmation that chemical peel of a particular type and depth is the desired treatment of choice
- Confirm that the patient is a suitable candidate to undergo the chemical peel session; this includes ruling out contraindications and exercising precautions in special cases. Assessment of skin type

TABLE 1: Broad indications of medium-depth peels[13,14,16,17]

Medical indications	Cosmetic indications
• Actinic keratosis • Photodamaged skin—Glogau II grade • Pigmentary dyschromias—melasma, PIH, LPP • Acne scars (depressed): Mild to moderate • Special indications for phenol 88% as spot therapy[16,17]—vitiligo, alopecia areata, IGH	• Photoaging • Superficial to moderate rhytides • Solar lentigines

PIH, postinflammatory hyperpigmentation; LPP, lichen planus pigmentosus; IGH, idiopathic guttate hypomelanosis.

and ethnicity, history of delayed wound healing and hypertrophic or keloid scar formation, tendency to development of PIH, quantification of sun exposure, history of herpetic infection, previous facial procedures and their outcome, any concomitant physical procedures being taken elsewhere, oral medications, especially hormonal agents including combined oral contraceptive pills (COCs), and photosensitizing medications like tetracyclines. Cardiac history is important if deep phenol peel or medium-depth phenol peel over a large surface area is planned. History of recent oral isotretinoin intake should be taken, but the erstwhile dictum of not performing chemical peeling or any physical procedure during and within 6 months of oral isotretinoin therapy is now conjectural (*vide infra*). History of smoking is important in deeper peels as smoking may delay the healing process[14,18,19]

- *Counseling*: Evaluation of the psychological aspects to judge the motivation and

expectations of the patient is prudent. Explanation about the nature of treatment, prepeel protocol, expected outcome, expected time of recovery, importance of adherence to postpeel care protocol, and discussion about adverse effects (common as well as unlikely), including PIH and scarring, are of vital importance[7,14,18,19]
- *Documentation*: It is important to get a comprehensive consent form duly signed and counter-signed by the treating dermatologist and an eyewitness, typically a family member[20]
- Photographic documentation prior to the peel is mandatory. A full-face photograph and photos of areas of specific interest, e.g., side profiles, zoomed images of the forehead, chin, etc. and close and focused images of scars etc. must be taken on baseline and on each visit prior to the procedure
- The author also recommends taking dermoscopic images of the involved areas and recording them, as it may help in early recognition of improvement as well as complications[21]
- *Herpes simplex infection*: In patients with a history of herpes infection, medium-depth or deep peels are preceded with oral anti-herpes treatment started at least 2 days before the procedure and continued for 5 days thereafter[7,14]
- Prepeel priming (vide infra) and emphasis during counseling on meticulous use of broad-spectrum sunscreen, physical sun-protection methods and moisturization
- *Postpeel guidelines*: In the first 24–48 hours, only splashes of cold water, with no rubbing of the skin is advised, after which gentle cleansing, preferably with a nondrying cleanser may be resumed. Use of sunscreens and moisturizers should begin right on the day of peeling. Resumption of adjuvant skin lightening agents and/or collagen synthesis boosters such as vitamin C and hyaluronic acid preparations may be started 2–3 days after the peel session
- It is ideal if the peel-related information is given to the patient and family members beforehand; also, a detailed proforma containing details of pre- and postpeel management and precautions is given.

Patient Selection Criteria

- *Skin type*: Fitzpatrick skin types I to II are ideal. Darker skin types must be primed [hydroquinone (HQ)-based and retinoic acid formulation] and also evaluated by a patch test before the full session. Despite that, PIH remains a possible complication
- Patients with Glogau II photoaging are excellent candidates; however, patients with more severe Glogau staging are also expected to note some benefit from a medium-depth peel
- Patients with more sebaceous thick skin can tolerate deeper peel compared with thinner skin
- *Downtime*: Patients should be ready to accept a downtime of 5–7 days and committed to remain indoors and follow strict sun protection and hydration for at least 7 days. Patients who want instant results are not good candidates for medium-depth peels
- Patients with realistic expectations.

CONTRAINDICATIONS AND PRECAUTIONS

- Active bacterial, viral, fungal or herpetic infection, or open wounds at the peel site
- History of concomitant or recently taken drugs with photosensitizing potential
- Known allergy to the peel component(s)

- Preexisting inflammatory dermatoses such as psoriasis, atopic dermatitis
- Unreliable and uncooperative patient
- Patient with unrealistic expectations
- Known history of abnormal scarring, keloids, atrophic skin
- Known or suspected cardiac disease, arrhythmias, renal or hepatic disease (for patients planned for phenol peels)
- Oral isotretinoin use in the 6 months (Read the discussion on this controversial issue in the ensuing paragraph).

ORAL ISOTRETINOIN AND MEDIUM-DEPTH PEELING

As per conventional recommendation, physical procedure or cutaneous surgery over the face should be delayed during and for up to 6–12 months of therapy with oral isotretinoin, due to the long-held notion of the possibility of abnormal scarring or delayed wound healing. However, this concept was based on countable case series published in mid-80s, with technical lacunae in the study design.[22] However, the results from a pilot study on 10 patients with acne scars demonstrated safety of manual chemabrasion of depressed acne scars (combination of medium-depth peel and sandpaper dermabrasion) conducted within 1–3 months after oral isotretinoin treatment.[23] A recent systematic review and consensus recommendations on isotretinoin treatment and timing of physical procedures revealed that there was insufficient evidence to support delaying manual dermabrasion, superficial chemical peels, cutaneous surgery, laser hair removal and fractional ablative and nonablative laser procedures for patients currently receiving or having recently completed isotretinoin therapy. However, mechanical dermabrasion and fully ablative laser were not recommended in the setting of systemic isotretinoin treatment.[22] Since medium-depth peel is definitely deeper than superficial peels, the decision of undertaking a patient on or within 6–12 months of oral isotretinoin treatment for medium-depth peel should be individualized as per the patient profile, skin condition and conducted only on receiving an informed consent from the patient, apprised of the risks and benefits.

PREPEELING: PRIMING

With increasing depth of the chemical peel, the risk of PIH becomes higher in SOC. Thus, to attain cosmetically good outcome and avoid such complications, every peel, in particular deeper peels, must be used on primed skins. The purpose of priming agents is multifold—enhance the peel penetration, accelerate the postpeel healing process, and avoid PIH and scarring. Apart from meticulous use of a broad-spectrum sunscreen, priming involves use of specific agents such as topical tretinoin, HQ, triple combination (TC), alpha-hydroxy acids (AHA), azelaic acid, among others. The commonly employed duration of prepeel priming ranges from 2–12 weeks, and the priming agent should be stopped for at least 2–3 days prior to the chemical peel session. Topical tretinoin, although enhances peel penetration and accelerates post-procedure healing,[14,24] suffers the disadvantage of poor tolerance in patients with ethnic skin, especially Indians.[25] A HQ-based priming agent is essential in patients with dark complexion, to reduce or prevent PIH.[19] However, the choice of the priming agent practically depends on the individual physician's preference and individualized patient requirements.

METHODOLOGY OF MEDIUM-DEPTH PEELING (TCA, AUGMENTED TCA, JESSNER'S SOLUTION)

1. Follow the prepeel protocols, including patient counseling, record maintenance, consent, priming and advice on postpeel care
2. *Test peel*: In darker skin types (due to risk of PIH), and those with history of abnormal scarring, a small test spot with the chemical peel agent may be performed over the postauricular area and outcome evaluated after 10–15 days. Test sites are not routinely necessary for specialists with more experience
3. *Analgesia*: The patients tolerate the medium-depth chemical peel (TCA 35%, JS) without any need for any analgesia. Although, use of an anxiolytic or analgesic, as well as topical EMLA have been suggested by some authors,[26] the author has never required them in his practice and does not recommend their use. Reassurance, a cooling fan and ice-cooling are more than sufficient to ensure patient comfort
4. A typical peel tray (Fig. 1) for a medium-depth chemical peel should include alcohol swabs, acetone, bottles containing appropriate concentrations of the peeling agents, cotton-tipped applicators, peel brushes, small cotton gauze pieces, glass vials or beakers to pour the peeling agent, vaseline, spray bottle with cold water, ice, cooling fan, digital timer and some extra water (to rinse the eyes in the event of an accidental splash)
5. *Cleansing*: Any topical application (sunscreen/moisturizing cream/makeup etc.) should be removed with a gentle cleanser. The face should be cleansed with spirit (alcohol) to remove any residual cosmetics or debris, followed by acetone to degrease the skin
6. *Protection of sensitive sites*: Vaseline or petroleum jelly should be applied to the corner of mouth and nose. Make the patient wear the disposable hair cap and put cotton plugs in the ears
7. *Peel application*: An even coat of the medium-depth peeling agent is applied on the entire face by a cotton-tipped applicator or peeling brush, moistened with the chemical by firmly rubbing the moistened applicator in a circular or linear fashion. The acid may also be applied with folded gauze pads, which decrease total time but also decreases precision of application. If multiple coats are applied (e.g., in JS solution), let the previous coat dry up, before applying the next one. If augmented TCA technique is employed, the first coat of GA 70% or JS should be left for 3–5 minutes followed by neutralization with a cold solution

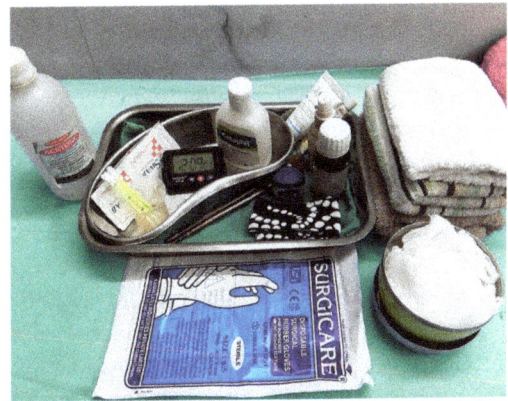

FIG. 1: A typical peeling tray demonstrating the essentials for a medium-depth peeling procedure. The tray contents include alcohol swabs, acetone, cleansing lotion, vaseline, the peel bottle (Jessner's solution in this case), digital timer, hair band, cotton gauze pieces, peel brush, cotton-tipped applicators, cold-water spray bottle for neutralization, towels, sunscreen lotion, and a pair of gloves (if needed).

containing bicarbonate salt, and then TCA 35% should be applied

8. *Sequence of peel application*: A typical sequence is usually advisable, beginning with the forehead, moving to the cheeks, then perioral and nasal region. Finally, each periocular unit can be addressed. In one approach, known as the "strip method," the face is divided into sections called strips.[27] The goal is to move across the face in a calculated fashion when applying the acid. The concentration of TCA (35–40%), number of passes per strip, and the directions of such passes (the strokes with the wet cotton gauze) per strip are kept identical (horizontal and vertical in each strip). Some specialists follow a specific concentration—location pattern of application, dividing the face into different units; e.g., TCA 40% over the forehead, cheeks, chin and jawline; TCA 30% for jawline and perioral area; and TCA 18% in the periorbital region

9. *Frosting*: Once the skin has been treated, it slowly changes color, becoming whitish-gray as a result of chemical coagulation of the epidermis (Fig. 2). This color change is called a "frost" and represents coagulation of keratin. Frosting induced by medium-depth peels is considered grade II frosting, which refers to a light-to-medium white frost with surrounding erythema. The frost appears more rapidly with higher concentrations of TCA and may take more time with low concentrations. A uniform crust is desirable; a patchy frost indicates uneven application of the peeling agent or inadequate degreasing of certain areas. The frost induced by JS is usually lighter than that of TCA

10. Feathering, along the scalp and jaw lines (as in superficial peels) is desirable, to prevent formation of demarcation lines

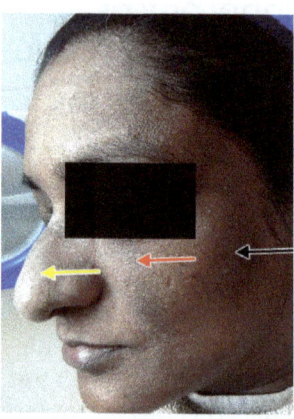

FIG. 2: Appearance of frosting after full-face peeling for melasma with augmented trichloroacetic acid (TCA), using one coat of Jessner's solution followed by a coat of 35% TCA. The frosting is in early formation (black arrow), nicely coalesced (red arrow) and fully established till grade II (yellow arrow).

11. Peel termination and duration: The total time taken in one complete session of medium-depth peeling ranges from 15–30 minutes. Peel termination for JS can be done with plain or bicarbonate containing cold-water spray; the same is ideally unnecessary for TCA. However, cold-water spray can still help reduce the peri-peeling discomfort. TCA stings moderately when applied and the pain correlates with the concentration of acid. The pain crescendos, normally peaking approximately halfway through the procedure. When multiple coats of JS are applied, the mild stinging sensation experienced after the first coat increases mildly with each additional coat. Use of a hand-held fan and dry cool ice compresses are helpful to soothe the discomfort

12. *Touch-up*: In areas that show a lack of frost 3–4 minutes after application, the TCA should be reapplied. Avoid reapplying the TCA peel to already frosted areas as this is likely to result in an unpredictable level of deeper peeling effect

Medium-depth Peeling with Special Consideration to Ethnic Skin

13. *Hot spots*: During this procedure, the specialist must be on the lookout for appearance of what we call "hot spots" that are areas of intense redness (associated with severe burning sensation and/or pain), which indicate a superficial burn or a deep peel. Prolonged application of ice packs topped up with the application of a recombinant epidermal growth factor-based skin repair gel (e.g., REGEN-D gel) over the hot spots may prevent the unintended damage (author's personal observation).

EXPECTED POSTPEEL EVENTS

- An initial inflammatory response is erythematous and edematous reaction that may last from 1 day to 2 days. In patients with sensitive or thinner skin, it may persist longer
- This is followed by formation of thin skin crusts and visible peeling of skin over the next week
- Recovery process, i.e., peeling and re-epithelialization of skin beneath with normalization of external appearance can take 5–14 days.

POSTPEEL INSTRUCTIONS

- Meticulous sun protection with repeated application of a broad-spectrum sunscreen with a high SPF and SPA factor is a must. The patient should be instructed to avoid any outdoor activity that may involve direct or strong sun exposure, at least for the first 7–10 days. Additional use of mechanical barriers like stoles, goggles and umbrellas should be advised
- Soothing gentle barrier repair creams in an emollient base must be used frequently
- Nondrying and preferably nonfoaming face washes should be used. Scrubs and harsh soaps have to be strictly avoided
- Home-based application creams containing AHA, vitamin C, etc. can be slowly reintroduced once healing is good
- Repeat sessions can be done at an interval of 4 weeks
- Makeup may be allowed after 5–7 days.

POTENTIAL COMPLICATIONS WITH MEDIUM-DEPTH PEELING IN SOC

- Delayed wound healing secondary to bacterial or fungal infections. It can be avoided by premedication with antivirals and delaying of the peel procedure till the infection heals
- *Pigmentary abnormalities*: Medium-depth peeling in ethnic skin may result in PIH (Fig. 3A) (more common), but may occasionally result in hypo- or depigmentation (Fig. 3B) also. Use of HQ and other depigmenting topicals, and a short course of topical and/or oral corticosteroids are helpful in reducing PIH, if treatment is started early. Hypo- or depigmentation may be permanent and may warrant cosmetic camouflage
- *Persistent erythema*: Persistent erythema is a syndrome where the skin remains erythematous beyond what is normal for the individual peel (1 month for medium-depth peel). Although it may stem from contact dermatitis, contact sensitization, re-exacerbation of prior skin disease, or a genetic susceptibility to erythema, it is also a sign of potential scarring. Thus, it should be treated promptly and appropriately with topical steroids, systemic steroids and intralesional steroids (if thickening is occurring). Topical and/or oral low-dose tranexamic acid may help in some cases (author's personal observation). In some cases, a pulsed dye vascular laser treatment may be required

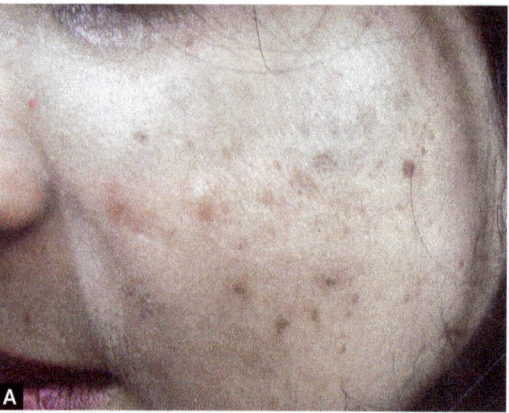 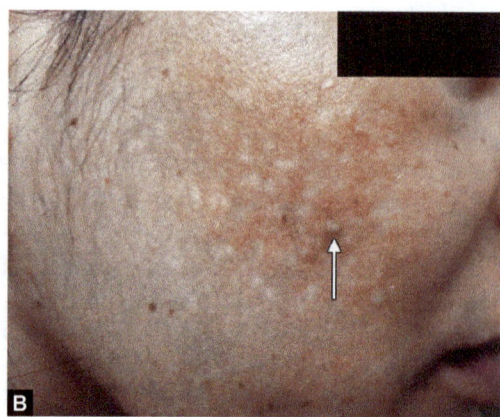

FIG. 3: Pigmentary complications of medium-depth peeling observed in two Indian women. **A,** Spotty hyperpigmentation that developed 1 month after the fourth session with multi-coat Jessner's solution; **B,** Patchy hypopigmentation developing within an otherwise improving melasma in a lady, 3 weeks after the second session with glycolic acid-trichloroacetic acid 35% medium-depth peel. The arrow is pointing towards milia formation as a minor complication.

- *Scarring*: If peel penetrates deeper, the recovery may occur with abnormal scarring—hypertrophic, keloidal or atrophic. The risk is considered to be increased in patients on concomitant oral isotretinoin
- *Milia*: These also develop as a result of inadvertent deep peeling (Fig. 3B), typically associated with a scar in the vicinity and may need mechanical extraction
- Lines of demarcation may form due to nonuniform peel application, and is best avoided by feathering during the procedure (*vide supra*)
- Textural changes such as temporary enlargement of facial pores and unevenness may be experienced by few patients, but these usually subside automatically
- *Blistering and skin burns*: They are typically encountered if a more concentrated peel (e.g., TCA 50%) is used, and in sensitive areas like the peri-orbital and peri-oral region and nasolabial folds. Appearance of "hot spots" during the procedure may predict the possibility of their occurrence. If not treated early, these complications may eventuate into PIH. Early use of repair creams like REGEN-D, HA-based creams or gels, vitamin C serum over the hot spots or the blistered or burnt areas may expedite healing and prevent pigmentary sequelae
- *Ocular complications*: Accidental spillage of any chemical peel agents in the eyes can cause eye injuries in the form of corneal damage. In cases of accidental spillage, the eyes should be flushed copiously with normal saline to prevent corneal damage. If phenol peels have been used, flushing should be done with mineral oil instead of saline. Urgent referral to an ophthalmologist for thorough evaluation including slit-lamp examination is warranted. This catastrophic complication may be avoided by following extreme care while peeling the periorbital area and strict avoidance of passing the peeling agent over the patient's eyes
- Contact allergic reactions are rare but may be encountered, and may be immediate

or delayed. They manifest as postpeel itchy, red papular eruptions. They need to be differentiated from allergic reaction to ingredients of other facial applications like sunscreen. If a particular peeling agent is confirmed to be the cause, it should not be used again for that patient
- *Systemic complications*: Cardiac and hepatorenal complications are typical of phenol peels, which are discussed is a separate chapter.

A detailed analysis on the possible complications of medium-depth peeling in ethnic skin, their risk factors, prevention and treatment has been described by Nikalji et al.[28]

topical tretinoin for 6 weeks.[31] They reported no additional benefit of topical retinoid pretreatment. In a split face study involving 15 patients with widespread facial AKs, a single application of JS-TCA medium-depth peel was found to be as efficacious as 3-weeks treatment with twice-daily application of 5% fluorouracil cream, in terms of net reduction in the number of visible AKs (75% by both modalities) as well as reductions in keratinocyte atypia, hyperkeratosis, parakeratosis and inflammation.[32] They reported that majority of patients preferred the peel over fluorouracil because of the single application and less morbidity.

EVIDENCE-BASED FACTS ON THE EFFICACY AND SAFETY OF MEDIUM-DEPTH PEELING

Studies of JS-TCA (Monheit's combination) in medium-depth peels have shown benefit in acne scarring in dark-skinned individuals.[29,30] Humphreys et al. reported improvement in solar lentigines, AKs and skin texture but minimal effect on wrinkles with single treatment using 40% TCA (a borderline medium-depth peel) in 16 white-skinned men, of which 8 had been pretreated with

AUTHOR'S EXPERIENCE WITH TCA AND JS-BASED MEDIUM-DEPTH PEELING IN SOC

- Acne scars: The author has successfully used medium-depth peel GA-TCA in patients of acne scars (6-7 sessions, 2 weeks apart) with skin types IV and V with excellent results and no PIH (Fig. 4). However, all of them were primed for at least 2-4 weeks with 4% HQ, which was stopped 3 days prior to the peel session. Meticulous sun protection with proper

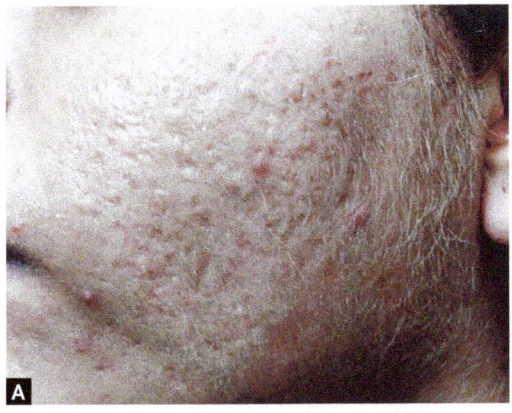
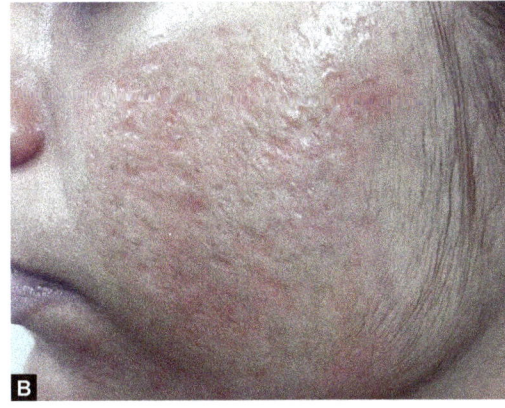

FIG. 4: Significant improvement in moderate-severe acne scars in a young Indian lady. **A,** Baseline and **B,** after 6 sessions of glycolic acid-trichloroacetic acid 35% medium-depth peel.

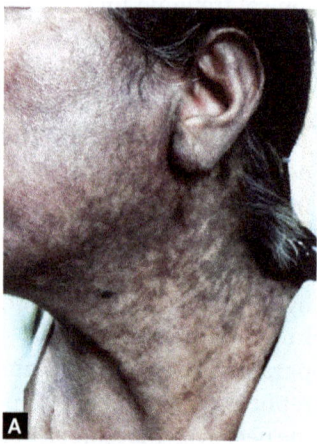 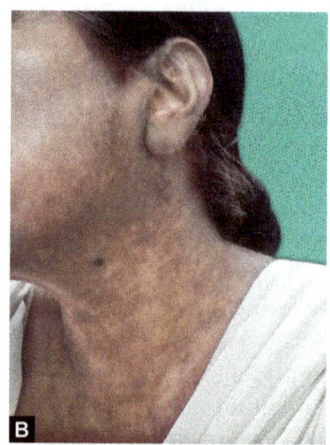

FIG. 5: Significant improvement in the hyperpigmentation of lichen planus pigmentosus in a 54-year-old Indian lady with medium-depth peeling after 4 weeks of priming with 5% hydroquinone. **A,** Baseline and **B,** after 6 sessions of Jessner's solution-trichloroacetic acid 35% medium-depth peel. The right face/neck of the lady was treated with 6 sessions of croton oil-free phenol combination (CFPC) peel, which also delivered excellent improvement.

use of broad-spectrum sunscreens and generous use of emollients were also followed by the treated patients
- *Lichen planus pigmentosus*: The hyperpigmentation of this condition is well known to be relatively resistant to any physical modality, owing to the presence of melanophages in deeper layers of the dermis. Although the author prefers modified low concentration phenol-combination peels for this condition (discussed in the chapter on phenol peels), he has also used JS-TCA with excellent outcomes in few patients with inactive treatment-refractory lichen planus pigmentosus (LPP) (Fig. 5)
- *Postinflammatory hyperpigmentation*: Treatment of PIH is difficult. However, the author has found good results with medium-depth peeling in patients with postacne PIH with multiple coat JS peeling (Fig. 6). Three coats of JS solution are applied on the entire face using gauze pieces, followed by 2-3 overlay coats over the PIH regions as spot therapy using cotton-tipped applicator. Priming with 4-5% HQ for at least 4-6 weeks and postpeel maintenance of effect with sunscreen and a topical depigmenting agent like kojic acid–alpha arbutin-based gel at night are essential
- *Solar lentigines*: The author found moderate to good results in few patients with solar lentigines by applying one full-face coat of TCA 35% followed by TCA 45% as a spot therapy (Fig. 7). Priming with HQ was done in all cases and postpeel protocol consisted of sunscreen and topical AHA-based maintenance gel (GA 20% solution at night was advised for 3 months after the sixth peel session.

COMBINATION OF CHEMICAL PEELS WITH OTHER RESURFACING PROCEDURES: AN EVIDENCE-BASED RECOMMENDATION

Combination of medium-depth peeling with other rejuvenation or resurfacing procedures is being actively explored. In a

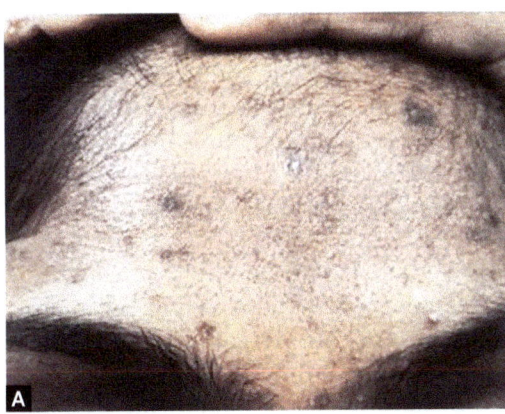 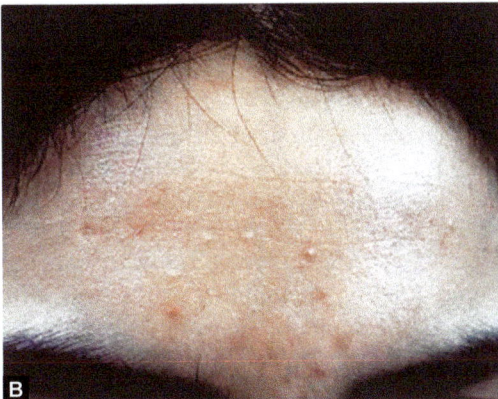

FIG. 6: Significant improvement in long-standing postacne postinflammatory hyperpigmentation of a 20-year-old Indian girl with medium-depth peeling, resistant to multiple previous treatments including superficial peels and Q-switched lasers. **A,** Baseline and **B,** after 8 sessions of multicoat Jessner's solution peeling in which three coats were applied on full face followed by 2–3 spot applications over the pigmented areas.

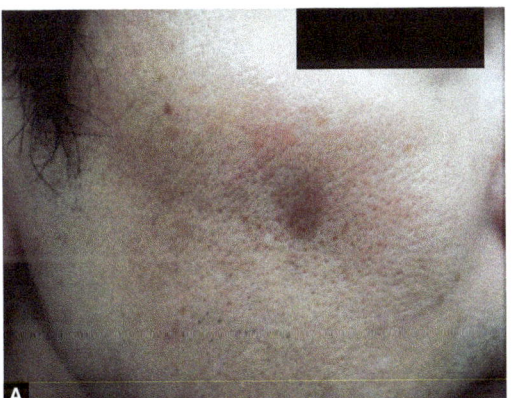 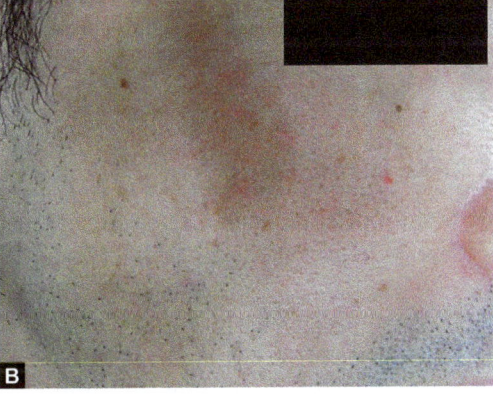

FIG. 7: Significant improvement in solar lentigines in a 50-year-old Japanese man with a trichloroacetic acid (TCA)-based medium-depth peel protocol. **A,** Baseline and **B,** after 5 sessions of one full-face coat of TCA 35% followed by TCA 45% as a spot therapy. Additional improvement in the facial pore size is also appreciable in this picture.

randomized single-blinded study involving 26 subjects (Fitzpatrick skin types I–III) with lateral canthal rhytides, improvement was significantly higher in the group that received pretreatment with botulinum toxin A before a single session of JS-TCA 35% peel, compared to the peel group without pretreatment.[33] Better improvement in acne scars and PIH by combining chemical peels with other modalities like regional dermabrasion, fractionated radiofrequency, microneedling, fractional CO_2 laser, pulsed dye laser and iontophoresis has been reported by many authors.[34-37] However, these studies were conducted either in "less risky" skin types (I–III) and/or employed a superficial chemical peel like GA or salicylic acid. Thus, based on these reports, currently it would be unadvisable to recommend combining a medium-depth peel with another resurfacing modality, at least in the darker skin types.

CONCLUSION

Despite the risks involved with medium-depth peeling in patients with SOC, the therapeutic outcome can be optimized while ensuring safety with careful patient selection, effective priming, patch testing, selection of optimum peel protocol, meticulous postpeel care and urgent intervention at the earliest hint of an impending complication. The availability of agents such as recombinant epidermal growth factor-based topicals and oral/topical tranexamic acid have added another dimension to safeguarding the treated skin in the event of overzealous epidermal damage or persistent erythema, respectively.

TAKE HOME POINTS

- Medium-depth peels penetrate till the level of upper reticular dermis (skin depth of 200 μm)
- A 'chemical peel agent' cannot be simply classified as a medium-depth peel. Various factors determine the ultimate depth reached by a peel protocol – the active ingredient, its concentration, pH of the solution, number of coats applied and the leave-on duration of the peel over the skin
- The list of agents and protocols that generally qualify as medium depth peeling is long, including glycolic acid (GA) 70% (3–15 min), pyruvic acid 60% (3–5 min), TCA 35–50%, Augmented TCA (TCA 35% combined with Jessner's solution (JS) or GA 70% or solid carbon dioxide), multiple coats of JS, 88% phenol and croton oil-free phenol combination (CFPC) peels
- The most commonly preferred peeling agents/combinations to provide safe medium-depth peeling in darker skin types include GA 70%, augmented TCA (combined with JS or GA) and multi-coat JS
- Medium-depth peeling can provide gratifying results in active acne, post-acne and postinflammatory hyperpigmentation, melasma, LPP and other facial melanoses, early photoaging and fine rhytides, open pores, uneven skin tone, freckles and post-acne scarring
- Careful patient selection, effective priming, peel patch testing, selection of optimum peel protocol, meticulous post-peel hydration and sun-protection, and urgent intervention at the earliest hint of an impending complication constitute the key to safe and successful outcome of medium-depth peels in darker skin types
- The availability of agents such as recombinant epidermal growth factor-based topicals and oral/topical tranexamic acid have added another dimension to safeguarding the treated skin in the event of overzealous epidermal damage or persistent erythema, respectively.

REFERENCES

1. Brody HJ, Monheit GD, Resnik SS, et al. A history of chemical peeling. Dermatol Surg. 2000;26:405-9.
2. Stuzin JM. Phenol peeling and the history of phenol peeling. Clin Plast Surg. 1998;25:1-19.
3. Eller JJ, Wolff S. Skin peeling and scarification. JAMA. 1941;116:934-8.
4. MacKee G, Karp F. The treatment of post-acne scars with phenol. Br J Dermatol. 1952;64:456-9.
5. Baker TJ, Gordon HL. The ablation of rhytides by chemical means—a preliminary report. J Fla Med Assoc. 1961;48:541.
6. Ayres S. Superficial chemosurgery in treating aging skin. Arch Dermatol 1962;85:125-33.

7. Monheit GD, Chastain MA. Chemical peels. Facial Plast Surg Clin North Am. 2001;9:239-55.
8. Brody HJ. Chemical peeling. St. Louis, MO: Mosby Year-Book; 1992.
9. Monheit GD. The Jessner's + TCA peel: a medium depth chemical peel. J Dermatol Surg Oncol. 1989;15:945-50.
10. Coleman III WP, Futrell JM. The glycolic acid trichloroacetic acid peel. J Dermatol Surg Oncol. 1994;20:76-90.
11. Tse Y, Ostad A, Lee HS, et al. A clinical and histologic evaluation of two medium-depth peels. Dermatol Surg. 1996;22:781-6.
12. Moy LS, Peace S, Moy RL. Comparison of the effect of various chemical peeling agents in a mini-pig model. Dermatol Surg. 1996;22:429-32.
13. Monheit GD. The Jessner's trichloroacetic acid peel. An enhanced medium-depth chemical peel. Dermatol Clin. 1995;3:277-83.
14. Roberts WE. Chemical peeling in ethnic/dark skin. Dermatol Ther. 2004;17:196-205.
15. Stegman SJ. A comparative histologic study of the effects of three peeling agents and dermabrasion on normal and sun damaged skin. Aesthetic Plast Surg. 1982;6:123-35.
16. Savant SS, Shenoy S. Chemical peeling with phenol: For the treatment of stable vitiligo and alopecia areata. Indian J Dermatol Venereol Leprol. 1999;65:93-8.
17. Ravikiran SP, Sacchidanand S, Leelavathy B. Therapeutic wounding - 88% phenol in idiopathic guttate hypomelanosis. Indian Dermatol Online J. 2014;5:14-8.
18. Otley CC, Roenigk RK. Medium-depth chemical peeling. Semin Cutan Med Surg. 1996;15:145-54.
19. Khunger N; IADVL Task Force. Standard guidelines of care for chemical peels. Indian J Dermatol Venereol Leprol. 2008;74 Suppl:S5-12.
20. Duffy DM. Informed consent for chemical peels and dermabrasion. Dermatol Clin. 1989;7:183-5.
21. Sonthalia S. Errichetti E. Dermoscopy: Not just for Diagnosis, Not Just for Dermatologists. Kathmandu Univ Med J (KUMJ). 2017;15(57):1-2.
22. Spring LK, Krakowski AC, Alam M, et al. Isotretinoin and Timing of Procedural Interventions: A Systematic Review with Consensus Recommendations. JAMA Dermatol. 2017;153:802-9.
23. Picosse FR, Yarak S, Cabral NC, et al. Early chemabrasion for acne scars after treatment with oral isotretinoin. Dermatol Surg. 2012;38:1521-6.
24. Monheit GD. Skin preparation: An essential step before chemical peeling or laser resurfacing. Cosmet Dermatol. 1996;9:13-4.
25. Garg VK, Sarkar R, Agarwal R. Comparative evaluation of beneficiary effects of priming agents (2% hydroquinone and 0.025% retinoic acid) in the treatment of melasma with glycolic acid peels. Dermatol Surg. 2008;34:1032-9.
26. Halaas YP. Medium depth peels. Facial Plast Surg Clin North Am. 2004;12:297-303.
27. Fanous N, Zari S. Universal Trichloroacetic Acid Peel Technique for Light and Dark Skin. JAMA Facial Plast Surg. 2017;19:212-9.
28. Nikalji N, Godse K, Sakhiya J, et al. Complications of medium depth and deep chemical peels. J Cutan Aesthet Surg. 2012;5:254-60.
29. Al-Waiz MM, Al-Sharqi AI. Medium-depth chemical peels in the treatment of acne scars in dark-skinned individuals. Dermatol Surg. 2002;28:383-7.
30. Monheit GD. Medium-depth chemical peels. Dermatol Clin. 2001;19:413-25.
31. Humphreys TR, Werth V, Dzubow L, et al. Treatment of photodamaged skin with trichloroacetic acid and topical tretinoin. J Am Acad Dermatol. 1996;34:638-44.
32. Lawrence N, Cox SE, Cockerell CJ, et al. A comparison of the efficacy and safety of Jessner's solution and 35% trichloroacetic acid vs. 5% fluorouracil in the treatment of widespread facial actinic keratoses. Arch Dermatol. 1995;131:176-81.
33. Tung R, Mahoney AM, Novice K, et al. Treatment of lateral canthal rhytides with a medium depth chemical peel with or without pretreatment with onabotulinum toxin type A: A randomized control trial. Int J Womens Dermatol. 2016;2:31-4.
34. Kroepfl L, Emer JJ. Combination Therapy for Acne Scarring: Personal Experience and Clinical Suggestions. J Drugs Dermatol. 2016;15:1413-9.
35. Kurokawa I, Oiso N, Kawada A. Adjuvant alternative treatment with chemical peeling and subsequent iontophoresis for postinflammatory hyperpigmentation, erosion with inflamed red papules and non-inflamed atrophic scars in acne vulgaris. J Dermatol. 2017;44:401-5.
36. Lekakh O, Mahoney AM, Novice K, et al. Treatment of Acne Vulgaris With Salicylic Acid Chemical Peel and Pulsed Dye Laser: A Split Face, Rater-Blinded, Randomized Controlled Trial. J Lasers Med Sci. 2015;6:167-70.
37. Sharad J. Combination of microneedling and glycolic acid peels for the treatment of acne scars in dark skin. J Cosmet Dermatol. 2011;10:317-23.

CHAPTER 18

Phenol Peels and Its Modifications for Skin of Color

Sidharth Sonthalia

INTRODUCTION AND HISTORICAL PERSPECTIVE

The use of phenol on the skin was for the first time comprehensively described by Unna in 1882, which was developed further in France after World War I.[1] In 1867, Lister first noted the germicidal effects of phenol.[2] The first systematic description on the use of phenol and other peeling agents for scar treatment was provided by Eller and Wolff in 1940s, which was followed by publication of results on the use of phenol for scars by Mackee in 1952.[3,4] The popularity of phenol as a peeling agent can be linked to the work done by French physicist Lagasse and his daughter.[2] Finally in the 1960s, two events marked the commencement of the modern era of peeling—the development of modified phenol solutions [specifically, the addition of croton oil (CO) by Baker and Gordon[5]], and histological assessment of peeling results of phenol and trichloroacetic acid (TCA) peels.[6] The Baker–Gordon (BG) formula has 2.1% CO, the highest concentration of CO, rendering it a very powerful and deep dermal peel. Modified light phenol formulas with CO in the range of 0.1–0.7% were popularized by lay peelers in the 1920s through the 1990s.[7] These formulas were analyzed in detail over by Hetter and Stone.[8-13]

In this chapter, the author discusses the properties, techniques of application and practical utility of phenol-based peels, with special emphasis on their role in the peeling armamentarium for patients with skin of color (SOC).

PHENOL: PHYSICAL CHARACTERISTICS[7-15]

- Phenol (C_5H_5OH) or carbolic acid is an aromatic hydrocarbon derived from coal tar that can be made from the partial oxidation of benzene
- Molecular weight = 94.11 g
- Needle-shaped crystals, colorless to pink, with a characteristic pungent "phenolic" odor
- Its color darkens when exposed to air and light
- Ninety-eight percent phenol appears as transparent crystals, while liquefied phenol consists of 88% USP solution of phenol in water
- Fusion point is approximately 39°C
- Boiling point = 182°C
- Phenol disrupts sulfide bonds, resulting in keratolysis and protein coagulation
- Phenol is a well-known melanotoxic chemical

- Phenol has additional antiseptic, ablative and analgesic properties.

Unique Properties of Phenol as a Peeling Agent

At 88%, phenol causes immediate coagulation of epidermal keratin and penetrates only to the level of the upper reticular dermis, thereby qualifying as a medium-depth peeling agent. However, when diluted to 45–55%, phenol becomes a keratolytic, disrupts sulfur bonds and attains the power to penetrate deeper to the mid-reticular dermis, behaving like a deep dermal peel.[16,17]

Phenol as a Deep Peeling Agent: Major Hazards of Deep to "Standard" Medium-depth Peeling by Phenol in Skin of Color

Phenol peels have conventionally been employed as deep dermal peels. The skin changes induced after a session of deep peel with phenol can be observed up to 20 years, and include normalization of epidermal architecture, uniform redistribution of basal melanocytes, homogenization of the basement membrane thickness, neocollagenosis with formation of compact bundles of collagen and neoelastogenesis.[16] Deep peeling with phenol solution is very painful and requires general anesthesia or at least deep sedation with topical anesthesia. The risk of cardiac arrhythmias and precipitation of heart failure requires cardiac monitoring; therefore, hospitalization is obligatory.

The prototypical phenol solution used for deep dermal peeling in skin types I and II is the Baker-Gordon solution, which consists of diluted phenol (45-55%) in addition to liquid hexachlorophene soap in alcohol, distilled water and croton oil (an epidermolytic vesicant that enhances penetration of phenol to the mid-reticular dermis).[2,5] Although deep peeling with this solution can provide gratifying results in deep coarse rhytides in patients with skin types I and II, the whole process of deep peeling needs intensive perioperative care, with special emphasis on maintaining hydration through intravenous fluids and close cardiac monitoring. It is clearly unsuitable for the darker skin types due to a high probability of delayed, and often irreversible adverse effects most common being persistent postinflammatory hyperpigmentation (PIH), followed by possible occurrence of depigmentation, which is sometimes referred to as "alabaster statue appearance" and scarring.[18]

Further, phenol may be absorbed systemically and result in hepatorenal and cardiac abnormalities, including cardiac arrhythmias.[19,20] To avoid these side effects, the peels should be administered slowly in a subunit approach. Typically, peel administration should span 60–90 minutes.[14] A further discussion on the unsuitability of phenol-based deep peels for darker skin types is beyond the scope of this chapter. Interested readers may refer to the exhaustive review article on "Deep Chemical Peeling" by Matarasso and Brody.[2]

MODIFIED PHENOL PEELS

Approach 1: Enhancing the Safety of Medium-depth to Deep Peeling with Phenol by Altering the Concentration of Phenol and Croton Oil

In view of the systemic adverse effects of concentrated phenol, and the risk of pigmentary dyschromias and scarring in darker skin types, many approaches have been explored to render phenol-based solutions safer for the ethnic skin. Such modified phenol–croton oil-based formulas are commercially available in many countries

TABLE 1: Some commercial phenol-croton oil peel solutions available in certain countries such as the United States

Formula	Phenol content (%)	Croton oil content (%)
Baker–Gordon	50	2.1
Exoderm-lift	64	0.6–0.7
Hetter (range 0.1–1.0%)	50	0.7
Hetter all around	35	0.4
Stone-2 (Stone 100/Grade II)	60	0.2
Hetter VL (neck/eyelid)	30	0.1

including the United States (Table 1).[12] The basic modification over the erstwhile Baker–Gordon solution involves the use of a similar or lesser concentration of phenol with dramatic reduction in the concentration of CO. Croton oil, an epidermal vesicant, enhances the penetration of phenol deeper into the dermis. The highest concentration of croton oil (2.1%) is present in the Baker–Gordon formula, therefore, results in deep dermal peeling (*vide supra*). These modified phenol formulas have been used for deep acne scars, photoaging, rhytides and melasma.[7-14] Two application protocols have been employed for these peels:

- Chemical reconstruction of skin scars (CROSS) technique (that has typically been described for high concentrations of TCA peel), using chemabrasion by one of the modified phenol–croton peels like the stone phenol (into the scars), topped up with full-face application of Jessner's solution (JS), or some other superficial to medium-depth peel. This approach has been suggested for moderately depressed scars and has a little downtime
- *Two-day chemabrasion of full face with a modified phenol-croton peel*:[7] This is performed for deep acne scars and needs an average downtime of 10–14 days for healing and strict sun protection for 1–3 months. The procedure is conducted under intravenous access with either oral or intravenous conscious sedation using agents like diazepam, midazolam, fentanyl, propofol and ketamine. The use of facial nerve blocks is effective at reducing the need for systemic medications. The formula is applied to five anatomic areas (forehead, two cheeks, perioral and chin, and periorbital and nose), spending 10–15 minutes per area so that the peel application takes approximately 60 minutes. A uniform frost and yellowish edematous appearance indicating epidermolysis is noted after 15–30 minutes. The patient is discharged after occluding the face with a waterproof tape and covering with a surgical face net. On day 2, the necrotic coagulum is debrided followed by pasting a mask of bismuth subgallate, an antiseptic and anti-inflammatory substance. Vigorous postpeel care of hydration and sun protection have to be followed for the next 2–3 months. A touch-up peel may be done with a lighter peel after 2–3 months.

Special prephenol-croton oil peel evaluation: Patients preparing to have a phenol-based peel require a full laboratory work-up, including hepatic, renal and cardiac testing.[12,13]

Complications Reported with Modified Phenol Peels for Deep Peeling

- Prolonged erythema
- Scarring—including hypertrophic and keloidal
- Milia formation
- Hypopigmentation or depigmentation
- *Systemic complications*: Cardiac, renal and hepatic.

Contraindications to Phenol Peels (Deep Peeling and Medium-depth Peeling Using Modified Phenol Peels)

- Fitzpatrick skin types IV–VI
- Pregnancy
- Lactation
- Oral isotretinoin treatment—active as well as within 6 months of the treatment completion
- Cardiac disease, especially heart failure and arrhythmias
- Insufficient kidney and/or hepatic function
- Known allergy to phenol or any other ingredient of the combination
- Tendency of keloidal scarring.

Approach 2: Croton Oil-free–Phenol Combination Peels—Ensuring the Efficacy and Enhancing the Safety by using Combination Phenol Peels, Free of Croton Oil and Containing Low Concentration Phenol and Other Peeling Agents in Low Concentration

- In order to provide a suitable balance between the efficacy and safety of phenol-based peels in darker skin types, the best approach in Indian Peel Specialists' and my experience is the use of combination peels that contain a CO-free pH-optimized combination of low concentration of phenol, in addition to multiple other peeling agents. One such range of oil-free–phenol combination (CFPC) peel, which is very popular and *in vogue* is the *nomelan fenol* (NMFP) peels (MEDIDERMA/SESDERMA), that are available in different strengths (Fig. 1). All the nomelan fenol peels (by Mediderma/Sesderma, India) consist of TCA (15%) and glycolic acid or GA (2%), in addition to varying strengths

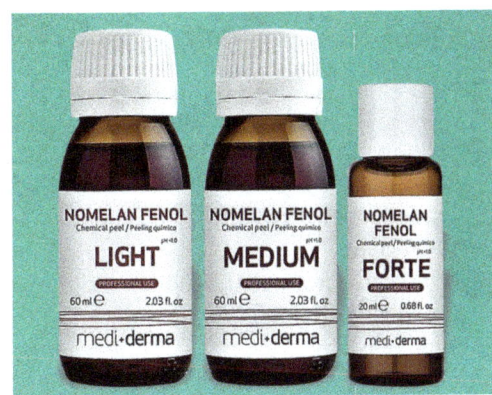

FIG. 1: Nomelan Fenol Peels (NMFP)—one of the most popular range of proprietary croton oil-free-phenol combination peels (CFPC) manufactured/marketed by MEDIDERMA/SESDERMA available in different strengths.

of phenol–8% (NMFP LIGHT), 15% (NMFP MEDIUM) and 25% (NMFP FORTE). The CFPC peels like the NMFP range are available as nonbuffered hydroalcoholic solutions with pH around 0.5. Since they are sensitive to sunlight, the peel bottles are dark brown and should be kept away from sunlight and heat. The bottle should be tightly secured with the cap after each use and shaken before use, since phenol tends to vaporize forming a concentrated layer on top of the solution.

Depth of Croton oil-free–Phenol Combination Peels

The final depth of penetration of these peels can be determined by altering factors like:
- Use of different strengths of the available proprietary peels
- Number of coats applied
- Duration of time for which the peel is left over.

This makes the CFPC peels highly versatile, efficacious and safe for use, especially in the darker skin types.

Indications of Croton Oil-free Phenol Combination Peels

- Photodamaged skin and superficial rhytides
- *Pigmentary dyschromias*: Melasma, PIH, lichen planus pigmentosus (LPP)
- Active acne
- *Acne scars (depressed)*: Mild to moderate
- Freckles and solar lentigines
- Stretch marks.

Advantages of Croton Oil-free Phenol–Combination Peels over Modified Phenol–Croton Oil Peels

- Minimal risk of postpeel pigmentary abnormalities and scarring, especially in darker skin types
- Better control of peel depth by alteration of factors like number of coats and leave-on duration of time
- No evidence of risk of any systemic adverse effects due to much lower phenol concentration
- Minimal to no pain and no need for parenteral hydration, analgesia, etc.
- *Total time taken*: 5–10 minutes during the session at the clinic, compared to 45–60 minutes essential for modified phenol-croton oil peels
- Postpeel care regimen—relatively more comfortable for the patients.

Technique of Application of Croton Oil-free–Phenol Combination Peels

Author's specific guidelines for CFPC peels, excluding the general guidelines applicable for any peeling methodology such as prepeel priming, counseling, photographic records, consent forms, etc.

- Cleansing and degreasing using alcohol swabs and acetone
- Application of a primer peel, e.g., GA 35% for 2–3 minutes (optional)
- Protection of sensitive sites with vaseline
- *First coat*: First coat of NMFP (Light/Medium/Forte—depending on condition, skin type and tolerance) peel should be applied all over the affected region, concentrating on the affected patches. It may be applied by two techniques:
  - Dabbing gauze soaked with the solution evenly and quickly without rubbing
  - Using a peel brush making sure of preventing double overlay.
- *Subsequent coats*: Allow every coat to dry (around 2–3 minutes) before applying the next one. The number of coats will depend on condition being treated and the skin type
  - For acne or light pigmentation: 2–4 coats may be applied in light skins (phototypes I-III)
  - Maximum of 2 coats in dark skins (phototypes IV-VI).
- *Full-face and spot coats*: In darker skin types with hyperpigmentation like melasma, LPP, PIH, etc., two coats may be applied on full face and subsequent 1–2 coats can be applied over the pigmented areas as spot peel
- *Frosting*: A uniform frost appears within seconds of the first coat (Fig. 2)
- Maximum application per session should not exceed 5 mL
- *Postapplication*: These are leave-on peels and are not to be washed, rather sealed off with a thin coat of a retinol-based cream, without rubbing the peel off. A coat of sunscreen is further dabbed after few minutes and the patient is sent back home with additional manual sun protection
- *Leave-on duration*: The peel may be left on for 2–10 hours (average 6–8 h). It is better to leave for not more than 2–4 hours after the first session. Graduated increment in leave-on duration time, e.g.,

Phenol Peels and Its Modifications for Skin of Color

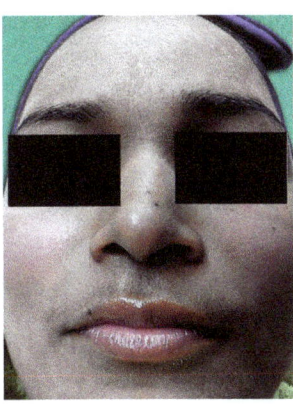

FIG. 2: Uniform frosting on the face of a young Indian girl with lichen planus pigmentosus, on the 3rd day of treatment with two full-face coats of a Nomelan fenol MEDIUM peel containing 15% phenol, 15% TCA and 2% GA with a leave-on time of 6 hours.

2-4-6-8-10 hours in subsequent sessions is a safe approach. Patient is instructed to gently rinse it off with cold water, avoiding the use of any harsh cleanser
- *Number of peel sessions and interval*: 4-8 peel sessions (every 2-3 weeks) may have to be given to achieve the desired improvement.

Postpeel Care Regimen
- Icing 2-3 times a day for 2-3 days
- Generous use of moisturizers: Vitamin C-based serum once a day aids in better healing and provides additional moisturization
- Strict sun protection with sunscreen of SPF 50+ three times a day
- Add-on depigmenting, scar-repair or anti-wrinkle creams locally over the patches starting 3-5 days after the session and stopped 1-2 days prior to next peel session.

Postpeel Expectations
- Erythema, superficial crusting and excessive dryness often occur
- In contrast to other peels, these appear on third or fourth day of the peel and may continue for another 2-3 days
- In almost all patients, adequate hydration and sun protection settles down these events
- Some patients complain of a temporary "bronzing" effect—it subsides within 3-5 days.

Adverse Effects Experienced with Croton Oil-free–Phenol Combination Peels
- Temporary burning
- *Phenolic odor*: Transient
- Postpeel—erythema, scaling and mild crusting—self-subsiding
- Temporary "bronzing" effect that simulates PIH.

Author's Personal Experience in the Use of Croton Oil-free–Phenol Combination in Patients with Lichen Planus Pigmentosus

In a prospective pilot study undertaken by the author, 11 patients (age range 23-52 years; skin type IV or V) with stable or inactive LPP with residual pigmentation were treated with 6 sessions of NMFP MEDIUM peel (2-weekly) with 2 coats on full face or neck and 2 spot coats on darkly pigmented areas, with leave-on time of 6 hours in each session. Final evaluation (patient-graded improvement) done 1 month after the last session revealed excellent (76% or more), moderate (51-75%), good (26-50%), mild (<25%) and nil improvement in 3, 3, 3, 1 and 1 patient, respectively.[21] Overall, good to excellent improvement (26-76% or more) was reported by 82% patients (Figs. 3 and 4). Adverse effects were mild and transient.

The results of a retrospective analysis of the efficacy and safety of six sessions of croton-oil free phenol combination (CFPC) peel done every 3 weeks, for inactive LPP-associated hyperpigmentation in 17 patients conducted

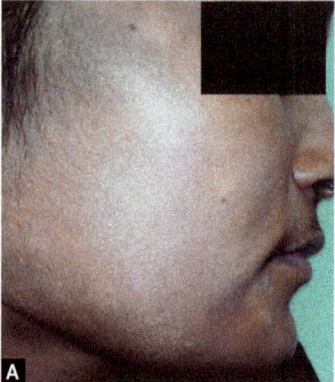 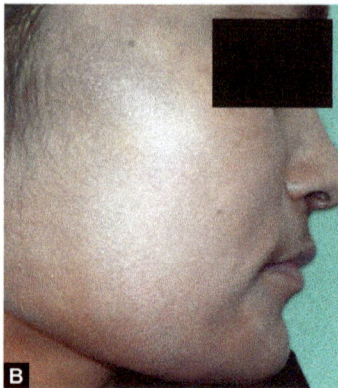

FIG. 3: More than 76% improvement in the residual pigmentation of stable lichen planus pigmentosus in a young Indian lady. **A,** Baseline and **B,** 1 month after 6 fortnightly sessions of Nomelan Fenol Medium peel.

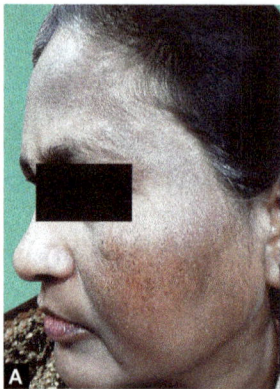 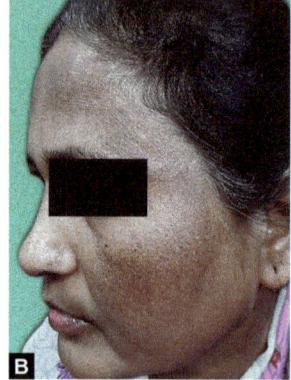

FIG. 4: More than 50% improvement in the residual pigmentation of stable lichen planus pigmentosus in an old Indian lady. **A,** Baseline and **B,** 1 month after 6 fortnightly sessions of Nomelan Fenol Medium peel.

by the author and his team, revealed excellent improvement with >75% reduction of pigmentation in around 1/3rd of the patients, moderate-to-excellent improvement (>25% reduction in pigmentation) in 3/4th of the patients. The treatment outcome was evaluated clinically as well dermoscopically. The treatment was well as tolerated with no serious local/systemic adverse effects.[22]

The author has also experienced gratifying results with CFPC peels in melasma, active acne with mild acne scars, as well as superficial rhytides. Thus, CFPC peels appear to be efficacious, convenient and much safer than modified phenol–CO peels for patients with darker skin types.

Approach 3: Therapeutic Wounding with 88% Phenol

As mentioned earlier, undiluted pure phenol 88% acts as a medium-depth peel, which has been utilized in medical conditions like vitiligo, alopecia areata (AA) and idiopathic guttate hypomelanosis (IGH), based upon the principle of controlled therapeutic wounding.[23,24] Therapeutic wounding refers to wounding the skin to induce pigment cells or hair follicles with the goal of producing pigmentation in depigmented skin patches (vitiligo, IGH) or hair regrowth in AA, that was earlier used for repigmenting small patches of stable vitiligo. In the study conducted in Indian patients by Savant and Shenoy, peeling with 88% phenol was carried out on 142 sites of stable vitiligo and on 69 sites of AA.[23] Phenol 88% was applied on affected areas till a uniform frost, after cleansing and degreasing. After healing, perifollicular and/or perilesional repigmentation was reported in all the lesions of vitiligo, and good hair regrowth in 72.5% patients with AA. Adverse effects reported were hypopigmentation (58 AA), hyperpigmentation (11 AA), persistent erythema (42 vitiligo, 28 AA), demarcation lines (4 AA) and secondary bacterial infection (2 vitiligo, 5 AA).

In the study by Ravikiran et al., 20 Indian patients with 139 IGH macules were subjected to spot phenol 88% peel, applied with an ear bud once a month for two sittings.[24] Repigmentation was noted in 64% of IGH macules. More than 75% improvement was seen in 45% of the total IGH macules at the end of 3 months. Persistent scabbing (17.26% of lesions) was reported to be the most common adverse effect.

The author has also successfully employed this approach in achieving repigmentation of stable refractory lesions of vitiligo (Fig. 5).

CONCLUSION

Phenol is a unique molecule with pleiotropic effects. The peeling power of this agent can be harnessed with efficacious results and safety, only by understanding its properties and utilizing modified protocols, which should be decided on the basis of skin type, indication and tolerance among others. If used carefully, phenol-based peels provide gratifying results in disorders of hyperpigmentation, acne and acne scars, photorejuvenation and medical conditions like vitiligo.

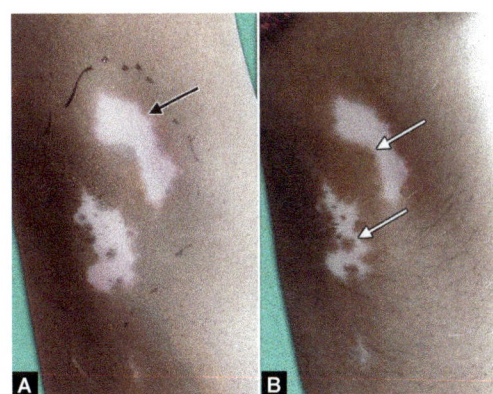

FIG. 5: Repigmentation in treatment-refractory lesions of vitiligo with 88% phenol spot peel. **A,** Immediately postphenol application (note the frosting indicated by black arrow) and **B,** 3 weeks after that single session (white arrows indicating perilesional and intralesional repigmentation).

TAKE HOME POINTS

- Phenol-based peels have been in use since the late 18th century
- Phenol is a pleiotropic molecule with properties like keratolysis, protein coagulation, antiseptic, ablative, analgesic, collagen remodeling, melanotoxic as well as pigment stimulatory. Its properties can be customized by varying its concentration, combining with other hydroxy acids, altering the pH, and modulating protocols of using it as a peel
- Unlike most of the other peels that penetrate deeper as their concentration goes up, phenol penetrates deeper till the mid-reticular dermis on dilution to 50% while its penetration gets restricted to upper reticular dermis when used at 88% concentration

- Conventional medium-depth and deep peeling regimes using phenol and croton oil-based peels need a dedicated set-up, careful monitoring and are suitable only for skin types I and II. Even then, cardiac, renal and other systemic adverse effects may occur
- Such peel protocols are unsuitable for darker skin types owing to the high risk of post-procedure dyschromic changes and scarring
- The new generation of phenol-based peels suitable for darker skin types are free of croton oil, i.e., CFPC peels that typically contain a mix of 8% phenol, 15% TCA and multiple alpha-and beta-hydroxy acids in low concentration (1–2%); available as nonbuffered hydroalcoholic solutions with a pH of 0.5
- Many proprietary preparations of CFPC peels with varying strengths are available in India, and are being used with good to excellent outcomes for dyschromias, photoaging, acne and acne-associated scarring, stretch marks, etc.
- The author's self-developed and fine-tuned protocol of using CFPC peels for residual pigmentation of LPP has shown excellent outcome and demonstrates the potential of these 'newgen' phenol peels in providing efficacious and safe outcome in cosmetic issues amenable to other chemical peels.

REFERENCES

1. Stuzin JM. Phenol peeling and the history of phenol peeling. Clin Plast Surg. 1998;25:1-19.
2. Matarasso SL, Brody HJ. Deep chemical peeling. Semin Cutan Med Surg 1996;15:155-61.
3. Eller JJ, Wolff S. Skin peeling and scarification. JAMA. 1941;116:934-8.
4. MacKee G, Karp F. The treatment of post-acne scars with phenol. Br J Dermatol 1952;64:456-9.
5. Baker TJ, Gordon HL. The ablation of rhytides by chemical means: A preliminary report. J Fla Med Assoc. 1961;48:541.
6. Ayres S. Superficial chemosurgery in treating aging skin. Arch Dermatol. 1962;85:125-33.
7. Rullan P, Lemmon J, Rullan JM. The 2-day phenol chemabrasion technique for deep wrinkles and acne scars. Am J Cosmet Surg. 2004;21:199-210.
8. Hetter GP. An examination of the phenol-croton oil peel: Part I. Dissecting the formula. Plast Reconstr Surg. 2000;105:227-39.
9. Hetter GP. An examination of the phenol-croton oil peel: Part II. The lay peelers and their croton oil formulas. Plast Reconstr Surg. 2000;105:240-8.
10. Hetter GP. An examination of the phenol-croton oil peel: Part III. The plastic surgeons' role. Plast Reconstr Surg. 2000;105:752-63.
11. Hetter GP. An examination of the phenol-croton oil peel: part IV. Face peel results with different concentrations of phenol and croton oil. Plast Reconstr Surg. 2000;105:1061-83.
12. Stone PA. The use of modified phenol for chemical face peeling. Clin Plast Surg. 1998;25:21-44.
13. Stone PA, Lefer LG. Modified phenol chemical face peels: recognizing the role of application technique. Clin Plast Surg. 2001;28:13-36.
14. Rullan P, Karam AM. Chemical peels for darker skin types. Facial Plast Surg Clin North Am. 2010;18:111-31.
15. Monheit GD, Chastain MA. Chemical peels. Facial Plast Surg Clin North Am. 2001;9:239-55.
16. Brown A, Kaplan L, Brown M. Phenol induced histologic changes: Hazards, techniques and uses. Br J Plast Surg. 1960;13:158-69.
17. Matarasso SL, Glogau RG. Chemical face peels. Dermatol Clin. 1991;9:131-50.
18. Coleman WP 3rd. Dermal peels. Dermatol Clin. 2001;19: 405-11.
19. Price NM. EKG changes in relationship to the chemical peel. J Dermatol Surg Oncol. 1990;16:37-42.
20. Stagnone GJ, Orgel MG, Stagnone JJ. Cardiovascular effects of topical 50% trichloroacetic acid and Baker's phenol solution. J Dermatol Surg Oncol. 1987;13:999-1002.
21. Sonthalia S. Phenol Based Peels on Refractory Lichen Planus- A New Hope! Singapore: International Pigment Cell Conference (IPCC) and 27th ASM of Dermatological Society of Singapore; 2014.
22. Sonthalia S, Vedamurthy M, Goldust M, et al. Modified Phenol peels for treatment-refractory hyperpigmentation of Lichen planus pigmentosus: A retrospective clinico-dermoscopic analysis. J Cosmetic Dermatol. [In Print]
23. Savant SS, Shenoy S. Chemical peeling with phenol: For the treatment of stable vitiligo and alopecia areata. Indian J Dermatol Venereol Leprol. 1999;65:93-8.
24. Ravikiran SP, Sacchidanand S, Leelavathy B. Therapeutic wounding - 88% phenol in idiopathic guttate hypomelanosis. Indian Dermatol Online J. 2014;5:14-8.

CHAPTER 19

Medium-depth Peels

Fischer Sabrina, Borelli Claudia

INTRODUCTION

Chemical peelings are classified by the level of injury (light/superficial, medium-depth and deep) and the mechanism of action (caustic, metabolic and toxic). They induce a controlled destruction of parts or the whole epidermis with or without the dermis, producing exfoliation with ablation of superficial lesions. The ablation is followed by regeneration of new epidermal and dermal tissue. Medium-depth peels are used to treat pigmentary disturbances like lentigines, acne scars and photoaged skin, as well as provide skin toning. Medium-depth peels penetrate in the epidermis and papillary dermis (Fig. 1). They lead to necrosis up to the upper reticular dermis. According to the severity of wrinkling, laxity and the patient's downtime the type of peel is selected. To receive an acceptable cosmetic improvement a complementary therapy with rejuvenating creams and dermal fillers may be added. Chemical peelings should be repeated to achieve the best possible cosmetic improvement and to obviate recurrence. Medium-depth peels can usually be repeated in 3 months. Premature peeling result in an increased risk of complications, in particular persistent erythema, postinflammatory hyperpigmentation, infections and following scarring. Because of the simplicity, the low morbidity, cost-effectiveness and simple availability, chemical peels still play an important role to treat photoaging and pigmentary disturbances, even though there are more modern techniques available like lasers.[1,2]

In sun-damaged skin with deeper wrinkles combined peels are often used, e.g., medium-depth peel for periorbital and upper-neck skin, and superficial peels for less sun-damaged skin, like lateral cheeks, lower neck, chest and forehead. In dark skinned patients medium-depth peels are not generally recommended as the risk for complications, especially of prolonged hyperpigmentation is clearly increased. In dark skinned patients especially medium-depth and deep peels should be performed with great caution.[1,4,5]

Especially in patients with dark skin, careful diagnosis regarding brown lesions at the initial evaluation is very important. They need to be distinguished as hyperkeratotic nonmelanocytic pigmented lesions, e.g., seborrheic keratoses versus truly melanocytic (e.g., lentigines). Wrong diagnosis or misclassification may result in ineffective ablative treatments and worsen the

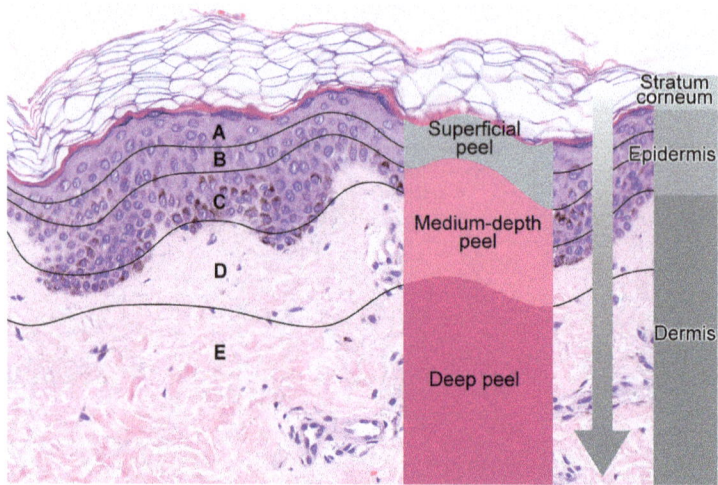

FIG. 1: Classification of the depth of peeling in five levels according to Schürer and Wiest.[3] **A,** Very superficial chemical peeling; **B,** Superficial chemical peeling; **C,** Peeling to stratum basale; **D,** Middle-depth chemical peeling to stratum papillare; **E,** Deep chemical peeling to stratum reticulare.

complexion. In medium-depth peels the face-neck skin color will be not as discordant as in a deep peel. Strict avoidance of the sun and chronic use of skin lighteners on the neck are necessary.[1,4]

CHEMISTRY AND CHEMICAL FORMULATIONS USED

Wound healing is modified according to pH, concentration, quantity applied, concomitant use, other chemicals and chemical ingredients of peels.[4]

In the 1960s trichloroacetic acid (TCA) peels became popular. TCA peels are manifold and can be used as superficial, to medium, to deep peel. For medium-depth peels on face and hands TCA at 35–40% is used as a standard solution. TCA can be used alone or as a combined peel. TCA in concentrations up to 35% has a low risk of side effects. TCA (50%) is used as a single frost medium-depth peel. Because of the high risk of side effects, in particular scarring, TCA is more often used in combined peels with a lower concentration and thus a lower risk of side effects. Combined peels, e.g., after the use of glycolic acid or Jessner's solution, are used to achieve a deeper peel by reducing the cohesion of the epidermal cells allowing a more even and better penetration of TCA. Combined peels are very practical in mild to moderate photoaging with pigmentary changes, hyperpigmentations, lentigines, superficial acne scars and rhytides. In areas like neck, arms and décolleté with low adnexal structures, Jessner's solution with 20% TCA is sufficient (Fig. 2). To increase a peel more coats are applied.[1-6]

Combination Peels

Combination peels (Table 1) are used to combine caustic, metabolic and toxic effects. TCA, denatures protein and precipitates epidermal proteins, leading to scaling and

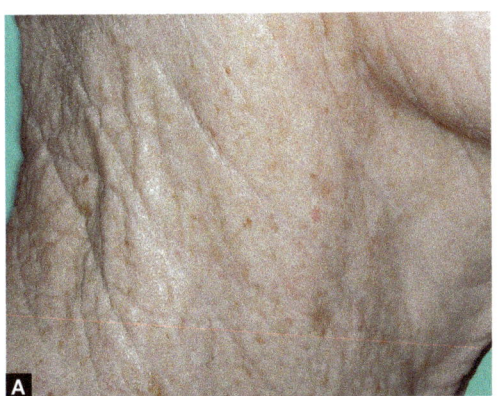 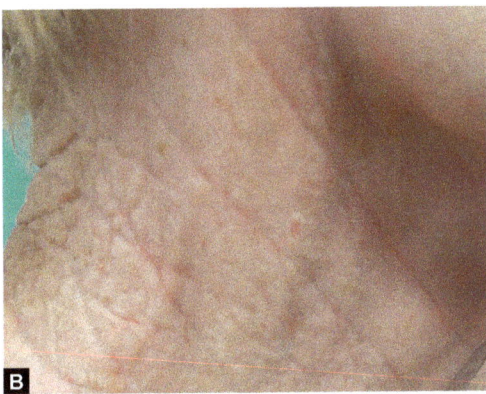

FIG. 2: **A,** Skin of the neck before chemical peeling; **B,** Skin of the neck after chemical peeling with 20% trichloroacetic acid.

TABLE 1: **Medium-depth peel agents** [1,4,6,10-12]

Name	Composition
Trichloroacetic acid (TCA)	Solid TCA 35–50%
Pyruvic acid	40–60%
Phenol	88% phenol unoccluded
Common combination peels	
Monheit's peel	Jessner's solution with 20–35% TCA
Coleman's peel	Glycolic acid (70%) combined with 35% TCA
Brody's peel	Solid CO_2 combined with 35% TCA
Obagi's blue peel (radiant peel)	20–30% TCA and a color-sensitive reaction (glycerin, saponins, and a nonionic blue indicator)
Wiest-Walker peel	Salicylic acid (25%) with glycolic acid (50%), combined with 35% TCA
Habig peel	Microdermabrasion with 35% TCA and dermasanding
Other medium-depth peels	
Light phenol peels	Light phenol peels with croton oil 0.1%
Hetter Very Light VL	30% Phenol
VI Precision	30% Phenol, 7% TCA with salicylic acid + tretinoin, but no croton oil
Universal peel x 2 days	30% Phenol plus proprietary ingredients
Chemical reconstruction of skin scares	Ice-pick scars treated with precise intralesional application of, e.g., 30% TCA

necrosis and dermal inflammation which appears as white frosting on the skin, is often used in combined peels.

The advantage of combined peel agents is an enhanced depth of the peel without using a higher concentration of the peel. They should be used carefully especially in dark skinned patients, as combined medium-depth peels may result in an uneven depth of peeling, leading to a higher risk for complications, e.g., pigmentary disturbances or scarring. According to the studies from Rullan et al. and Sarkar et al., TCA can also be safely used in dark skin types. A longer preconditioning of the skin, as well as the use of the lowest effective strength of TCA and immediate care for occurrence of postinflammatory hyperpigmentation are required for the safe use of TCA.[1,4,7,8]

Jessner's Peel

Jessner's TCA (20–35%) is a keratolytic peel combining 14 g salicylic acid, 14 g lactic acid (85%) and 14 g resorcinol, mixed in ethanol (96%) for a final volume of 100 mL.[1,4]

To achieve a medium-depth peel pretreatment of the stratum corneum by application of Jessner's solution is required. Only 1-2 coats of Jessner's solution are applied to avoid postinflammatory hyperpigmentation. The pretreatment is followed by an application of 20–35% TCA.[1,4,9]

Obagi's Blue Peel

Obagi's blue peel contains a fixed concentration of TCA (recommended 20–35%), as well as a blue peel base containing glycerin, saponins and a nonionic blue indicator which allows to estimate the depth of the peel.[1,4]

Pyruvic Acid

Pyruvic acid normally at 40–60% concentration is used to treat moderate acne, photoaging and melasma. It is physiologically converted from an α-ketoacid to a lactic acid. A pretreatment with topical retinoids is important.

Chemical Reconstruction of Skin Scares

Especially in pigmented skin ice-pick scars can be treated by dint of, e.g., a toothpick or very fine brush with precise intralesional application of, e.g., 30% TCA in thin skin.

To smoothen the demarcation lines and optimize the cosmetic outcome chemical peeling can be also combined with dermabrasion, laser resurfacing, e.g., with pulsed carbon dioxide laser for skin rejuvenation, dermasanding, botulinum toxin and fillers (Table 1).[1,2]

INDICATIONS[1,2,4,9,10,13]

Photoaging/aging skin changes:
- Solar lentigines
- Flat actinic keratoses
- Beginning solar elastosis
- Superficial fine wrinkling/elastotic rhytide.

Pigmentary disturbances/disorders/changes:
- Poikiloderma
- Lentigines
- Freckles
- Melasma.

Acne:
- Superficial acne scars
- Comedonal acne
- Acne excoriée
- Dilated pores.

Other/benign epidermal growth:
- Seborrheic keratoses
- Actinic keratoses
- Milia.

CONTRAINDICATIONS

- Recent (2–6 month) facial surgery or open wounds in the area to be treated
- Patients with active infections (bacterial, viral or fungal), facial dermatitis, e.g., atopic dermatitis or psoriasis

- A history of delayed wound healing or tendency to keloids, atrophic skin
- Treatment with isotretinoin in the last 6 months
- History of drugs with photosensitizing potential, previous facial radiation and smoking or imunocompromising diseases leading to a potential delayed wound healing
- Uncooperative patient (careless about sun exposure or application of medicine) and unrealistic expectations
- Another relative contraindication for medium-depth peels is Fitzpatrick skin type IV-VI, as they have a high risk of complications, particularly postinflammatory hyperpigmentation.[1,2]

PATIENT PREPARATION

A detailed medical examination including a detailed general, personal and medical history, in particular the degree of sun exposure and occupation to judge an augmented sun exposure, cutaneous malignancy, a history of hypertrophic or acne scars, previous surgical treatment, immunocompromising conditions, postinflammatory hyperpigmentation and herpes simplex outbreaks, as well as a therapy with isotretinoin in the last 12 months is essential. Active dermatosis, e.g., acne should be treated before the peel. It is also important to rate the available downtime and a possible influence that may affect the healing, e.g., sun exposure. Patient with a high intensity of exercise and other temperature-increasing activities or smoking may also lead to a delayed wound healing, especially in medium-depth and deep peels. A detailed medical examination, with physical and cutaneous examination including skin type, degree of photoaging and sebaceous activity (dry or oily skin), as well as the presence of postinflammatory hyperpigmentation, hypertrophic scars or keloids, and pre-existing inflammation or infection should be obtained. Additionally a photographic documentation with direct lighting and shadows should be taken.[1,4]

A precise consent is very important and should include details about the procedure, a discussion of likely and unlikely complications and side effects especially pigmentation changes, information about the recovery time and the significance of maintenance regimes, as well as the expected outcome and explanation of the nature of treatment. It is recommended to downplay the level of improvement expected and warn the patients that they will look terrible for a minimum of 10 days after the medium-depth peel. A proper consent form should also outline the limitations of the treatment, clearly mention the number of treatments or if more procedures are needed for a proper result and should be signed by the patient. The physician should also estimate the patient's motivation and expectations, and explain that patients should have realistic expectations. The patients should have the opportunity to seek information through brochures, presentations and personal discussions. Because of the high risk of side effects, particularly prolonged hyperpigmentation, medium-depth peels should be practiced with great caution in patients with dark skin. Besides the peel will be much stronger than expected if the skin is dry, has an abrasion or is retinized.[1,5,14]

The patients should be explained that pigmentary disturbances like solar lentigines may disappear initially after the peel, but then return as the melanocytes which are responsible for the pigmentation are below the level of the chemical peeling. To improve the cosmetic outcome those patients need to use sunscreen, hydroquinone or other bleaching agents and retinoids.[5]

Prepeel conditioning is obligatory to improve the peel outcome and to reduce the risk of side-effects, especially the risk of postinflammatory hyperpigmentation. A prepeel priming involving broad-spectrum sunscreen is essential for the patient's skin. Patients susceptible to postinflammatory hyperpigmentation receive a priming with hydroquinone (2-4%). It is important to control any active pre-existing dermatoses or infection.[4]

Topical agents/priming are recommended for a minimum of 2-4 weeks prior to the procedure. It thins out the stratum corneum, facilitates the peel to penetrate rapidly through the stratum corneum, detects intolerance to any agent, enforces the patient compliance, and also improves re-epithelialization and wound healing but decreases the risk of complications, especially postinflammatory hyperpigmentation. In patients with a history of herpes simplex infection or bacterial infections, antiviral or antibacterial prophylaxis starting two days before the procedure until 7-10 days or until complete re-epithelialization is needed. Patients without prophylaxis need to be treated at the slightest sign of herpes simplex or bacterial infection.[1,4]

PEEL TECHNIQUE

Preparation

It's recommended to place the peeling solution in a labelled small glass or disposable plastic cup. For a face or neck peeling usually 2-4 mL solution is sufficient. For application two wooden handled Q-tips are used. Further equipment including a head band for the patient, gloves, 2" × 2" cotton gauze pieces and a timer is needed. You may also offer a portable personal fan for cooling to the patient (not in case of salicylic acid chemical peeling).[1,3,4]

Anesthesia is not generally required in medium-depth peels. In anxious patients anxiolytics, mild tranquilizers or sedatives like diazepam, β-blocker (orally administered clonidin), may be used. Peripheral nerve blockage with, e.g., prilocaine 0.5%, mepivacaine 0.5% and bupivacaine 0.25% or ketorolac intramuscularly may be necessary for TCA peels. For nerve-blocks normally 0.5-1 mL is used per nerve (supratrochlear, infraorbital or mental nerve).[1,3,4,6]

Arrangements

- Different concentrations of labelled peeling solutions
- Alcohol for skin cleaning
- Acetone for skin degreasing
- Cold water
- Saline for irrigation of the eyes in case of accidental spillage
- Neutralizing solution.

To avoid accidental spillage, the soaked applicator should never be passed over the patients face. A syringe filled with saline or water should always kept ready for irrigation of the eyes in case of accidental spillage. Always double check the label of the peeling agent before applying the peel.[1,4]

Before starting the peel, the patient needs to take off the jewelry (necklace, earrings) and take out their contact lenses. They are asked to wash the face with soap and water, wrap their hair back with a hair cap or band and to lay down with their head elevated to 45° with their eyes closed. Afterwards the skin is cleaned with alcohol and degreased with acetone using 2" × 2" gauze pieces. More the pressure used to apply the peel with the wooden handles Q-tip, deeper is the penetration of the peeling. According to the numbers of applied coats the penetration depth increases as well.[1,3,4]

For the application of the peel a 2" × 2" gauze is dipped into the solution containing cup, and squeezed dry carefully before the application. It is first applied to the lateral regions, then carefully centrofacially, and lastly to the perioral and periorbital regions. The depth of the peel results from the applied numbers of the peel. Multiple applied coats of Jessner's solution on dry, retinized skin can cause a medium-depth injury by reaching the upper reticular dermis. More the pressure used to apply the peel with the wooden handles Q-tip, deeper is the penetration of the peeling. The frost will appear more slowly in less porous or leathery skin, e.g., along the mandible. The end-point of the medium depth peel is frosting. Starting from the eyelids and then the entire face the peel is neutralized with neutralizing agent or cold water. Occlusive dressings after TCA peels are described to reduce the risk of dermal necrosis.[1,3,9]

Analgesia and sedation, e.g., with oral sedatives like diazepam, β-blocker (orally administered clonidin), nerve-blocks or ketorolac intramuscularly may be necessary for TCA peels.[1,4]

Jessner's Solution

To achieve a medium-depth peel a pretreatment of the stratum corneum, e.g., by application of Jessner's solution until a frost appears is required. The skin is first cleansed with hexachlorophene, alcohol, and degreased with acetone. Only one to two coats of Jessner's solution are applied to avoid postinflammatory hyperpigmentation until a spotty frosting is achieved and a slight drying of acne lesions is achieved.

The pretreatment is followed by an application of 20–35% TCA. For the application of TCA a 2″ × 2″ gauze is dipped into the TCA solution, and squeeze dry carefully before the application. It is first applied to the lateral regions, then carefully centrofacially, and lastly to the perioral and periorbital regions. The peel is applied up to the hairline, neckline, and right below the mandibular border. One coat of TCA is sufficient. Avoid over coating with TCA. For a complete frost, the solution is left on the skin for 5 minutes.

Jessner's peel leads to a burning pain for the first 1–3 minutes which can be reduced by a fan or cool-pack. Within 24 hours, exfoliation with edema, redness, blistering, and crusting will be observed. To reduce the swelling a dose of 20 mg triamcinolon intramuscularly may be used. The healing takes generally 7–10 days.[2-4]

Blue Peel

Blue Peel is also used as a medium-depth peel, containing 20–30% TCA and a color sensitive reaction, allowing to estimate the depth of the peel. For a medium-depth peel to the papillary dermis the TCA solution is applied until the appearance of an organized white layer with a pink background. For a deep peel, the pink background successively diminishes and the layer will appear white.[1,4]

Pyruvic Acid

Pyruvic acid normally at 40–60% concentration is used to treat moderate acne, photoaging and melasma. It is physiologically converted from an α-ketoacid to lactic acid. A pretreatment with topical retinoids is important. It penetrates to the papillary dermis and increases the production of collagen and elastic tissue. An adequate frosting will be observed after approximately 2–5 minutes. The face is then soaked with water. Some authors recommend a neutralization with 10% sodium bicarbonate and water. It takes 1–2 weeks for the re-epithelialization. The erythema may stay for 2 months. For the treatment of warts and actinic keratoses pyruvic acid is used in combination with 5-fluorouracil.[5]

POSTPEEL CARE

Minimizing complications and ensuring an early recovery is the aim of good postoperative care. This is even more important in dark skinned patients who are more susceptible to pigmentary alterations. A reliable and careful maintenance care including sunscreens and moisturizers is crucial to secure the result of chemical peeling in most patients.[1,4,5]

For the postpeel period, clear instructions must be given to the patient. For the first 2 days the skin appears light pink. Then the skin darkens on day 3 and day 4. Afterwards the skin starts peeling off in sheets by day 5. Although, the erythema may last till day 14, the peeling should be complete by day 10.[4,5]

In medium-depth peels erythema, edema, and desquamation occur for 5-10 days. Nonsoap or mild soap cleansers may be used. To prevent bacterial infection a topical antibacterial ointment should be used in case of crusting. To soothe the skin cold compresses may be used. Patient needs to be told to strictly wear broad-spectrum sunscreens and only bald moisturizers until the completion of peeling. The patients should strictly avoid peeling or scratching the skin, because of an increased risk of scarring. In case of burning sensation analgesics can be used.[1,2,13]

For patients treated only with TCA the healing time is between 5-7 days. Patients with combined peels of TCA and either glycolic acid or Jessner's solution need 7-10 days healing time.[5]

In case of open wounds at the peeled skin, cool compresses of water with some drops of white vinegar can be used to treat the burning sensations. Appropriate oral analgesia is necessary. To reduce the risk of postinflammatory hyperpigmentation and persistent redness, sun and heat exposure should be strictly avoided. Exercise may also lead to an increased body heat and enhance the risk of redness on the face. It's allowed to use mineral sunscreen powder. A postpeel care with clear zinc oxide sunscreen, gentle cleansers, and barrier repair cream is recommended.[4]

COMPLICATIONS

Detecting patients at risk and using lighter peels is important to prevent complications. Especially patients with a history of postinflammatory hyperpigmentation, delayed wound healing and keloids, sensitive skin that doesn't tolerate the postpeel regimes, particularly sunscreen and hydroquinone, patients with a high sun exposure, e.g., construction worker and incompliant patients, are at a high risk for complications.[1]

For optimal and satisfactory cosmetic results an adequate patient selection, proper counseling, a solid priming of the skin, supportive medical therapy, as well as appropriate intraoperative and postoperative care is essential.[1]

Be very careful using medium-depth peels on the mandible, neck, and chest, as the risk of scarring is greatest in these areas.[5]

Complications do affect all skin types and can be classified as major and minor complications (Box 1).

Postinflammatory Hyperpigmentation or Hypopigmentation

Aggressive treatment should be neglected. Darker skin types are mostly affected. Postinflammatory hyperpigmentations occur

---

BOX 1 Complications

- Pigmentary disturbances
- Infection
- Scarring
- Allergic reactions
- Milia
- Acneiform eruptions
- Lines of dermacation
- Textural changes
- Persistent erythema
- Toxicity

when the pink inflammatory stage starts to pale out. It is often persistent and difficult to treat. An early treatment with class V or VI steroid creams can reverse early signs of postinflammatory hyperpigmentation. In general postinflammatory hyperpigmentation is treated with retinoids, hydroquinones, steroids, antioxidants or azelaic acid in combination or alone. Light peels are also effective. The use of hydroquinones by itself or in combination with glycolic or retinol cream is recommended in aggravated hyperpigmentation. Aggressive treatments such as treatment with tretinoin or laser treatments are not recommended as it can cause more postinflammatory hyperpigmentation.[1,4]

Infections

Infections are mostly caused by virus (*Herpes simplex*), bacteria (*Staphylococcus, Streptococcus* or *Pseudomonas*) or mycoses (*Candida*). The risk of scarring and infections is more common in medium and deep peels. To avoid scarring the patients should be immediately treated with topical or oral antiviral, antibiotics or antifungal agents. A prophylactic therapy with acyclovir or valacyclovir is indicated in patients with recurrent herpes simplex infections starting 2 days before the procedure until 7–10 days or until complete re-epithelialization is accomplished.[1,4]

Scarring

Scarring is the worst complication. Scarring is classified as hypertrophic, atrophic, and keloidal scarring. Especially, patients with a history of keloids or poor wound healing, who develop infections during peeling, who undergo surgery without waiting for appropriate skin healing, patients with a too short interval between the second peel and the first peel, patients with medium-depth and deep peels, or patients who have been treated particularly in the last 12 months with isotretinoin, are at a high risk of scarring. The risk of scarring can be minimized through priming the skin, the proper choice of peeling agent and a consistent postpeel care.[1,2,4]

Persistent redness and a delayed wound healing are first signs of potential scarring. A solid prepeel treatment is very important to reduce the risk of scarring.[4]

Besides, more rare complications like ectropion, allergic reactions, milia, acneiform eruptions, lines of demarcation, textural changes, toxicity (e.g., in resorcinol, salicylic acid, and phenol), and persistent erythema may occur. Persistent erythema is defined by an erythema for 3 weeks after the peel and can be an early sign of potential scarring. It should be immediately treated with potent topical corticosteroids for approximately 2 weeks, to prevent scarring.[1,2]

PRACTICAL TIPS

- To increase a peel more coats are applied
- More the pressure used to apply the peel with the wooden handles Q-tip, deeper is the penetration of the peeling[3]
- The peel will be much stronger than expected if the skin is dry, has an abrasion or is retinized
- The frost will appear more slowly in less porous or leathery skin, e.g., along the mandible
- Be very careful using medium-depth peels on the mandible, neck, and chest, as the risk of scarring is increased in these areas[5]
- Multiple applied coats of Jessner's solution on dry, retinized skin can cause a medium-depth injury by reaching the upper reticular dermis
- To avoid accidental spillage, the soaked applicator should never be passed over

the patients face. Patients have to close their eyes, the whole time during chemical peeling. A syringe filled with saline or water should always kept ready for irrigation of the eyes in case of accidental spillage
- Detecting patients at risk and using lighter peels is important to prevent complications
- The face-neck skin color will be not as discordant as in a deep peel, still a strict avoidance of the sun and chronic use of skin lighteners on the neck is necessary
- To avoid complications, aggressive treatment should be neglected.[1]

CONCLUSION

Middle depth chemical peelings are good option of treatment for a variety of skin conditions or skin problems. Prior to the chemical peeling priming of the skin is crucial to receive the best possible and safest results. The risk of side effects is higher in darker skin types and not all sorts of chemical peelings should be performed in darker skin types. The knowledge of how to treat complications is very important for those performing chemical peelings. Through combinations of different peeling ingredients or different procedures stronger results can be achieved.

TAKE HOME POINTS

- A reliable and strict prepeel and postpeel care including adequate sunscreen is essential for a satisfying cosmetic result
- Priming the skin is necessary for at least 2-4 weeks prior to the peeling
- The peel is first applied to the lateral regions, then carefully centrofacially, and lastly to the perioral and periorbital regions
- To avoid accidental spillage, the soaked applicator should never be passed over the patients face. A syringe filled with saline or water should always kept ready for irrigation of the eyes in case of accidental spillage
- Avoid over coating, as it may result in a higher risk of complications
- In pigmentary disturbances and dark skinned patients aggressive treatment should be neglected.

REFERENCES

1. Khunger N. Standard guidelines of care for chemical peels. Indian J Dermatol Venereol Leprol. 2008;74:5-12.
2. Drake LA, Dinehart SM, Goltz RW, et al. Guidelines of care for chemical peeling. Guidelines/Outcomes Committee: American Academy of Dermatology. J Am Acad Dermatol. 1995;33(3):497-503.
3. Schürer NY, Wiest LG. Picture Atlas Scrub Basics I Practice I Indications I. Germany: KVM - The medical publisher; 2011.
4. Rullan PP. Karam AM. Chemical peels for the aging faces of all skin types. International Peeling Society; 2017 [cited 2017 Nov 27]. Available from: http://www.peelingsociety.com/fileadmin/user_upload/Press/Member_Area/Chemical_peels_for_the_aging_faces_of_all_skin_types.pdf
5. Baumann L. Cosmetic Dermatology: Principles and Practice. Second Edition. United States: McGraw-Hill Education/Medical; 2009.
6. Wiest LG, Habig J. Chemical peel treatments in dermatology. Hautarzt. 2015;66(10):744-7.
7. Rullan P, Karam AM. Chemical peels for darker skin types. Facial Plastic Surgery Clinics. 2010;18(1):111-31.
8. Sarkar R, Bansal S, Garg VK. Chemical peels for melasma in dark-skinned patients. J Cutan Aesthet Surg. 2012;5(4):247-53.
9. Schurer NY, Wiest L. Chemical peels. Hautarzt. 2006;57(1):61-77.
10. Reserva J, Champlain A, Soon SL, et al. Chemical peels: Indications and special considerations for the male patient. Dermatol Surg. 2017;43 Suppl 2:163-73.
11. Coleman WP 3rd, Futrell JM. The glycolic acid trichloroacetic acid peel. J Dermatol Surg Oncol. 1994;20(1):76-80.
12. Monheit GD. The Jessner's + TCA peel: A medium-depth chemical peel. J Dermatol Surg Oncol. 1989;15(9):945-50.
13. Committee for Guidelines of Care for Chemical Peeling. Guidelines for chemical peeling in Japan (3rd edition). J Dermatol. 2012;39(4):321-5.
14. Al-Waiz MM, Al-Sharqi AI. Medium-depth chemical peels in the treatment of acne scars in dark-skinned individuals. Dermatol Surg. 2002;28(5):383-7.

20
CHAPTER

Deep Peels: A Review of Chemical Peels for All Skin Types

Peter P Rullan

INTRODUCTION

This chapter will focus on deep chemical peels for all skin color types, including darker skin color types. It is commonly accepted in cosmetic dermatology that deep peels are not typically performed in Fitzpatrick skin types IV–VI. The author's opinion, however, is that these can be done successfully by experienced physicians who have been trained in peels. They are especially effective for the treatment of challenging acne scars in all skin color types and, as in the case of lighter skin types, for skin laxity and deep wrinkles. Physicians who perform both ablative laser peels as well as croton oil–phenol peels, all feel that the later is the "gold standard" for resurfacing.[1,2] The depth of a peel must be adjusted to the depth of the pathological process to be treated, so in cases of Glogau level III–IV photoaging, or deep ice-pick scars, where the pathology extends into the mid-reticular dermis, deep peels are required. The new lower croton oil formulas have allowed deep peels without the alabaster hypopigmentation that characterized the Baker-Gordon phenol peels.[1,2]

The new global "melting pot" of mixed cultures and races has resulted in African Americans, Asians, Middle Easterners and Latinos with skin types III and IV; whites with skin type IV; and European Hispanics with skin types I–III. When evaluating a patient for a skin resurfacing procedure, information on family lineage will assist the clinician in estimating a patient's response to treatment, for example a tendency to get postinflammatory hyperpigmentation (PIH) from skin burns, as well as creating an appropriate pre and postpeel regimen to manage variables such as inflammation, infection and sebum.

PRECONDITIONING AND CLINICAL EVALUATION

All patients require a full personal, family and medical history. Special consideration should be given to history of cutaneous malignancy, history of acne scarring or PIH and herpes simplex outbreaks. The timing of superficial peels following the use of isotretinoin was previously believed to be an issue, but has been recently shown to be a manageable risk.[3] Performing a deep chemical peel on a patient on isotretinoin or within 6 months of discontinuation of isotretinoin is still contraindicated, and requires that normal pilosebaceous activity of the skin has been regained in the area of the peel.

Chemical Peels: A Global Perspective

TABLE 1: Peel selection

Indication	Chemical peel	Comments
PIH, Melasma	• SA 20–30% (series of 3–6 peels)	• Low cost, safe, good for acne-prone patients, somewhat effective
	• GA buffered (series of 3–6 peels)	• Low cost, safe, good for dry skin types, somewhat effective
Ice-pick acne scars	• CROSS with 30–100% TCA or 88% Carbolic, plus a full-face superficial-medium peel or microneedling	• Good for localized scars, little downtime; always consider subcision with either 18G Nokor or Cannula
Box acne scars	• CROSS with 88% Carbolic acid plus superficial-medium peel	• Good for more severe scars, little downtime
	• Full-face 2-day 0.35% croton oil/phenol chemabrasion	• Good for more severe scars, 10–14 days of downtime, must avoid sun exposure for 1 month
Photoaging	• Jessner or Jessner + 15% TCA	• For mild cases
	• Dry ice CO_2 plus 20–35% TCA, or Jessner + 20–30% TCA	• For moderate cases
	• Hetter peels or 2-day taped 0.35–0.7% croton oil/phenol chemabrasion	• For moderate to severe cases, 2 weeks of downtime, must avoid sun exposure for 1 month

PIH, postinflammatory hyperpigmentation; TCA, trichloroacetic acid; GA, glycolic acid; SA, salicylic acid; CROSS, chemical reconstruction of skin scars.

Patients preparing to have a phenol-based peel require a full laboratory work-up, including hepatic, renal and cardiac testing. During the initial evaluation, the clinician should assess elements that can help predict healing, such as the presence of a suntan, the level of exercise (or other temperature-increasing activities), use of makeup, tendency to heal with PIH, parents' skin colors and available downtime. Guidance for peel selection is shown in table 1.

Preconditioning the Skin

To reduce the risk of PIH and to improve the efficacy of the peel outcome, preparation of the skin for chemical peels requires preconditioning of the skin for 2–12 weeks (Table 2).[4,5] Topical agents are used to reduce seborrhea and thin the epidermis. These agents allow rapid penetration of the peel, accelerate re-epithelialization and wound healing, and decrease the risk of PIH due to the bleaching effect that results from dispersion of melanin granules. Prevention of bacterial infections and herpes simplex flares during healing requires antibacterial and antiviral prophylaxis. The status of the skin on the day of the peel is critical. If the skin is dry, has an abrasion, or is retinized, the peel will be much stronger than expected, which can be an advantage (in patients with thick, sebaceous or scarred skin) or detrimental (in patients with melasma or PIH, especially over thin skin).

The use of tretinoin, hydroquinone (HQ) or a glycolic-hydroquinone cream is recommended 4–12 weeks before the peel. Treating active acne before the peel leads to better cosmetic results and may require the use of retinoid creams, acne surgery and isotretinoin pills. The peel should be delayed until isotretinoin has been discontinued for 6 months or until the skin has regained its normal sebaceous activity and healing capacity.

Deep Peels: A Review of Chemical Peels for All Skin Types

TABLE 2: Preconditioning treatments

Indication	Drug and dose
Antiviral	Famciclovir (500 mg twice daily), valacyclovir (500 mg twice daily), or acyclovir (400 mg twice daily) for 7–10 days starting 1–2 days before peel
Prevention of PIH and enhanced peel quality	Retinoid creams applied for up to 12 weeks for medium-depth peels, to be restarted after skin peeling and irritation subsides; discontinue 1–2 days before peel if photodamage is evident and 1–2 weeks before peel if treating melasma or PIH
Retinoid sensitivity	Glycolic creams can be used with 2–8% HQ at bedtime
Preexisting PIH	Fluocinolone cream (0.01–0.025%) twice daily for 2–12 weeks
PIH, acne scars	Tazarotene cream (0.05%) at bedtime
Ultraviolet radiation protection	Physical sunblocks, e.g., zinc or titanium oxide creams, ColoreScience™ or mineral makeup, visors

PIH, postinflammatory hyperpigmentation; HQ, hydroquinone.

TYPES OF CHEMICAL PEELS AND FORMULAS

Deep peels penetrate to the upper and mid-reticular dermis (400–600 mm). Skin thickness, how oily is the skin and how well it is degreased, the pH of the selected peel, the concentration of the active ingredients [trichloroacetic acid (TCA), phenol, croton oil], the quantity applied, the number of coats and how aggressive it is applied, can all affect the depth of the peel.

Jessner's or Dry Ice Plus Trichloroacetic Acid Peel[6]

Jessner's peel is a keratolytic, which combines salicylic acid (SA) (14 g), resorcinol (14 g) and lactic acid 85% (14 g) mixed in ethanol for a final volume of 100 mL. Lactic acid is an alpha-hydroxy acid (AHA) that causes epidermolysis. Resorcinol is structurally similar to phenol, and disrupts the weak hydrogen bonds of keratin.

Trichloroacetic acid is a protein denaturant that precipitates epidermal proteins, causing sloughing, necrosis and dermal inflammation. These processes appear as white frosting (coagulation of epidermal keratinocyte proteins) on the skin surface. This versatile peel can be used to achieve superficial, medium or deep peels, depending on the skin conditioning, the strength of the acid and the number of coats applied. The recommended strength of TCA is 20% for neck and superficial face peels, and 35% for medium-to-deep peels when augmented with Jessner's, glycolic or solid CO_2 (dry ice) (see later). TCA (available from Delasco™) is formulated commercially or in the clinic as a weight-volume preparation from 10–100%.

Multiple studies in the past 40 years have shown that TCA can be safely used in nonwhite dark skin types. Safe use of TCA requires longer preconditioning of the skin, use of the lowest effective strength of TCA, and strategies for dealing with potential cases of PIH.[7,8] A study of Korean patients by Lee et al. showed that applying TCA (the author prefers 88% carbolic) in a smaller area, for example inside an ice-pick scar [using CROSS (chemical reconstruction of skin scars)], significantly reduces the risk of PIH and facilitates correction of PIH.[9]

To achieve a medium-to-deep peel, Jessner's is applied as multiple coats until the skin is lightly and evenly frosted, followed by multiple coats of 35% TCA. The goal is to produce an organized white sheet without a pink background. When the peel reaches the deepest safest level, (the immediate reticular dermis) the pink background gradually diminishes because of the coagulation of blood vessels, and the sheet appears pure white.[10]

Sedation and analgesia are usually necessary with TCA peels that are not performed with solid CO_2. Sedatives (oral diazepam), beta-blockers (oral clonidine) and nerve blocks or ketorolac administered intramuscularly (IM), are used routinely in my practice. Immediate postoperative procedures and medications can be used to reduce burning, such as an ice-water compress, 10% sodium bicarbonate rinse, cold aloe vera lotion, a Zimmer cooler or topical lidocaine ointment.

Performing a mixed peel, where the upper face is peeled with a medium to deep TCA peel, and the perioral region is peeled with a taped croton oil–phenol peel, allows the physician to use only oral sedation or analgesia, and nerve blocks for the mouth region. This is particularly useful when the perioral wrinkles are deep and the upper face is only photodamaged and without much laxity (Fig. 1). The upper and lower eyelids can be peeled with the Hetter VL formula.

Solid CO_2 and Trichloroacetic Acid Technique (Fig. 2)

Dr Harold Brody[10] has elegantly described the use of solid CO_2 (dry ice) and 35% TCA to achieve a medium-to-deep peel.[11] Solid CO_2 is less destructive than liquid nitrogen, and the margin of safety of solid CO_2 is well accepted in dermatology. Dr Brody wraps the solid CO_2 in a small hand towel and dips it in a solution of ~3:1 acetone:alcohol, which facilitates application and kills surface bacteria. An individual lesion or the entire

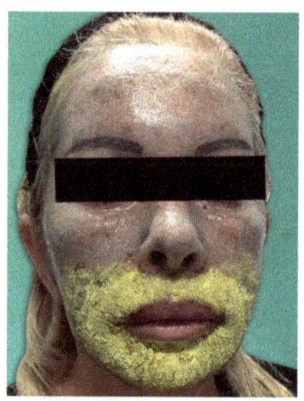

FIG. 1: Combination Jessner's plus 35% trichloroacetic acid to upper face, and Hetter 0.35%, taped, for perioral region, with bismuth subgallate powder postoperative. Only oral sedation and nerve block needed.

face may be easily slushed by using slow and even strokes. The epidermal depth is affected by the pressure of application, so a heavier application technique creates a deeper peel. The skin reaction ranges from mild erythema to vesiculo-bullae formation. Next, the skin is lightly wiped with dry gauze, and 35% TCA is applied with either two cotton-tipped applicators (for a lighter application) or with a 4" × 4" gauze pad (for a heavier application). A cotton-tipped applicator can be used to apply 35% TCA under the eyes, and a 4" × 4" gauze pad can be applied to the remainder of the face.

Croton Oil–Phenol Peels

Phenol formulas typically consist of 88% phenol (carbolic acid), croton oil, hexachlorophene, olive oil or distilled water (Table 3). Phenol disrupts sulfide bonds, which causes keratolysis and protein coagulation. Phenol is also melanotoxic. Hexachlorophene is an antiseptic with surfactant properties, which allows a uniform and deep penetration by decreasing surface tension. Croton oil is now considered the most important ingredient in

Deep Peels: A Review of Chemical Peels for All Skin Types

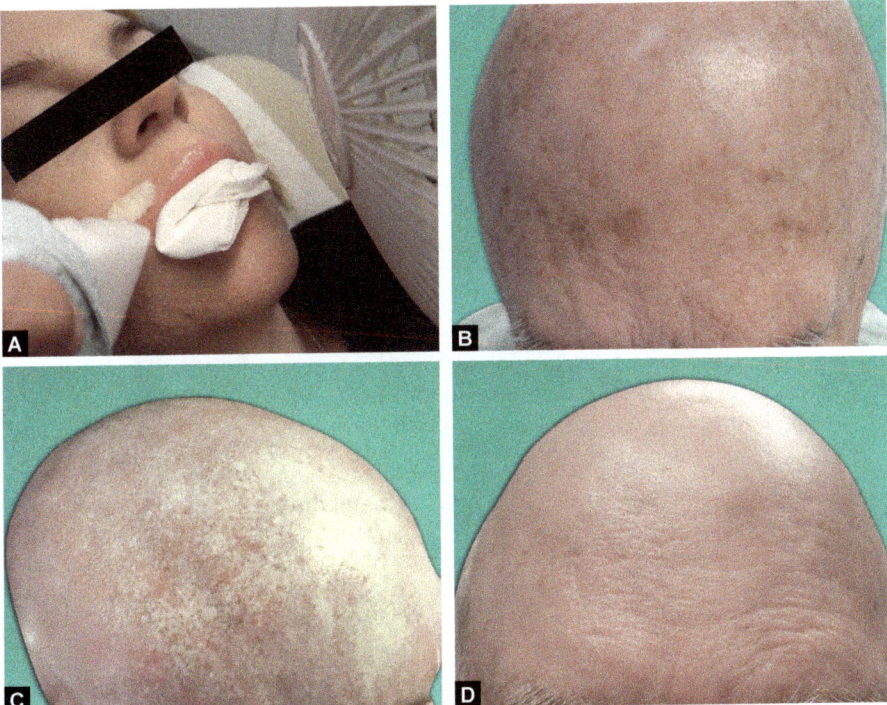

FIG. 2: **A,** Dr Brody applying dry ice before applying 35% trichloroacetic acid, achieving both increased penetration and anesthesia; **B,** Patient with photodamage, before Dr Brody's dry ice and trichloroacetic acid peel; **C,** Intense frost after rubbing dry ice and then applying 35% trichloroacetic acid; **D,** After photograph showing excellent correction.

TABLE 3: Hetter's Heresy croton oil–phenol peel formulas

Peel	Formula
Medium light peel 0.35% croton oil	• 6 cc water • 4 cc phenol 88% • 16 drops Septisol • 1 drop croton oil
Medium peel 0.7% croton oil	Add 1 drop croton oil to medium light peel formula
Medium heavy peel 1.1% croton oil	Add 1 drop croton oil to 0.7% croton oil in medium light peel formula
Very light peel 0.1% croton oil and 30% phenol	• 3 cc medium light peel formula • 5 cc water • 2 cc phenol 88%
PIH, acne scars	Tazarotene cream (0.05%) at bedtime
Stone's grade II 0.2% croton oil and 44% phenol	Includes glycerin, olive oil and water

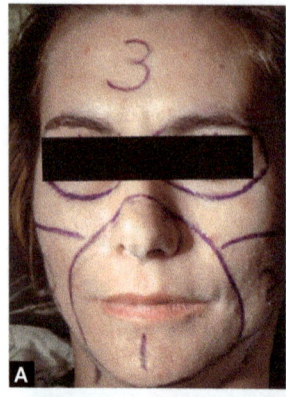
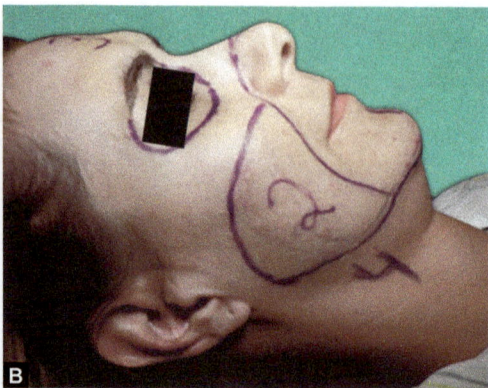
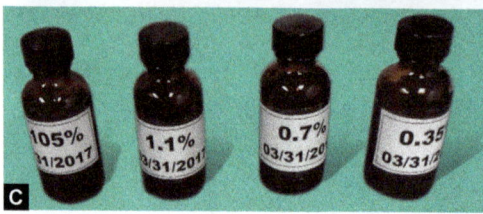

FIG. 3: **A,** Frontal view of regions; **B,** Hetter's regions, strongest percentage in region 1, mildest in region 4. Technique used for only one day and does not tape for occlusion; **C,** Hetter 1.1% (region 1), 0.7% (region 2), 0.35% (region 3), 0.105 (region 4).

phenol formulas.[12-15] Croton oil is a vesicant (and therefore epidermolytic) that greatly enhances the absorption of phenol. In some formulas, olive oil is added to slow the cutaneous absorption rate of these agents to reduce potential systemic toxicity.

Croton oil–phenol peels are useful for correcting skin laxity, deep wrinkles and acne scars. If, however, facial wrinkling is accompanied by significant laxity or volume deficiency, dermal or periosteal fillers with cosmetic surgery (lower and upper rhytidectomy) may also be necessary to achieve optimal results. The patient must have family or nursing support for the first 3 days. A selling point of this "only once-in-a-lifetime" procedure is the peel's well-documented life-long rejuvenation of the skin.

Commonly used phenol formulas include Hetter's Heresy formulas, which have 33% phenol, and croton oil concentration that range from 1.1% (perioral and tip of nose), 0.7% (for mid-cheeks), 0.35% (forehead, temples, upper cheeks) and 0.1% (also known as very light), used for eyelids and neck. One drop of croton oil is added to the phenol to prepare the 0.35% formula, two drops for the 0.7% formula and 3 drops for the 1.1% (Table 3 and Fig. 3). Dr Phil Stone has used "lay peeler's formulas," and suggested that application technique, phenol concentration and croton oil are also important variables to achieve an optimal peel, and has noted these peels are safe for use in patients with darker skin color.[16,17] Dr Yoram Finsti and Dr Marina Landau popularized the Exoderm formula and technique.[18,19] Finally, Baker–Gordon's formula (2.1% croton oil, phenol 50%) has been largely replaced by Hetter's and Stone's formulas.

Phenol peels have the potential for cardio-toxicity and renal toxicity. The preoperative procedure for this technique requires a full laboratory work-up, with hepatic, renal and cardiac tests [10-lead electrocardiography (EKG)], including a letter from their physician clearing them for the peel. Dr Carlos Wambier has reported that phenol may cause a corrected QT (QTc) prolongation, especially under some conditions such as use of certain medications (erythromycin, fluconazole, antimalarials, amiodarone, antidepressants, antipsychotics, terfenadine, hydrochlorothiazide and others) or electrolytic abnormalities (hypomagnesemia, hypokalemia).[20] According to Dr Wambier, when two or more of these conditions are present, the risk for QTc interval prolongation occurs (dangerous if above 480 ms), triggering a potentially fatal "Torsade de Pointes" ventricular arrhythmia during a phenol peel.

Patients should be hydrated during the peripeel period and monitored for cardiac arrhythmias. To avoid these cardiac side effects, the peels should be administered slowly in a subunit approach. Typically, peel administration should span 60 minutes (15 minutes per section).

Rullan's 2-day Croton Oil/Phenol Chemabrasion Technique

Anesthesia, Medications and Monitoring

Intravenous (IV) access is always required, as well as constant cardiac monitoring to comply with Advanced Cardiac Life Support (ACLS) guidelines for conscious sedation. Sedation can be accomplished with oral (diazepam, triazolam or hydromorphone), IM (ketorolac 30–60 mg) or IV agents (midazolam, fentanyl, propofol or ketamine). I routinely use midazolam and fentanyl in my practice. Dr Larry Kass has established a sedation strategy of 1 mg of alprazolam at 4 hours, 2 hours and 1 hour administered orally before the peel, and 10 mg of zolpidem upon arrival at the clinic.[21] This strategy provides real amnesia and sedation. Clonidine (0.1–0.2 mg) orally can also be used as a preoperative medication to reduce the likelihood of hypertension and tachycardia in addition to providing mild sedation.

The use of facial nerve blocks is effective at reducing the need for or quantity required of systemic medication. The use of epinephrine is avoided or minimized in these blocks to reduce the risk of tachycardia and arrhythmias. General anesthesia is not recommended because of respiratory and pH issues. The oxygen partial pressure (pO_2) must be more than 90% throughout the procedure, and sinus tachycardia must be brief and minimized. The patient is discharged home with diazepam, hydromorphone, triazolam and ondansetron for nausea. Acyclovir is started one day before the peel (400 mg TID × 10 days) but if antibiotics are prescribed, they should not be used until the third day to avoid nausea access should be maintained overnight and the nurse or family member must be trained in assisting with oral medications.

Day 1 (Figs. 4A and B)

Ringer lactate (1–2 L) is infused for 2 hours. The face is thoroughly cleansed and degreased as described previously. IV sedation is given. Nerve blocks are performed just prior to peeling of each anatomic area. For a full-face peel, Stone's Gradé II with 0.2% croton oil and 44% phenol, with glycerin and olive oil formula; Hetter's "all around-stock" formula of 0.35% croton oil and 33% phenol can be used; or Dr Rullan's modification of the Gradé II formula (with 0.35% croton oil). These are slowly applied with regular Q-tips, which are rolled against the edge of the stainless-steel cup to remove excess fluid. The formula is applied to five anatomic areas (forehead, two cheeks, perioral and chin, and periorbital and nose), spending 10–15 minutes per area; application of the peel takes approximately 60 minutes. Ice-pick scars receive an additional peel application with a fine paintbrush to ensure complete wetting of the lesion. A complete, organized frost must be achieved

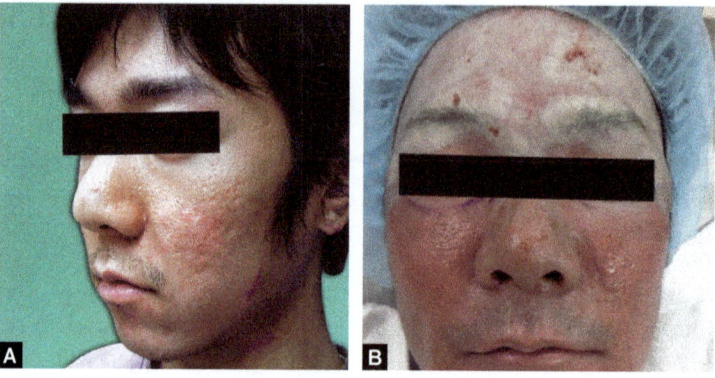

FIG. 4: A, Asian male skin type IV, with acne scars (ice-pick, box, rolling and hypertrophic); **B,** Full face 0.35% croton oil and 44% phenol, doing second region (forehead) after doing perioral and nose.

in each area, and a yellowish edematous appearance (indicating epidermolysis) should be noted after 15–30 minutes. The face is completely taped (except the upper lids) with 1-inch to 2-inch strips of waterproof Hy-Tape (Hy-Tape International, Patterson, New York, the United States of America) and covered with a surgical face net. Patients can only drink fluids that can be squeezed into the mouth through a long-tipped bottle for the next 7–8 days.

For regional acne scars, I suggest applying these phenol formulas only into ice-pick and box scars (CROSS technique), using a toothpick with TCA (or with fine brush if 88% carbolic) to deliver the solution directly into the scars. The rest of the face can then be peeled with a lighter acid, microneedeling or with fractional CO_2 ablative resurfacing. Subcision can also be performed at this visit.

Day 2 (Figs. 4C and D)

The patient is usually groggy but pain-free when returning to the clinic. The Hy-Tape is easily removed. Additional sedation and analgesia are sometimes given if the condition is severe and aggressive abrasion is expected. The necrotic coagulum is debrided using a tongue blade or a large 6 mm Fox curette. Ice-pick scars and box scars or deep wrinkles are debrided using 1–2 mm chalazion-type curettes to achieve punctate bleeding inside the scars to ensure de-epithelialization of these types of lesions. The goal is to create a true open wound within the lesions to induce secondary healing and wound closure. An antiseptic, anti-inflammatory powder, bismuth subgallate (Delasco or Spectrum Pharmaceuticals, Irvine, California, the United States of America) is applied to the entire face except the upper lid and the patient is discharged home. The mask dries out and stays in place for the next 7–8 days. I call it the protective "green mask cocoon."

Days 3 to 8 (Fig. 4E)

The patient is restricted to home and is not allowed to shower until the mask is removed. On approximately the eighth day, the mask separates because of skin re-epithelialization. Vaseline is then applied over the entire mask, allowed to soak in and left on overnight. The mask is gently removed the next morning by applying more Vaseline while showering, under the slowly separating mask. Medical barrier creams (Epionce™) or Aquaphor™

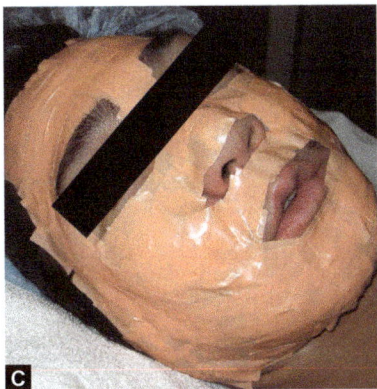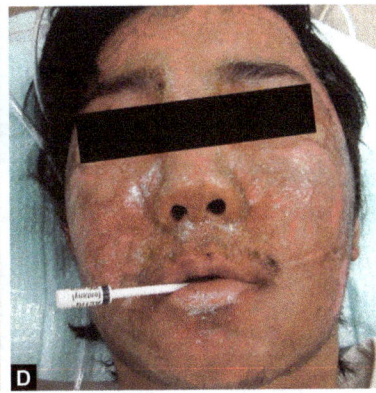

FIG. 4: **C,** Hy-Tape waterproof occlusive dressing, secured with surgical net, for 24 hours (do not tape eyelids); **D,** Immediately after removing tape, showing liquefied epidermis (coagulum), where even gentle debridement creates punctate bleeding. Entire face is debrided to reduce risk of infection and inflammation.

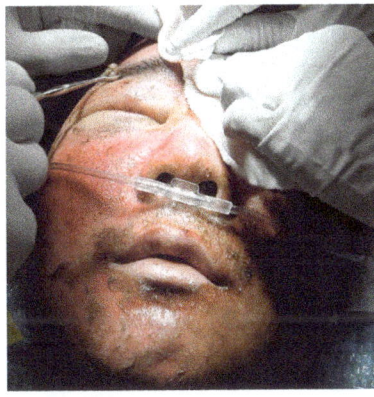

FIG. 4E: Debridement using tongue depressor and curettes of different diameters.

ointment (Eucerin, Beiersdorf AG, Hamburg, Germany) are used until the skin is no longer tender or red. Most patients are 99% re-epithelialized by day 9. There has been no occurrence of infections following this procedure in my clinic. Using white vinegar compresses as described can be very soothing and reduces the risk of infection.

Days 8–30 and beyond (Figs. 4F to H)

The skin is fragile and sensitive, and in general using gentle cleansers and light noncomedogenic and hypoallergenic creams and lotions is recommended. For patients with oily skin with active acne, a short course of isotretinoin 10–20 mg a day for 2–4 weeks may help prevent acneiform eruptions, milia and PIH, especially in darker skin types. Other sebolytic measures, including spironolactone and acne medications, are also effective. Sun and heat avoidance is required for 30 days, but many patients return to their normal lifestyle by slowly increasing their activity in measure with how red their skin gets when hot. Camouflage makeup that can be easily removed is recommended. The least understood and feared wound healing phenomenon after a deep peel in a darker skin type (Fig. 5) is the gradual return of normal skin color.

Touch-ups

Two to three months after the peel has healed, a regional or lesional (CROSS) peel can be repeated for persistent acne scars or perioral wrinkles, even in skin types IV-VI. These lighter skin types can tolerate a regional peel. The intent is to create an open wound inside the ice-pick scars or wrinkles, adding new collagen so they eventually fill in almost completely.

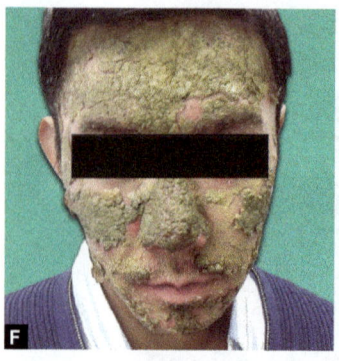
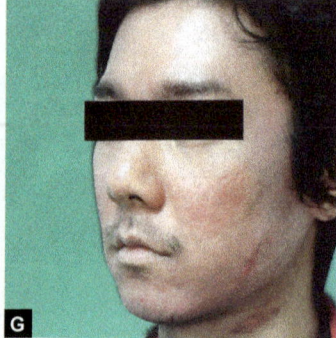
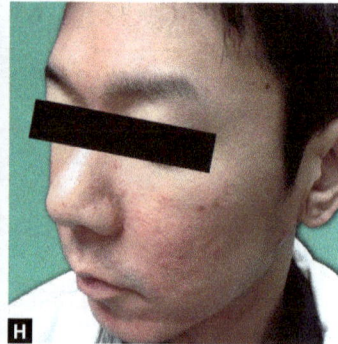

FIG. 4: F, Day 8 of peel, showing powder mask almost completely removed, and skin being almost 100% re-epithelialized; **G,** Day 10 of peel, with fully healed skin. Hypertrophic scars were injected with triamcinolone and 5 fluorouracil; **H,** 3 years after peel, showing normal skin color and no contrast with neck color.

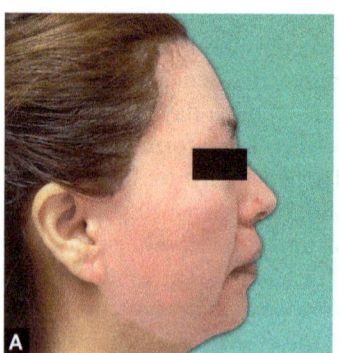
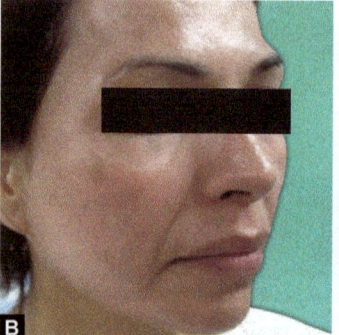
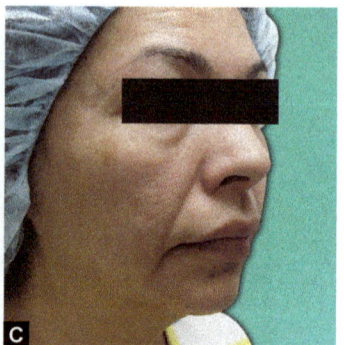

FIG. 5: A, Latina woman with acne scars, skin type IV–V, 10 days after full-face 2-day 0.35% taped croton oil–phenol chemabrasion, showing dramatic color contrast between neck and face; **B,** 30 days postoperatively, showing early return of skin color; **C,** 2 months after peel, showing normal return of skin color. Skin may appear slightly lighter because it is not sun damaged.

APPROACHES TO COMMON CLINICAL INDICATIONS

Acne Scars

Acne scars are categorized as ice-pick, box scar, rolling scar, atrophic or hypertrophic types.[22] In all skin colors, improvement of acne scars is best accomplished by learning to identify the different types and combining treatments best suited for those types. For severe and widespread acne scars for all skin types, I use the 2-day 0.35% croton oil and 44% phenol chemabrasion technique (Figs. 6 and 7). For localized ice-pick scars, this is best achieved with either punch-excisions or with CROSS using a pointed toothpick or very fine paintbrush to apply the acid only within the scarred pore, sometimes abrading the internal edges with the toothpick.[9,23] Shallower lesions such as box scars respond to either ablative lasers or to medium-to-deep peels. I use 30% TCA for patients with thin skin or on isotretinoin; 60% TCA for medium thickness or darker skin; and 95–100% TCA for those with thick sebaceous lighter skin. I prefer using 0.2% croton oil and 60% phenol

Deep Peels: A Review of Chemical Peels for All Skin Types

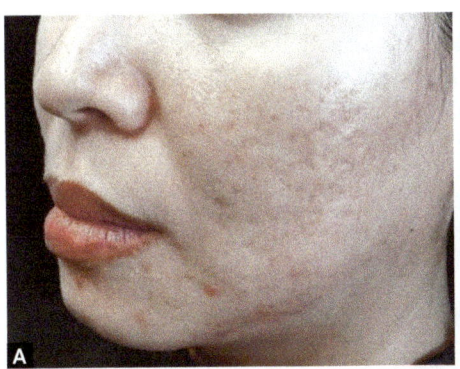
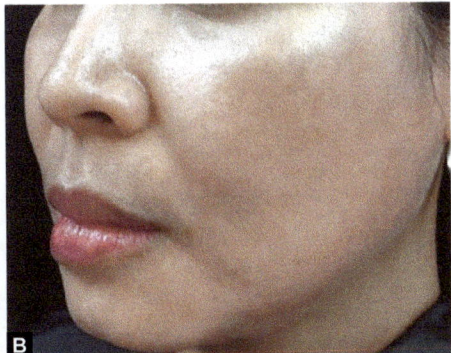
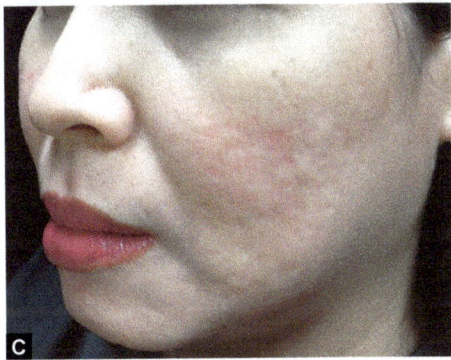

FIG. 6: **A,** Filipino woman with acne scars, skin type IV; had previously undergone CO_2 laser ablation; **B,** 1 month post peel with 2-day taped 0.35% croton oil–44% phenol chemabrasion. Received 2 weeks of 20 mg a day of isotretinoin to reduce postinflammatory hyperpigmentation and acneiform eruption; **C,** One year after peel, with slightly lighter but normal skin color. Would benefit from filler injections into atrophic acne scars as will most acne scar patients. These scars are now distensible and responsive to fillers.

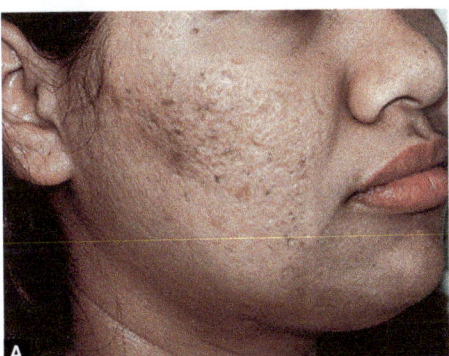
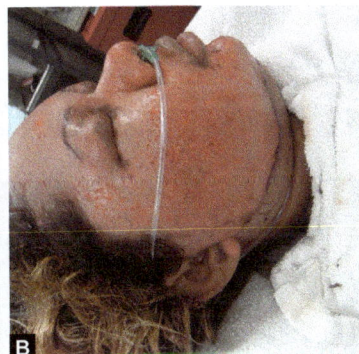
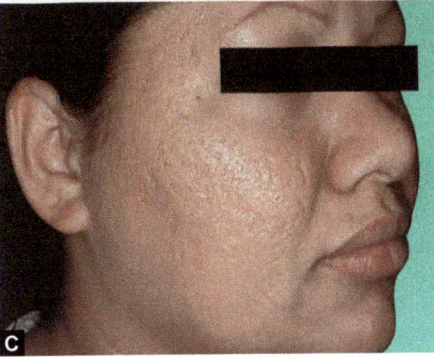

FIG. 7: **A,** Afro-Caribbean woman with skin type VI, with deep acne scars; **B,** Immediately after debridement on day 2 of 0.35% croton oil–44% phenol taped peel. We use large 6 mm curettes to debride full face, followed by 1–2 mm chalazion curette to debride inside ice-pick and box scars to de-epithelialize all the walls of scars. This allows for effective secondary healing and filling of scars; **C,** 2 years after peel, showing lighter but normal skin color, and no contrast with color of neck.

formula for CROSS when box scars are large (Fig. 8). Any resurfacing procedure can be done immediately afterwards depending on skin thickness and color, requiring caution over bony prominences, dark skin and thin skin. I use fractional erbium or microneedling for resurfacing over CROSS (Fig. 9). Rolling scars (with tethered adhesions) respond

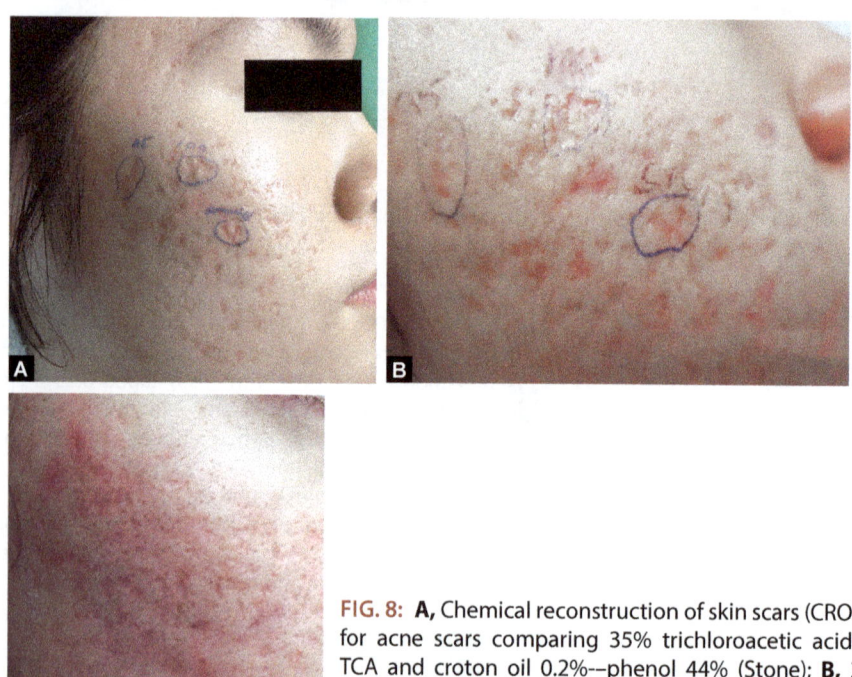

FIG. 8: **A,** Chemical reconstruction of skin scars (CROSS) technique for acne scars comparing 35% trichloroacetic acid (TCA), 100% TCA and croton oil 0.2%--phenol 44% (Stone); **B,** 30 days after, showing better blunting of sharp edges of scar treated with croton oil–phenol; **C,** Overall improvement following fullface croton oil–phenol 2-day chemabrasion.

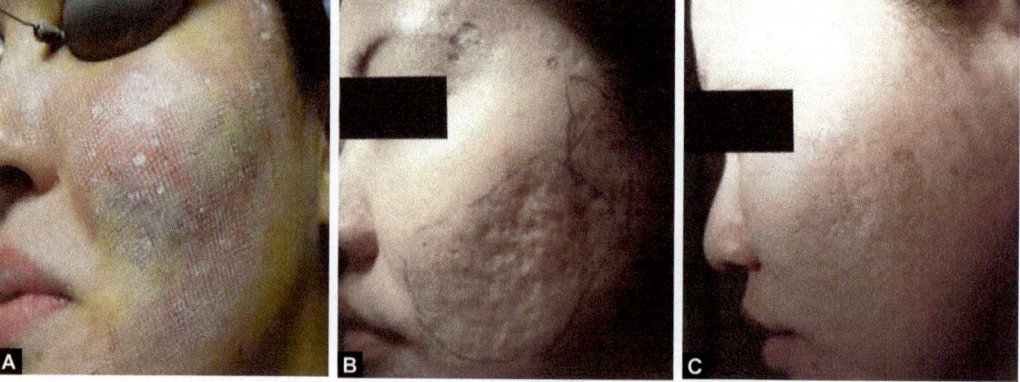

FIG. 9: **A,** Combination technique for acne scars in Asian skin, to reduce demarcation and postinflammatory hyperpigmentation, by first doing chemical reconstruction of skin scars (CROSS), then subcision, and then fractional erbium laser only to region with scars; **B,** Before combination, using shadow photography to more honestly evaluate results; **C,** One month after, with shadow photography, showing improvement yet maintaining normal skin color and no demarcation lines.

to a series of subcisions or microneedling. Atrophic scars best improve with dermal fillers. Hypertrophic scars require repeated intralesional steroids (sometimes with additional 5-fluorouracil or hyaluronidase) and pulsed-dye laser therapy.

Postinflammatory Hyperpigmentation

The treatment of PIH is more effective than that for melasma. As noted by Grimes, retinoids, hydroquinones (HQ 2-4%), topical steroids (class VI, e.g., fluocinolone 0.01%), azelaic acid and antioxidants (alone or in combinations) are used in the treatment of PIH.[24] When used for 2-6 weeks before and after a peel, these agents provide preventive and recuperative benefit. 30% SA (30%) peels (1-2 coats) can be repeated every 1-2 weeks and are useful for treating PIH. An almost complete response can be seen within 2-3 months (see section on complications).

Photoaging

Glogau's stage 4 (wrinkles at rest) requires medium-to-deep peels, and the clinician is advised to attend live workshops to develop an expertise in the peels. Most chemical peel experts agree that the croton oil–phenol peel, especially if taped for 24 hours, provides the most dramatic improvement for deep wrinkles in the perioral region. Well done Monheit or Brody TCA peels can be very effective in the rest of the face, but if you want to achieve periorbital tightening, the lighter Hetter peels, (with 0.1-0.35% croton oil) are more effective than TCA. I recommend the full-face croton oil–phenol peel rather than combinations with TCA because of the more even results in terms of skin color and texture (Figs. 10 and 11).

ALTERNATIVE POSTPEEL REGIMEN FOR DEEP PEELS

The 2-day Rullan peel's postoperative regimen has been discussed. The "open" croton oil–phenol peels (Fig. 12A) does not use bismuth subgallate powder, and prefers using a postoperative regimen that is very similar to that used for the medium-to-deep peels. These peels use dilute white

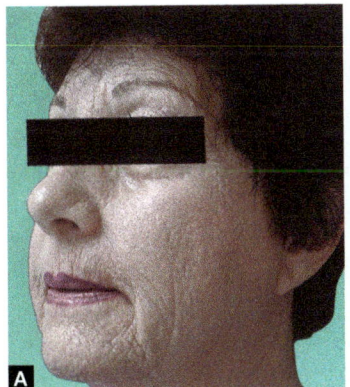
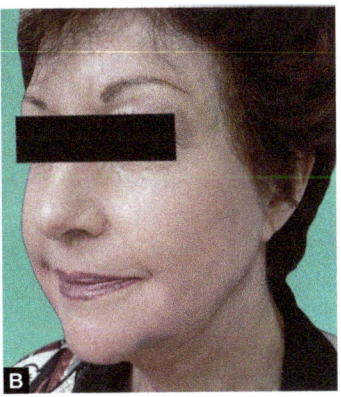

FIG. 10: A, 70-year-old woman with skin type II, with Glogau 4 photaging and deep perioral wrinkles; **B,** 6 months after 2-day taped 0.35% croton oil–phenol peel, with smoother skin and correction of challenging deep perioral wrinkle and marionette lines.

Chemical Peels: A Global Perspective

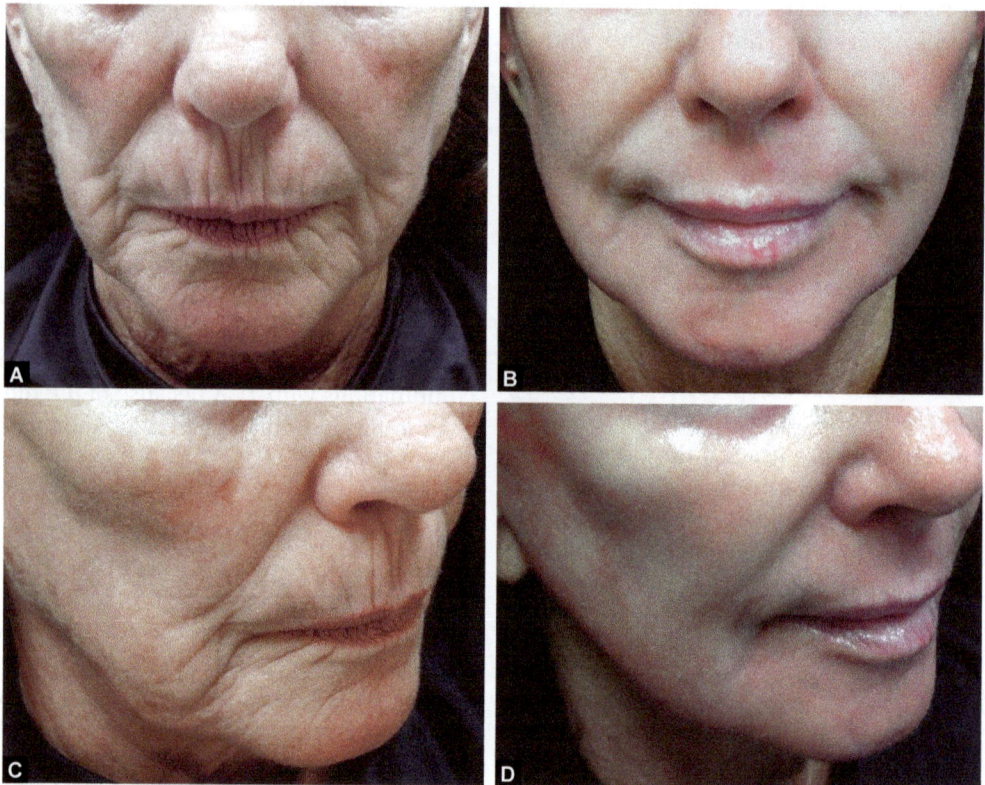

FIG. 11: A, 75-year-old woman with skin type II–III, with Glogau 4 photoaging, and deep perioral wrinkles; **B,** One month after taped 2-day 0.35% croton oil–phenol peel, with dramatic improvement of both texture and laxity. Patient did receive 0.5 cc of hyaluronic acid injection only into her vermillion one week before photo; **C,** Three-quarter angle photo of same patient, before; **D,** Before and after 1 month.

vinegar compresses (1 tablespoon in 1 cup of water) and petrolatum, and require daily gentle washing of the face and some gentle debridement, (usually by office staff if croton oil–phenol was used). For direct information on this, the reader can communicate with well-known peelers like Doctors Brody (Atlanta), Luitgard Wiest (Munich), Larry Kass (St. Petersburg, Florida) and Greg Hetter (retired). I prefer the use of bismuth subgallate powder "cocoon" (Fig. 12B) because it provides protection, and is antiseptic and provides anti-inflammatory benefits.

COMPLICATIONS

Chemical peeling complications can occur in any patient regardless of skin color. The early recognition and management of these complications is essential for a successful resolution. They are listed below along with suggestions for their management:

- *Herpes simplex infection*: Prevention of a herpes simplex outbreak is accomplished with oral antiviral medications beginning 1 day before peel and extending until re-epithelialization is completed; appears as erosions

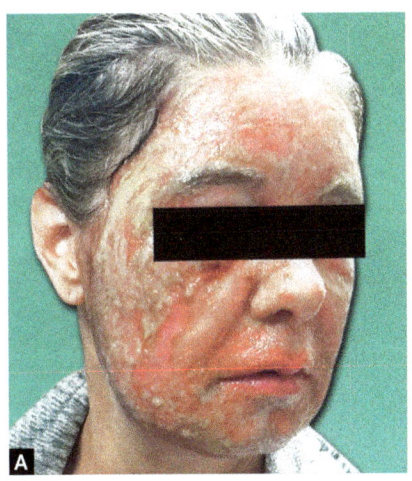 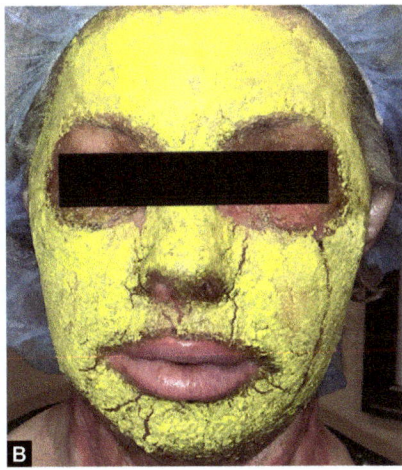

FIG. 12: **A,** Day 3 after a croton oil–phenol peel using petrolatum ointment and white vinegar compresses, known as the "open" technique which has visible draining exudate; **B,** Day 3 of full face, taped 0.35% croton oil–phenol 44%, using bismuth subgallate as a powder "dressing" to absorb the drainage and creates a protective "coccoon" for 7 days.

- *Bacterial or yeast infection*: Both bacterial infections and yeast infections have to be cultured and can be treated with white vinegar, if persistent. These infections are different in appearance than the acneiform eruption typically seen while using with the use of occlusive ointments post peels
- *Persistent erythema*: Erythema can be treated with topical steroids class VI (or stronger) BID, pulsed dye laser every 2 weeks, barrier creams or makeup. Treatment of prolonged erythema requires persistence but is effective
- *Contact dermatitis*: The risk of contact dermatitis can be recognized while reviewing what the patient is actually using at home. Once the offending chemical is identified and eliminated, you treat like any contact dermatitis and then return to petrolatum and white vinegar compresses
- *Scarring*: Scarring can be minimized with weekly-biweekly, low-dose intralesional triamcinolone 5 mg/cc or pulsed dye laser every 2 weeks. For resistant cases, it may be necessary to add 5-fluorouracil monthly to triamcinolone (equal parts), topical steroids and barrier creams
- *Postinflammatory hyperpigmentation*: In addition to being an indication for a peel, PIH can be a complication of a peel. To treat PIH, a 30% salicylic peel every 2-4 weeks can be safely used. The author likes to add 0.1% fluocinolone cream and a barrier cream BID to these areas. 2-4% hydroquinone is added after 1 month, if needed. Low-dose isotretinoin for 30 days should be used if widespread PIH appears in oily skin of color, especially in acne-prone patients that are still oily
- *Pseudo-hypopigmentation*: Hypopigmentation can have an insidious onset and creates lines of demarcation. To avoid hypopigmentation in patients deeply tanned, it is best to avoid medium-to-deep peels and just use a superficial-to-medium peel like 20% TCA. Hypopigmentation can be most obvious when peeling the chest and neck area [I prefer intense pulsed light (IPL)]. Normal skin color gradually

returns if patient gets "sun exposure" or targeted narrow band ultraviolet B (UVB) phototherapy.

CONCLUSION

Peel selection is determined by the depth of the peel required and the mechanism of action of the peel. Peels are commonly used in combinations, as a series, or as a component of a multimodal approach with laser ablation, electrocautery, surgery, dermal fillers and neurotoxins to correct multiple defects. Care must be taken to reduce the risk of peel and associated PIH. Preconditioning is required for all peels and a rigorous postoperative maintenance regimen ensures long-term satisfaction.

Long-term care and commitment are required from patients who have had peels. Patients may expect peels to control or shrink pores in a lasting manner, but this does not happen. Patients, particularly those with large pores or active acne, need to control the oiliness of their skin by the use of cleansers and drying agents and acne medications, such as spironolactone and especially isotretinoin. Lifestyle changes may also be required, including avoidance of sun and the reduction of exercise-induced heat (e.g., swimming rather than running). These measures will help to ensure patients' lifelong satisfaction with their appearance following a chemical peel.

TAKE HOME POINTS

- Using 30% salicylic acid for acne or melasma is really useful and easy
- Learn to use TCA or phenol formulas by applying them on actinic keratosis
- Join the International Peeling Society to learn hands-on peeling.

REFERENCES

1. Rullan P, Lemmon J, Rullan JM. The 2-day phenol chemabrasion technique for deep wrinkles and acne scars. Am J Cosmet Surg. 2004;21:199-210.
2. Rullan P, Karam AM. Chemical peels for darker skin types. Facial Plast Surg Clin North Am. 2010;18(1):111-31.
3. Spring LK, Krakowski AC, Alam M, et al. Isotretinoin and timing of procedural interventions: A systematic review with consensus recommendations. JAMA Dermatol. 2017;153(8):802-9.
4. Obagi S, Bridenstine JB. Lifetime skin care. Oral Maxillofac Surg Clin North Am. 2000;12(4):531-40.
5. Obagi S, Bridenstine JB. Chemical skin resurfacing. Oral Maxillofac Surg Clin North Am. 2000;12(4):541-53.
6. Monheit GD. The Jessner's 1 TCA peel: a medium-depth chemical peel. J Dermatol Surg Oncol. 1989;15(9):945-50.
7. Brody HJ, Monheit GD, Resnik SS, et al. A history of chemical peeling. Dermatol Surg. 2000;26(5):405-9.
8. Fanous N, Zari S. Universal trichloroacetic acid peel technique for light and dark skin. JAMA Facial Plastic Surgery. 2017;19(3):212-9.
9. Lee JB, Chung WG, Kwahck H, et al. Focal treatment of acne scars with trichloroacetic acid: chemical reconstruction of skin scars method. Dermatol Surg. 2002;28(11):1017-21; discussion 1021.
10. Obagi ZE. Obagi Skin Health Restoration and Rejuvenation, 1st Edition. New York: Springer; 1999.
11. Brody HJ. Chemical Peeling and Resurfacing, 3rd Edition. Atlanta, GA: Emory University; 2008.
12. Hetter GP. An examination of the phenol-croton oil peel: Part I. Dissecting the formula. Plast Reconstr Surg. 2000;105(1):227-39; discussion 249-51.
13. Hetter GP. An examination of the phenol-croton oil peel: part IV. Face peel results with different concentrations of phenol and croton oil. Plast Reconstr Surg. 2000;105(3):1061-83; discussion 1084-7.
14. Hetter GP. An examination of the phenol-croton oil peel: Part III. The plastic surgeons' role. Plast Reconstr Surg. 2000;105(2):752-63.
15. Hetter GP. An examination of the phenol-croton oil peel: Part II. The lay peelers and their croton oil formulas. Plast Reconstr Surg. 2000;105(1):240-8; discussion 249-51.
16. Stone PA. The use of modified phenol for chemical face peeling. Clin Plast Surg. 1998;25(1):21-44.
17. Stone PA, Lefer LG. Modified phenol chemical face peels: recognizing the role of application technique. Clin Plast Surg. 2001;28(1):13-36.

18. Fintsi Y. Exoderm - a novel, phenol-based peeling method resulting in improved safety. Int J Cosmet Surg. 2001;1(4):40-4.
19. Fintsi Y. Exoderm chemoabrasion original method for the treatment of facial acne scars. Int J Cosmet Surg. 2001;1(4):45-52.
20. Wambier C. QTc prolongation during phenol-croton oil peels. Letter to the Editor. J Am Acad Dermatol. 2017;Submitted.
21. Kass LG, Kass KS. The lost art of chemical peeling: My fifteen year experience with croton oil peels. Adv Ophthalmol Optometry. 2017;2:391-404.
22. Jacob CI, Dover JS, Kaminer MS. Acne scarring: a classification system and review of treatment options. J Am Acad Dermatol. 2001;45(1):109-17.
23. Yug A, Lane JE, Howard MS, et al. Histologic study of depressed acne scars treated with serial high-concentration (95%) trichloroacetic acid. Dermatol Surg. 2006;32(8):985-90; discussion 990.
24. Grimes PE. Aesthetics and Cosmetic Procedures in Darker Racial Ethnic Groups. Philadelphia: Lippincott Williams & Wilkins; 2008.

21 CHAPTER

Sequential Peels

Aarti Sarda, Abhishek De

INTRODUCTION

Chemical peel is a time tested and reliable procedure for different skin types and skin conditions. The body of scientific knowledge correlating the chemistry, histology, depth of penetration and clinical outcome studies for technique and methodology has reinforced the position of this procedure.[1]

With the availability of various peeling agents with differing mechanism of action, chemical peeling has become a versatile procedure. There are many new techniques of peeling like switch peeling, combination peels and sequential peeling.

Switch peel is a technique wherein different peels are used in subsequent sessions. For, e.g., salicylic or retinol peel in comedogenic or inflammatory acne switched over after clearance of acne to glycolic, mandelic peels in subsequent sessions to improve scars and texture. In combination peels, various peeling agents are used in a single formulation. These peeling agents act synergistically, enhance efficacy and depth of a peel. Salicylic with mandelic acid targets seborrhea, acne as well as postinflammatory hyperpigmentation. Mandelic acid has antibacterial properties and is safe for darker skin types.

Sequential peel is a technique in which peels are applied sequentially. The action of one peel is terminated followed sequentially with another peel, which is terminated or left on as a leave-on peel. Sequential peels are medium or deep peels mainly indicated for conditions that have a dermal component such as mixed melasma, lichenoid disorders, postinflammatory hyperpigmentation, etc. The idea behind sequential peel is that the first peel exfoliates the skin, thereby enhancing penetration of the second peel leading to greater depth of peeling. Another reason is that different chemicals have varying pKa; therefore, the use of optimal strength of each chemical in a single composition may not be practical.[2]

Sequential peels can be customized depending on the patients' skin condition. It should be used with special precautions and priming in dark-skinned individuals as they are at a risk of postinflammatory hyperpigmentation.[2]

Few of the well-known sequential peels are Coleman peel and Monheit peel.

Coleman peel is glycolic acid (GA) 70% combined with trichloroacetic acid (TCA) 35%. GA is applied first followed by application of TCA. GA 70% is applied for 2 minutes, the solution is washed off, and then TCA 35% is applied. This combination has been found to produce a deeper and more uniform peel than TCA used alone.[3]

Monheit peel is Jessner's solution with TCA 35%.[3,4] Sequential peels with TCA are strong medium-depth peels and should be avoided in dark skin.[4-6]

INDICATIONS

Sequential peels are deep peels mainly indicated for mixed melasma, lichenoid disorders, postinflammatory hyperpigmentation, etc. The authors use salicylic acid and GA in a sequence in case of acne vulgaris with postinflammatory hyperpigmentation. It is suggested that GA 70% peel might enhance the penetration of salicylic acid (SA) 20% leading to a greater depth of the peel, with less chances for postinflammatory hyperpigmentation, especially in ethnic skin groups.

Glycolic acid and TCA peels are performed sequentially in cases of postinflammatory hyperpigmentation, postacne pigmentation and melasma. This combination has been found to produce a deeper and more uniform peel than TCA used alone.[7]

Combining Jessner's solution and GA for the treatment of photoaged skin, actinic keratoses and rhytides resulted in a uniform GA peel, but the risk of overpeel and scarring are high, especially in dark-skinned individuals.[8]

CONTRAINDICATIONS[9-14]

- Active infection, open wound or dermatitis
- Sunburn or recent suntan
- Impaired healing
- Excessively dry skin
- Unrealistic patient expectations
- Pregnancy or lactation
- Body dysmorphic disorder.

PATIENT PREPARATION

Detailed history and cutaneous examination should be performed in all patients prior to chemical peeling. Note the patient's Fitzpatrick skin type, Glogau's score, skin thickness, dryness, acne scars, pigmentation, and vascular and pigmented lesions. Assessment of patients' expectations at the time of consultation and commitment to a series of treatment is essential to ensure success with these treatments. Obtain an informed consent. Standardized photography should be taken of all areas to be peeled, preferably full face, frontal and lateral areas.

Priming with topical retinoids should be started 2-6 weeks prior to the peel. This thins the stratum corneum, increasing the uniform penetration and depth of peel and enhances epidermal turnover. It also decreases the content of epidermal melanin and expedites the healing. Retinoids should be stopped 2 days prior to peeling.

Equipment required for peel are:
- Prepeel cleanser
- Headband or surgical cap
- Degreasing lotion
- *Applicators*: Cotton-tipped buds, brushes, gauze sponges
- Petroleum jelly
- Gloves
- Saline eyewash
- Timer
- Face towels
- Cotton
- Chemical peel
- Dispensing cups
- Moisturizer or sunscreen.

PEEL TECHNIQUE[11,15]

The patient should be comfortably placed in supine position. Apply a headband to pull hair away from the face and drape a towel on the neck. Set all the products required. After the skin is cleaned and degreased, and a suitable protectant is applied to sensitive areas, one coat of the first peel is applied into the skin. Application of peel may be started from the forehead followed by cheeks, chin, nose and upper lip. The first peel is terminated followed by application of the second peel in a similar fashion. The second peel is terminated or left on as a slow-release peel (Figs. 1–3).

POSTPEEL CARE

After approximately 12 hours, the patient can wash the area with a mild cleansing gel. Patients should not expose treated skin to the sun or high temperature for 3–7 days after the peel treatment. The procedure can be done every 15 days, and series of 6–12 treatments typically produce the best results.

COMPLICATIONS[16-18]

Complications are the same as can occur with the various peels, depending on the peel used. The following complications can occur:
- Pain or discomfort
- Blistering, crusting or desquamation
- Prolonged irritation or erythema
- Hyperpigmentation

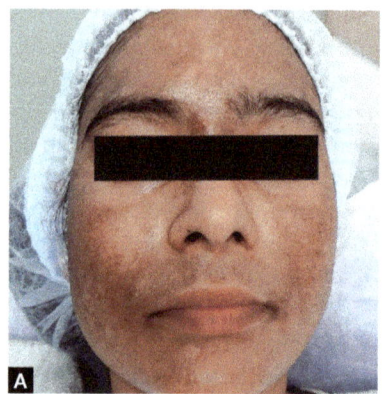
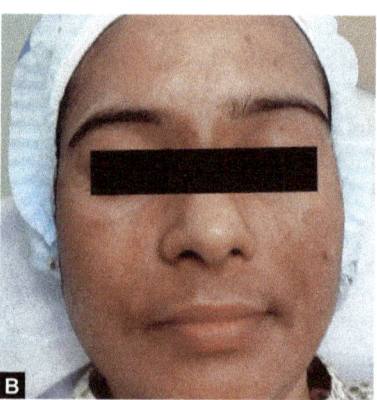

FIG. 1: A, Before; and **B,** after two sessions of sequential peel with 35% glycolic acid and kojic acid.

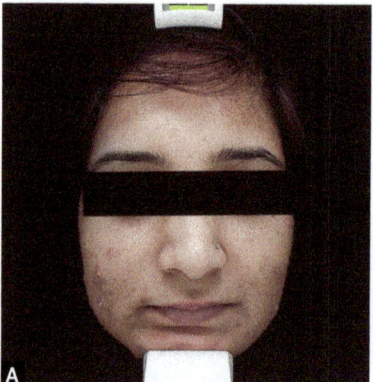
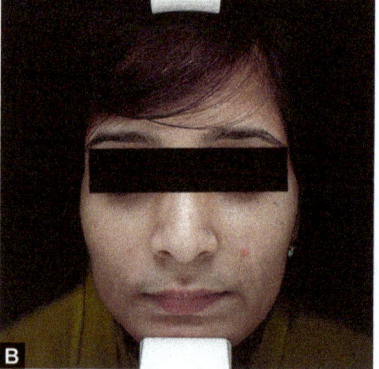

FIG. 2: A, Before; and **B,** after two sessions of sequential peel with glycolic acid and salicylic acid.

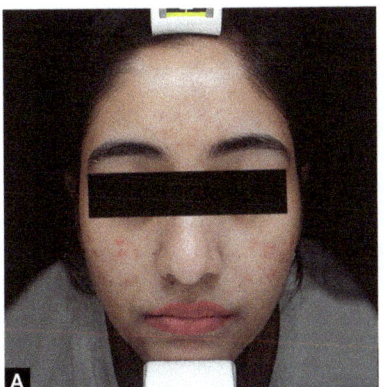 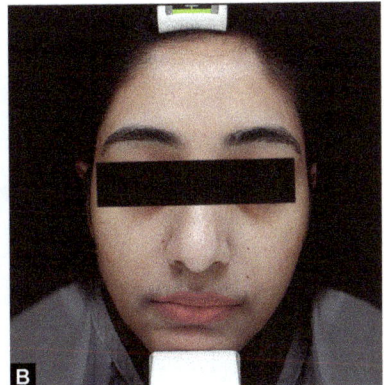

FIG. 3: **A,** Before; and **B,** after two sessions of sequential peel with glycolic acid and kojic acid.

- Hypopigmentation
- Excessive dryness
- Milia
- Infections
- Exacerbation of acne or dermatitis
- Allergic reaction
- Scarring
- Contact sensitization
- Salicylism (with salicylic acid).

PRACTICAL TIPS

- It should be remembered that combining two agents in a sequential manner can increase the concentration of second peeling agent and increase the depth of peel with increase in complications. Therefore, the concentration of second peeling agent should be lowered than what is normally used
- Sequential peels are useful for treating inflammatory acne with postinflammatory hyperpigmentation, wherein salicylic acid and GA are used in sequence
- The authors have tried 35% GA with kojic acid sequentially in melasma with good results.

CONCLUSION

Sequential peel is a technique of application of multiple peels in one session. The idea behind sequential peel is that the first peel exfoliates the skin, thereby enhancing penetration of the second peel leading to greater depth of peeling.

TAKE HOME POINTS

- Sequential peel is a versatile peeling technique in which more than one peel is used in a sequence depending on the indication
- Sequential peels can be medium-to-deep peels mainly indicated for conditions that have a dermal component
- The idea behind sequential peel is that the first peel exfoliates the skin, thereby enhancing penetration of the second peel leading to greater depth of peeling.

REFERENCES

1. Monheit GD. Chemical Peeling: Combinations of Therapy. In: Rubin MG, Tung R (Eds). Procedures in Cosmetic Dermatology Series: Chemical Peels. St Louis, MO: Elsevier; 2006. pp. 115-36.

2. Khunger N, Arsiwala S. Combination and sequential peel. In: Khunger N (Ed.) Step-by-Step Chemical Peels, 2nd Edition. New Delhi: Jaypee Brothers Medical Publishers. pp. 179-88.
3. Coleman WP 3rd, Futrell JM. The glycolic, trichloroacetic acid peel. J Dermatol Surg Oncol. 1994;20:76-80.
4. Monheit GD. Chemical peels. Skin Therapy Lett. 2004;9(2):6-11.
5. Monheit GD, Chastain MA. Chemical peels. Facial Plast Surg Clin North Am. 2001;9(2):239-55, viii.
6. Monheit GD. The Jessner's + TCA peel: A medium-depth chemical peel. J Dermatol Surg Oncol. 1989;15:953-63.
7. Moy LS. Superficial chemical peels with alpha-hydroxy acids. In: Robinson JK, Arndt KA, Le Boit PE, Wintroub BU (Eds). Atlas of Cutaneous Surgery. Philadelphia, PA: WB Saunders; 1996. pp. 345-50.
8. Monheit GD. How to select the appropriate peel for each patient. In: Rubin MG, Tung R (Eds). Procedures in Cosmetic Dermatology Series: Chemical Peels. St Louis, MO: Elsevier; 2006.
9. Grimes PE. Salicylic acid. In: Tosti A, Grimes PE, De Padova, Maria Pia. (Eds) Color Atlas of Chemical Peels, 2nd Edition. Berlin Heidelberg: Springer; 2012. pp.49-57.
10. Kinsley M, Metelitsa AI, Somani AK. Chemical peels. In: Wolverton SE (Ed.) Comprehensive Dermatologic Drug Therapy, 3rd Edition. New York: Elsevier Saunders; 2013. p. 579-82.
11. Small R, O'Hanlon K. Chemical Peels. In: Usatine R, Stulberg D, Pfenninger J, Small R. (Eds). Dermatologic and Cosmetic Procedures in Office Practice. Philadelphia: Saunders; 2012. pp. 259-73.
12. Small R. Aesthetic procedures in office practice. Am Fam Physician. 2009;80(11):1231-7.
13. Baumann L, Saghari S. Chemical Peels. In: Baumann LS (Ed.). Cosmetic Dermatology: Principles and Practice, 2nd Edition. New York: McGraw Hill, 2009. pp. 148-62.
14. Paula E, Angela J. Chemexfoliation and superficial skin resurfacing. In: Cheryl M Burgress (Eds). Cosmetic Dermatology. Springer; 2005. pp. 63-82.
15. Monheit GD, Chastian MA. Chemical and mechanical skin resurfacing. In: Bolognia JL, Jorizzo JL, Rapini RP (Eds.) Dermatology. Philadelphia, PA: Mosby; 2003.
16. Khunger N. Standard guidelines of care for chemical peels. Indian J Dermatol Venereol Leprol. 2008;74 Suppl S1:5-12.
17. Nikalji N, Godse K, Sakhiya J, et al. Complications of Medium Depth and Deep Chemical Peels. J Cutan Aesthet Surg. 2012;5(4):254-60.
18. Anitha B. Prevention of Complications in Chemical Peeling. J Cutan Aesthet Surg. 2010;3(3):186-8.

22 CHAPTER

Yellow Peels

Shehnaz Z Arsiwala

INTRODUCTION

The yellow peel or retinol peel has gained popularity in recent years due to its target specific and yet a multimodality action on epidermis, pigmentation, texture, comedogenic and inflammatory acne as well as early acne scars.

The techniques and formulation for retinol peels have evolved over time and are discussed herewith.

CHEMISTRY AND CHEMICAL FORMULATIONS OF YELLOW PEELS

Retinoids are a class of lipids including vitamin A retinol and its synthetic analogs.

Mode of action of retinol peels is metabolic and it modifies cell structure and synthesis resulting in keratinocyte dyscohesion, exfoliation, regeneration and remodeling. Retinoids act by specific or nonspecific binding with retinoid receptors which then influence keratinocyte regulation, regeneration and remodeling. The retinoid class constitutes the active tretinoin and isotretinoin, and mild forms of retinaldehyde and retinol; the active forms are used in a wide variety of topical agents in concentrations not above 0.1%.[1]

Clinically, due to their action on epidermis and dermis, retinol peels can cause regeneration of a thinner and more compact stratum corneum, regularization of atypical epidermal keratinocytes, elimination of epidermal melanin, action on dermal matrix metalloproteinases, causing neocollagenosis, increased deposition of glycosaminoglycans and increased dermal neovascularization.[1-4]

Retinoic acid peels are not only keratolytic but also sebolytic and thus express strong comedogenic and anti-inflammatory actions, and felicitating epidermal elimination, pigment lightening, textural regulation as well as helps in collagen remodeling with resultant anti-wrinkling effect.

Formulations

Retinoic acid peels are formulated using natural retinoid (retinol, all-trans retinal and retinoic acid). Peels are formulated with high concentration between 1% and 5% and some formulations in paste base have up to 10–12%. It is available as tinted gel, lotion, cream or propylene glycol vehicles. They are generally a slow release or a liquid peel and have synergistic actions when used along with ascorbyl glucoside.

TABLE 1: Formulations of yellow peels

Yellow peel—Geosmatic	Miami AR	Tryses—Cipla	Retises CT—Sesderma	I Image retinol
Retinol: 0.1% with resorcinol 14%, trichloroacetic acid 14%, lactic acid 13% and salicylic acid 5%	Stabilized retinol ester with linelonic acid	Retinol 4% with ascorbic acid	Liquid prepeel ampoule with antioxidants and 10% vitamin C, paste containing 4% retinol and 4% nicotinamide	Retinol 4% in combination with salicylic 20%, glycolic acid 10% in alcohol base

TABLE 2: Indications for yellow peels

Acne	Pigmentation	Texture
Comedogenic, papular, inflammatory acne, acne corporis, postacne pigmented marks, early acne scars	Postinflammatory hyperpigmentation, tanned skin, melasma, freckles, lentigines, actinic keratoses, perioral and periorbital hyperpigmentation, acanthosis nigricans	Dull skin, photodamage, fine lines, stretch marks

Some formulations have combinations with salicylic or glycolic acid, kojic acid, ascorbic acid, etc. to enhance the action of the peeling agent.

Various formulations of yellow peels are available and listed in table 1.

INDICATIONS

Main indication of yellow peels includes photodamaged skin with patchy pigmentation, freckles and hyperchromic spots, comedogenic or inflammatory acne, postacne marks, early superficial atrophic scars, traumatic scars, facial rejuvenation, fine wrinkles, stretch marks and dull complexion. It is indicated in cases of mild-to-moderate photoaging, melasma, acne, superficial scarring and postinflammatory hyperpigmentation[5-7] (Table 2).

Good results are seen, with retinol peels used sequentially at extra facial sites, especially when used for acne and scars in males, as in these regions, the skin is more seborrheic and thicker. Pigment elimination, textural improvements and photodamage correction are marked with this peel.

Photoaging

Retinol peels are excellent for improvement of photodamage. Fifteen patients were studied with biweekly 5 sessions and resulted in textural improvement of skin. Histopathology revealed thinning of stratum corneum and increased epidermal thickness.[8] When the peel is used for photoaging, it helps to improve pigment, texture and fine lines; however, the skin needs adequate hydration and sun protection during this process as risk of dryness and photosensitivity is high while on this peel. The improvement is more in mild photoaging while moderate to severe photoaging needs optical interventions according to the author; however, in moderate to severe cases of photoaging, yellow peels act as interventional priming before laser resurfacing techniques.

Acne and Postacne Pigmented Marks

Comedones, both open and closed, respond very well to retinol peels. In closed comedones, extraction of comedones is followed by application of retinol peel in a paste format to expedite clearance. Papular inflammatory acne responds well to yellow peels; also this peel has additional action on pigment reduction so helps in minimizing postacne, hyperpigmented marks. Early grade scars do get alleviated with series of yellow peels due to downregulation of MMPs. Action on closed comedones enables prevention of inflammatory lesions and textural improvement.

Retinol peels are now mainstay for acne in dark skin due to strong keratolytic, sebostatic and pigment elimination helpful for acne of any stage as well as postinflammatory hyperpigmented marks. Topical retinoids are recommended as first-line treatment for acne and are excellent priming agents; hence, retinol peels are a natural choice of intervention for postacne marks. It is also used for acne and scars in males as skin is more seborrheic and thicker. Pigment elimination, textural improvements and photodamage correction is marked with this peel. Retinol peels are relatively safer and often show good results when used sequentially at extra facial sites. Retinoic acid peel is useful as a slow-release peel as it can be used sequentially after salicylic acid or trichloroacetic acid (TCA) peels. In authors' experience, retinoic acid peel form an excellent priming peel before laser resurfacing.[9,10]

Pigmentation

All epidermal component of pigmentation can be improved with yellow peel.

In melasma, the slow release tretinoin peels help to reduce the epidermal pigmentation in addition to reduction of photodamage and improvement of texture. It is beneficial as the patients are already primed with topical tretinoin alone or in triple combination therapy. Tretinoin peels versus glycolic acid peels in the treatment of melasma in dark-skinned patients has been studied by Khunger N, Sarkar R and Jain RK, where tretinoin peel at 1% strength versus 70% glycolic acid peels was applied for melasma for 4 hours once a week, for 12 weeks and found to be of equal efficacy.[11-14]

Combinations in retinol peel formulations include nicotinamide, ascorbic acid, glycolic acid and ferulic acid. The combination formulas are actually either with pigment lighteners and antioxidants as adjuvants or synergistic alpha-hydroxy agents to improve the peel outcome.

Combinations with Other Peels

In some formulations, retinoic acid is available as a slow-release peel, when combined with alpha- or beta-hydroxy peels like salicylic acid, mandelic acid, glycolic or TCA, the yellow peels act synergistically to enhance the efficacy when layered with superficial peels. In the sequence, the terminative peels are applied first, washed off and then sealed by using paste form of slow-release yellow peels. This is done commonly after salicylic acid, glycolic acid or TCA peels. The choice of this combination is ideally suited for male skin, acne prone skin with comedones, papules mingled with early-pigmented scars and when acne and scars are associated with melasma. A sequential combination peel is best avoided in a sensitive skin as exacerbation of postpeel dryness and photosensitivity is high.[10]

Combinations with other procedures: The yellow peel is appropriate as a combination with other procedures and usually can be applied after the procedure. Post microdermabrasion yellow peel works for patients with advanced photodamage, papular amyloidosis and thick-skinned individuals, as well as acanthosis nigricans. A study revealed efficacy for photodamage post microdermabrasion and 5% retinol peels.[14,15]

Tretinoin peel should be conducted in a series of 3–5 sessions before laser resurfacing in pigmented acne scars in skin types 3–5 acne scars as well as photodamage skin.[9,16]

CONTRAINDICATIONS FOR YELLOW PEELS

The generally tolerable retinol peels are absolutely contraindicated in pregnancy and relatively in lactation phase. A dry sensitive or atopic skin is unsuitable for this peel. Probable contraindications for yellow peels include:[6]
- Pregnancy and lactation
- Dry skin conditions, atopic dermatitis, seborrheic dermatitis and sensitive skin
- Reactivity to any ingredients in the formulation
- Herpes or any active viral infections
- Photosensitive dermatoses
- Patients on other peels in last 1 month
- Unrealistic expectations.

PATIENT PREPARATION

Priming thins out stratum corneum and paves way for a slightly lighter and sun protected skin which can uniformly absorb the peel.

Priming with a broad-spectrum sunscreen is absolutely mandatory and should be started 2–3 weeks minimum and 6 weeks maximum before undertaking the peel. Also, an optimal priming agent like glycolic acid, kojic acid, ascorbic acid or a topical retinoid adapalene, tazarotene or tretinoin with emollient is mandatory in dark-skin types. This allows uniform penetration and absorption as well as no adverse effects. Priming agent before yellow peel can be chosen according to the indication, skin type and gender of patient. A photodamaged skin can be primed with topical retinoid with adequate emollients and withheld 3 days to a week (in sensitive skin patients) before; also use of retinoids as priming agents helps to unmask any retinoid dermatitis before peels and warrants anticipatory observation of skin for any untoward effects of retinol peels. Lactic acid with glycolic acid priming works well if textural improvement is desired and kojic acid with ascorbic acid priming for pigmentary conditions. Azelaic acid is a good priming agent for acne and acne marks before retinol peels. Patch testing is recommended to unmask potential retinoid dermatitis or a sensitive skin.[15]

PEEL TECHNIQUE (FIGS. 1–4)

Application technique is undertaken after an adequate informed valid consent and photographic documentation.
1. Remove any makeup and cleanse the skin; a headband used to secure hair away from face; patient should be in semi-recline position
2. Degreasing of skin with acetone and alcohol-based solution. Sensitive crevices of the face like corner of eyes and mouth may be protected with petrolatum jelly
3. Uniform application of the peel liquid-based formulations on the skin with slight rubbing in circular motion, in multiple coats 2 minutes apart based on skin type and indication. For paste-based formulations, the peeling agent can be evenly spread on skin and left on
4. Sequence of application is forehead, cheeks, chin, nose, perioral and periorbital area
5. The peel can be left on for minimum 1–4 hours up to 8 hours depending on the formulation, skin type and indication, and at stipulated time, washed off with neutral pH cleanser
6. This peel does not require neutralization
7. Post application, the liquid as well as the paste formulation leaves a yellow film on

Yellow Peels

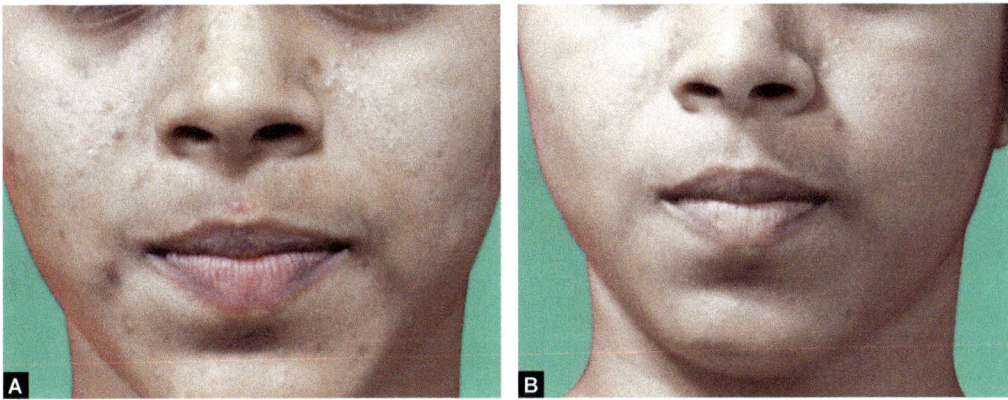

FIG. 1: Response of comedogenic, papular acne, marks, and textural enhancement after retinol peels. **A,** Before; **B,** After.

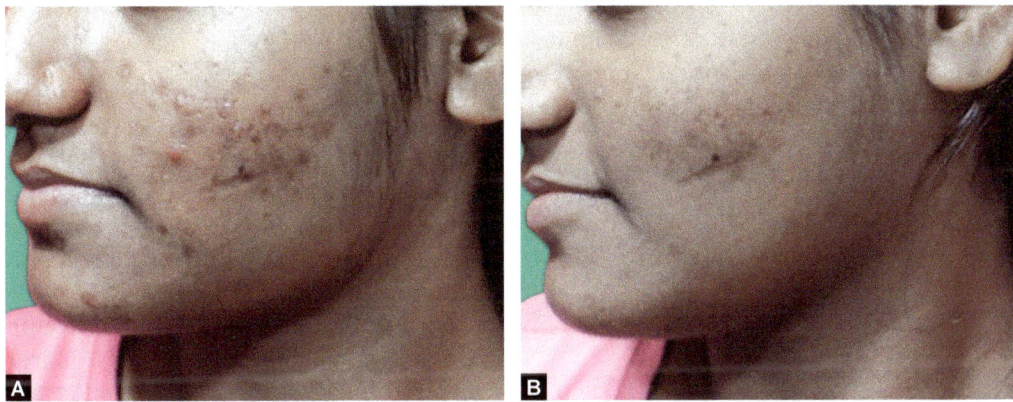

FIG. 2: Response of seborrhea, papular acne, and early-pigmented scars to leave-in retinol peels. **A,** Before; **B,** After.

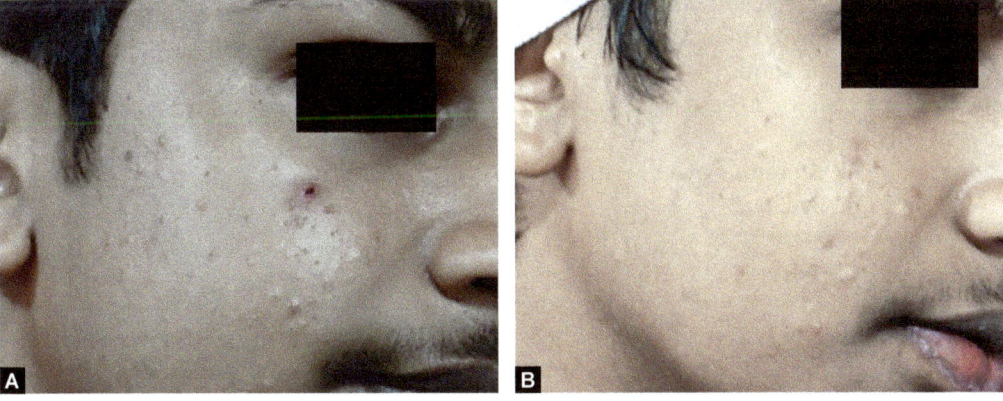

FIG. 3: Response to retinol peel in single session seen as marked reduction in oiliness and comedones along with improvement in photodamage. **A,** Before; **B,** After.

Chemical Peels: A Global Perspective

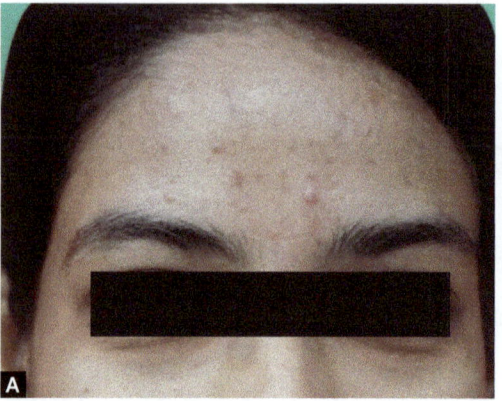
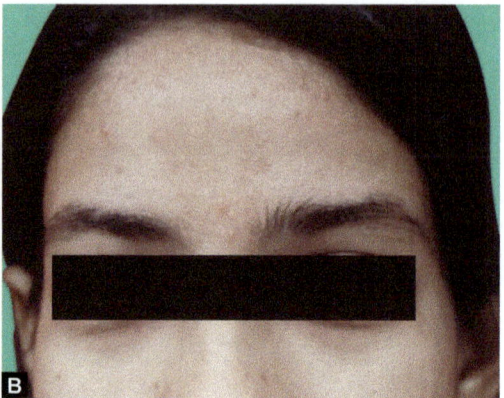

FIG. 4: Combination of retinol and salicylic peel to improve papular forehead acne, marks, and texture of the skin. **A,** Before; **B,** After.

the skin; the yellow tint stays for 20 minutes and disappears in paste form whereas in liquid form, the yellow tint stays longer sometimes until it is washed off
8. Patient can wash off the product at home with mild cleanser at time indicated. In cases of extreme burning or stinging, the peel may be terminated immediately
9. Sessions can be repeated at 10-15 days for a series of 5-6 sessions
10. Dryness and scaling at 2-3 days are expected endpoint of the yellow peel, often emollient
11. Sun protection is mandatory with a broad-spectrum sunscreen and unnecessary sun exposure to be avoided for 2-3 days
12. Picking of skin should be avoided and emollients where necessary should be suggested
13. Any topical therapies to be resumed 4-7 days after peel.

POSTPEEL CARE

All drying agents and retinoid to be withheld for 4-5 days after the peel. Drying face washes to be withheld. Reintroduction is advised after 3-5 days.

COMPLICATIONS

Complications from yellow peel are rare most of the untoward effects; these are transitory effect of retinol on the skin and generally manageable. Some of the milder side effects of retinol peels include excessive dryness, irritation, itching, persistent redness; photosensitivity is a well-known effect due to keratolytic action and thinner stratum corneum after exfoliating peels. Rarely increased postpeel hyperpigmentation may be seen with inadvertent sun exposure and poor sun protection modes while on peels.

Other complications like uniform eruption, telangiectasias and superficial keratitis are being cited in the literature.[8]

Complications of retinol peel are mild to moderate and can be easily managed with adequate emollients for hydration, sun protection, lightening agents and adequate postpeel care.

PRACTICAL TIPS

- Yellow peel is a one of the few peels, which has multimodality actions and is the only peel, which has epidermal, pigmentary and dermal actions

- It is used judiciously in sensitive skin
- It can be combined with other peels which can be terminated
- Retinol peels can be combined with other procedure like microdermabrasion, lasers, comedone extraction, etc.
- It is beneficial in extra facial sites and male skin
- It is great for comedolysis in combination with salicylic peels
- It is beneficial for pigmentary stretch marks and works well under occlusion
- One must watch for retinoid dermatitis with prolonged stay time in leave-in formulations
- Mandatory sunscreen creams and emollients are needed in the postpeel phase.

CONCLUSION

The retinol peels are the most gratifying peels for type 3–5 skin for multiple indications if patient selection is done well and yield very good results if thorough priming, optimum sessions and good postpeel care are ensured. Combinations with this peel are often synergistic, and side effects are mild and manageable.

TAKE HOME POINTS

- Yellow peels are retinol-based peels in various formulations
- Yellow peels are used for pigmentation, melasma, photodamage, etc.
- They are often used synergistically with other peels and techniques
- Adverse effects of yellow peels are transient and manageable.

REFERENCES

1. Creidi P, Humbert P. Clinical use of topical retinaldehyde on photoaged skin. Dermatology. 1999;199:49-52.
2. Draelos ZD. Retinoids in cosmetics. Cosmet Dermatol. 2005;18:3-5.
3. Araújo ALN, Pinto SFM, Sobrinho OAP, et al. Peeling químico: avaliação de ácido glicólico, ácido retinóico e ATA. Rev Cosmet Med Est. 1995;3(3):41-4.
4. Dréno B, Fischer TC, Perosino E, et al. Expert opinion: efficacy of superficial chemical peels in active acne management--what can we learn from the literature today? Evidence-based recommendations. J Eur Acad Dermatol Venereol. 2011;25(6):695-704.
5. Cucé LC, Bertino MC, Scattone L, et al. Tretinoin peeling. Dermatol Surg. 2001;27(1):12-4.
6. Langsdon PR, Rodwell DW 3rd, Velargo PA, et al. Latest chemical peel innovations. Facial Plast Surg Clin North Am. 2012;20(2):119-23.
7. Faghihi G, Shahingohar A, Siadat AH. Comparison between 1% tretinoin peeling versus 70% glycolic acid peeling in the treatment of female patients with melasma. J Drugs Dermatol. 2011;10(12):1439-42.
8. Gold MH, Hu JY, Biron JA, et al. Tolerability and Efficacy of Retinoic Acid Given after Full-face Peel Treatment of Photodamaged Skin. J Clin Aesthet Dermatol. 2011;4(10):40-8.
9. Shehnaz AZ. Chemical Peels for Post Acne Hyperpigmentation in Skin of Color. Pigmentary Disorders. 2015;2:162.
10. Khunger N, Arsiwala S. Combination and sequential peels. In: Khunger N (Ed.). Step-by-Step Chemical Peels, 2nd Edition. New Delhi: Jaypee Brothers Medical Publishers (P) Ltd.; 2014. pp. 179-94.
11. Khunger N, Sarkar R, Jain RK. Tretinoin peels versus glycolic acid peels in the treatment of Melasma in dark-skinned patients. Dermatol Surg. 2004;30:756-60; discussion.
12. Dewandre L, Tenenbaum A. The chemistry of peels: A hypothesis of action mechanisms and a proposal of a new classification of chemical peels. In: Tung RC, Rubin MG (Eds). Chemical Peels, 2nd Edition. Philadelphia: Elsevier/Saunders; 2011. pp. 1-16.
13. Jackson A. Chemical peels. Facial Plast Surg. 2014;30(1):26-34.
14. Kligman DE. Tretinoin peels versus glycolic acid peels. Dermatol Surg. 2004;30(12):1609.
15. Khunger N. Standard guidelines of care for chemical peels: IADVL task force. Indian J Dermatol Venereol Leprol. 2008;74:S5-12.
16. Arsiwala S. Acne Scars: Complications of treatment and their management. In: Khunger N (Ed.) Step-by-Step Treatment of Acne Scars, 1st Edition. New Delhi: Jaypee Brothers Medical Publishers (P) Ltd.; 2014. pp. 225-48.

Arginine Peel

Ishad Aggarwal, Manmit K Hora

INTRODUCTION

Chemical peeling of skin is a procedure which utilizes the regenerative properties of skin after inflicting a controlled injury to a desired depth by topical application of a peeling agent. The aim of the procedure is to improve the texture of the skin, reduce pigmentation and signs of aging such as superficial wrinkles and fine lines. Though the traditional agents of chemical peels are widely used, newer molecules are emerging and gaining popularity predominantly because of lesser side effects and increased number of indications for which they can be safely used. In this chapter we are going to discuss arginine as an agent of chemical peeling in dermatological and esthetic practice.

CHEMISTRY

Arginine (pKa −2.17), a 2-amino 5-guanidino-pentanoic acid is a basic amino acid containing universal properties (Fig. 1). It is produced in adult human body and can be obtained after fermentation of brown sugar and sugarcane.

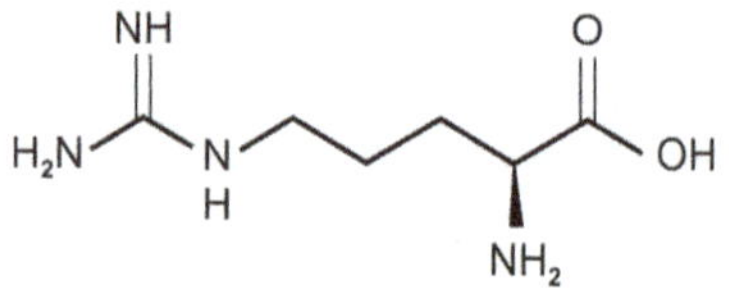

FIG. 1: Structure of arginine.

MECHANISM OF ACTION[1]

Arginine is a superficial peeling agent which works on the horny stratum corneum. Since most formulations of arginine peels contain pH of 4–6, it is very helpful for patients with hypersenstive skin. Since, arginine is a large molecule, after application on skin, the penetration of the molecule through the epidermis is very slow, therefore making it less prone to deleterious side effects, often seen with stronger peels. In addition, it is also known to have moisturizing owing to its amino acid group. Thus, it has an ability to hydrate the skin and provides it turgor. It is also said to enhance collagen production. It is also known to have antibacterial benefits. These qualities of arginine make it an excellent agent of chemical peels for patients with dry, sensitive and irritable skin.

FORMULATION

It is available as 20% arginine gel peel. Most of the formulations containing arginine are generally combination of different peeling agents (Table 1).

TABLE 1: Composition of various commercially available arginine peels

Name of the peel/name of the company	Composition
Leaderma	Aqua (water), lactic acid (20%), arginine HCl (20%), ethoxydiglycol, urea (5%), aloe barbadensis leaf juice (1%), allantoin, xanthan gum and disodium EDTA
Claze peel, cipla	Arginine HCl 20% + lactic acid 20% + kojic acid 5% + arbutin 2% + citric acid 2%
Argipeel, sesderma	Arginine 20% + lactic acid 20% + urea + allantoin + aloe vera

EDTA, ethylenediaminetetraacetic acid.

Most of the arginine peels are available in gel form. The combination of alpha-hydroxy peels along with arginine peels hastens the skin regeneration, improves the microtopography and homogenizes the pigmentation.

INDICATIONS

Arginine peel is a mild peel with remarkable properties which makes it an ideal peeling agent of choice for people with hyperirritable and sensitive skin types. It is very commonly used in esthetic practice to rejuvenate the periorbital region. Periorbital dullness due to hyperpigmentation, tear trough deformity and wrinkles is a very common concern that a lot of patients come with. However, the skin in this region is very thin and more prone to side effects by a stronger peel. The ability of arginine peel to hydrate the skin and its safety profile makes it an excellent candidate for periorbital rejuvenation (Fig. 2).[1,2] The same property can also be exploited to treat patients who often complain of dullness and tiredness of skin (Fig. 3). It is also a good peel for priming the skin, to prepare it for other stronger peel. Since it is known to induce production of collagen, it is also used as an anti-aging peel. However, one must note that the effect of arginine peel on signs of aging such as superficial fine lines and wrinkles may be more visible in younger patients than older patients, mainly because it is a superficial peeling agent. Therefore, it can be used an anti-aging peel for people in their mid-30s. For people above 40 years of age it should mainly be reserved to hydrate, provide luster and reduce sullenness from the face or as maintenance after stronger peels. In a single-blinded randomized control trial between glycolic acid peel versus amino fruit peel in treatment of melasma, patients

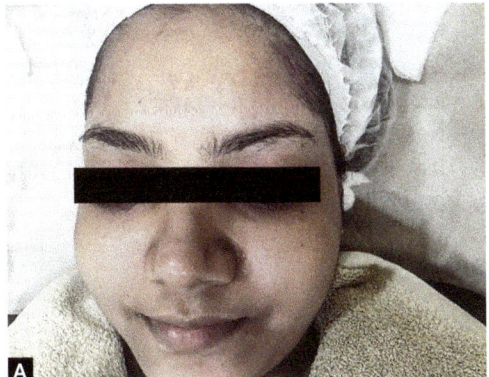 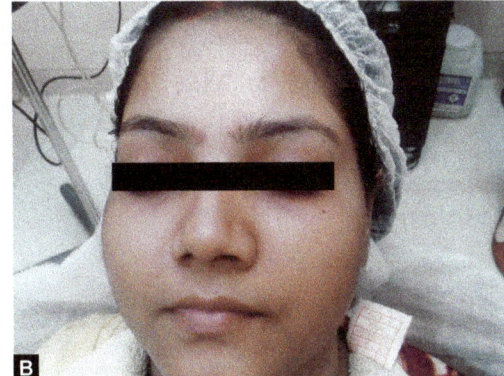

FIG. 2: Periorbital rejuvenation with arginine peel. A, Before; B, After single session of arginine peel.
Courtesy: Manmit K Hora, Consultant Dermatologist, Kolkata.

Chemical Peels: A Global Perspective

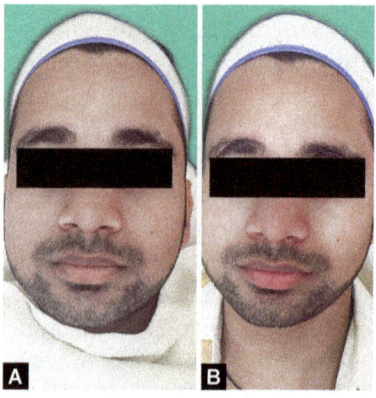

FIG. 3: Facial rejuvenation with arginine peel in a patient complaining of dullness and tiredness on the face. **A,** Before; **B,** After single session of arginine peel.

BOX 1	Indications of arginine peels

- Periorbital rejuvenation
- Sensitive skin
- Superficial pigmentation
- Aging skin
- As a priming peel

received serial peels on two halves of the face. There was statistical difference in the melasma area and severity index (MASI) score from baseline for both the agents and there was no statistical difference between glycolic peels and amino fruit peels in terms of regression of melasma.[3] When taken regularly arginine peel also improves superficial pigmentation and photoaging (Box 1).

CONTRAINDICATIONS

Absolute

- Idiosyncrasy to components
- Active viral or fungal infections
- Damage to skin
- Excessive exposure to sun
- Pregnancy.

Relative

- Use of microdermabrasion treatment within last 6 months
- Less than 1 week of hair epilation
- Intake of immunosuppressive drugs
- History of isotretinoin use in last 1 month
- Photosensitive disorders.

PREPEEL PRECAUTIONS

Skin preparation for arginine peel should begin at least 2 weeks prior to procedure. The patient should be told to avoid waxing, threading, bleaching or other parlor and beauty services. They should be told to stop vitamin A containing derivatives, retinoids or other exfoliating cosmetic and beauty products at least 3 days before the procedure. They should be advised to wear a sunscreen three times per day on a regular basis. Written informed consent forms and detailed medical history should always be taken. If a patient presents with herpes infection, acute sunburns or rashes, the procedure should be postponed.

Procedure

- Clean and degrease the skin
- Remove all the makeup
- Vaseline should be applied in all sensitive areas of the skin
- Cover the eyes with a wet cotton
- Apply the peel evenly with a peel brush and wait for 10–12 minutes
- Neutralize the skin with water
- If irritation occurs wash with cold water immediately.

POSTPEEL CARE

Although arginine peel is a very mild peel, but a meticulous postpeel care should always be advised to the patients after the peel.

- Sun protection is most important. Use of broad spectrum sunscreens, avoidance of direct exposure to sun, using physical sun protection can help minimize any untoward side effects
- The patient should also be told to avoid any depilatory, exfoliative, beauty or cosmetic treatment for at least 7 days after the peel.
- No decorative makeup should be applied for up to 24 hours postpeel.

COMPLICATIONS

Complications are part and parcel of esthetic practice. No matter how simple and safe a procedure might be, one should always have a watchful eye. Arginine peels are no exceptions. Although the rate of complications may be very low, following complications should be borne in mind.

Superficial burn, manifesting as hyperemia or erythema may be seen. These burns may leave postinflammatory hyperpigmentation. Idiosyncratic reactions to any of the component of the peel may occur. Sloughing of the skin is a temporary complication which resolves in 2–3 days.

CONCLUSION

Arginine peel is uniquely placed in our basket of chemical peels owing to its remarkable properties, making it suitable, even for people with hypersensitive skin. It is a relatively safer to use peel for a variety of indications and can thus help dermatologists to improve outcomes in tricky situations, where other peels might be more difficult to use.

TAKE HOME POINTS

- Arginine peel is a safe peel for irritable, sensitive skin types because it is a superficial peel with large molecule and a higher pH
- It has moisturizing and anti-aging properties like collagen induction, improvement of skin micro relief, reduction of superficial fine lines, pigmentation and improvement of skin microcirculation
- It is used mainly for periorbital rejuvenation, irritable skin like acne rosacea, maintenance of skin, as anti-aging peel and as priming peel
- It can be repeated once in 2 weeks.

REFERENCES

1. Talwar A, Talwar K. Newer superficial peels. In: Mysore V (Ed). ACS(I) Textbook on Cutaneous and Aesthetic Surgery, 2nd edition. New Delhi: Jaypee Brothers Medical Publishers (P) Ltd; 2013.
2. Kumarasinghe P, Hewitt D. Neoplasms with pigmentary changes or discolouration. In: Lahiri K, Chatterjee M, Sarkar R (Eds). Pigmentary Disorders: A Comprehensive Compendium, 1st edition. New Delhi: Jaypee Brothers Medical Publishers (P) Ltd; 2014. pp. 95-6.
3. Ilknur T, Biçak MU, Demirtaşoğlu M, et al. Glycolic acid peels versus amino fruit acid peels in the treatment of melasma. Dermatol Surg. 2010;36(4):490-5.

24 CHAPTER

Ferulac Peel

Aarti Sarda, Abhishek De

INTRODUCTION

With the market flooded with various combination peels, it becomes difficult to decide which new peel to incorporate in your practice to give maximum benefit to the patients. Since, all peeling agents ranging from superficial to medium depth to deep are derived from basic chemicals known to cause exfoliation, destruction and/or inflammation of skin in a controlled manner. The clinician must know what is new and better about the product.[1]

Ferulac peel is one of the latest liposomal peels which claims to have good results in photoaging and pigmentation. It is an antioxidant rich, superficial peel which provides multiple benefits with no irritation. Also, it is extremely safe with no risk of hyperpigmentation for any Fitzpatrick skin type.

CHEMISTRY AND CHEMICAL FORMULATIONS USED

Ferulac peel is a superficial chemical peel which contains ferulic acid, phloretin, fruit acids and retinoids. Ferulic acid (4-hydroxy-3-methoxycinnamic acid, FA) was isolated from *Ferula foetida* and thus its name was based on the botanical name of plant.[2] The structure of ferulic acid is shown in fig. 1. Ferulic acid is commonly found in commelinid plants, grasses, grains, vegetables, flowers, fruits, leaves, beans, seeds of coffee, peanuts and nuts.[3-8] Cell walls (1.4% of dry weight) of cereal grains and a variety of food contains extractable amount of FA, mostly in the trans-isomeric form which is esterified with the specific polysaccharides.[9-13]

Like several other phenols, FA has strong antioxidant activity in response to free radicals. The antioxidant activity is via donating one hydrogen atom from its phenolic hydroxyl group. Ferulac peel also shows strong anti-inflammatory activity.[14-15]

Ferulic acid is a strong ultraviolet (UV) rays absorber[15], and skin absorbs it at the same rate at acidic and neutral pH.[14] It gives a considerable protection to the skin against UVB-induced erythema in a time dependent manner. Thus, also increases protection

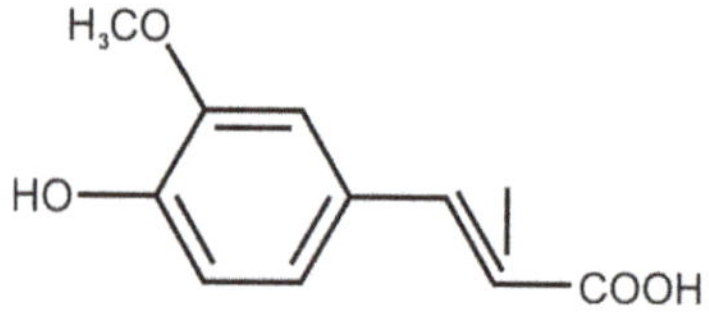

FIG. 1: Ferulic acid, a phenol derivative.

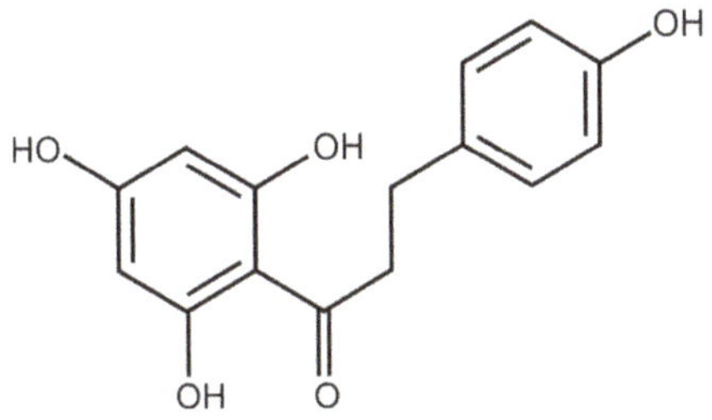

Ferulac Peel

FIG. 2: Phloretin.

against UV radiation. Ferulic acid alone or along with vitamin E and vitamin C provides protection against solar-simulated radiation damage. Ferulic acid structure is similar to tyrosine, and as it is a noncompetitive inhibitor of tyrosinase, it has depigmenting properties.[15]

Phloretin is a flavonoid found exclusively in apples and in apple-derived products, wherein it is present in the glucosidic form, namely, phloridzin (phloretin 2'-O-glucose). The structure of phloretin is shown in fig. 2. Phloretin, is also a powerful antioxidant which interacts with lipids of the stratum corneum, helping in better penetration of the peels and other active ingredients. In addition, phloretin inhibits matrix metalloproteinase-1, thereby decreasing the degradation of collagen and elastin.[16-19] The fruit acids, namely, malic, citric and lactic acids contribute to exfoliation properties; further enhance penetration of the ferulac peel's other active ingredients; and help in synergy between the ferulic acid and phloretin. The retinol gives antiaging and antiacne effects.

All of the ingredients in the Ferulac peel are encapsulated in nanosomes, tiny vesicles measuring 50-200 nm that are completely assimilable by the body. They are similar in composition and structure to that of cell membranes. The nanosomes themselves have resurfacing, anti-inflammatory, antibacterial, clarifying and sebum regulating properties; and given their size, are capable of selectively transporting the active ingredients to the appropriate layers of skin. They allow controlled release of the embedded active ingredients, which enhances their effects. Nanosomes also protect the embedded ingredients, bringing greater stability to the formulation. Finally, given their level of penetration and controlled release, smaller amounts of active ingredients can be used compared with other peel treatments, which reduces toxicity and other side effects.

FORMULATION

Ferulac peel works in a two-step system.

Step 1: Ferulac classic is comprised of high strength ferulic acid (12%) and phloretin (5%). Ferulac plus is comprised of a lower strength of ferulic acid (8%) and the same amount of phloretin (5%) plus a mix of fruit acids (5%) including malic, citric and lactic acid plus retinol (0.25-0.50%).

Step 2: A mix of liposomes of ferulic acid and phloretin, nicotinamide, azelaic acid, retinol, zinc and ceramides are presented as the Ferulac nanoadditive.

INDICATIONS

The main indication of this peel is photoaging with benefits in melasma, acne and rosacea. It is able to reduce signs of photoaging such as fine wrinkles, promote even skin tone by reducing hyperpigmentation, and return skin to its natural brightness by stimulating cell replacement. Overall skin texture is said to improve, and the treatment boosts hydration by increasing the level of ceramides in the skin to help prevent water loss. For patients with rosacea and acne, the treatment can reduce sebum production, improve the appearance of scars and diminish pore size. This peel is also indicated as a preparation for other aesthetic procedures.

CONTRAINDICATIONS[20-25]

- Active infection/open wound/dermatitis
- Sunburn or recent suntan
- Impaired healing
- Excessively dry skin
- Unrealistic patient expectations
- Pregancy/lactation
- Body dysmorphic disorder.

PATIENT PREPARATION[22,26,27]

Detailed history and cutaneous examination should be performed in all patients prior to chemical peeling. Note the patient's Fitzpatrick skin type, Glogau score, skin thickness, dryness, acne, scars, pigmentation, and vascular and pigmented lesions. Assessment of patient expectations at the time of consultation and commitment to a series of treatment is essential to ensure success with treatment. Obtain an informed consent. Standardized photographs should be taken of all areas to be peeled, preferably full face, frontal and lateral areas.

Priming with topical retinoids should be started 2-6 weeks prior to the peel. This thins the stratum corneum, increasing uniform penetration and depth of peel and enhances epidermal turnover. It also decreases the content of epidermal melanin and expedites healing. Retinoids should be stopped 2 days prior to peeling.

EQUIPMENT REQUIRED FOR PEEL

- Prepeel cleanser
- Head band or surgical cap
- Degreasing lotion
- Applicators—cotton tipped, brushes and gauze sponges
- Petroleum jelly
- Gloves
- Saline eyewash
- Timer
- Face towels
- Cotton
- Chemical peel
- Dispensing cups
- Moisturizer/sunscreen.

PEEL TECHNIQUE

The patient should be comfortably placed in supine position. Apply a head band to pull hair away from the face and drape a towel on the neck. Set all the products required. After the skin is cleaned and degreased and a suitable protectant is applied to sensitive areas, 2-3 coats of Ferulac Peel Classic solution are massaged into the skin. Application of peel may be started from the forehead followed by cheeks, chin, nose and upper lip.

When the solution has dried, appearing as a light white mask, two coats of Ferulac Peel Plus solution are applied, massaged between each coat, and allowed to dry. Ferulac peel does not need neutralization. The system is completed with high strength liposomal retinol (Figs. 3-7).

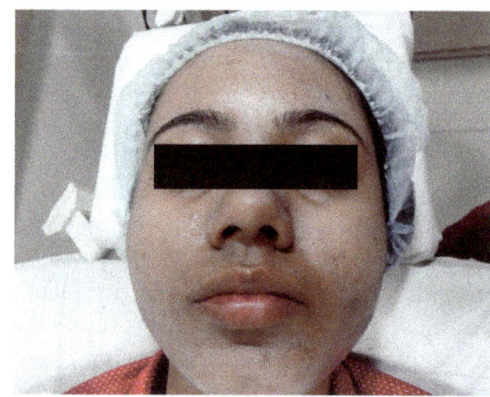

FIG. 3: Light white mask formed after application of ferulac peel.

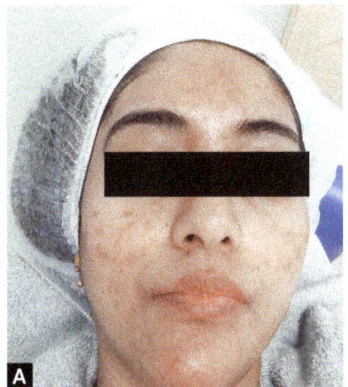 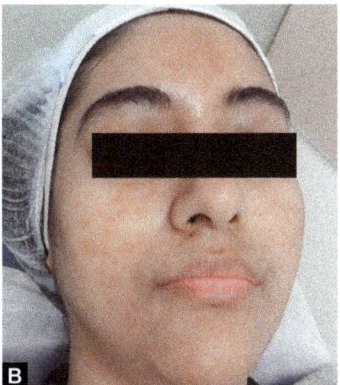

FIG. 4: **A,** Before; **B,** After one session of ferulac peel.

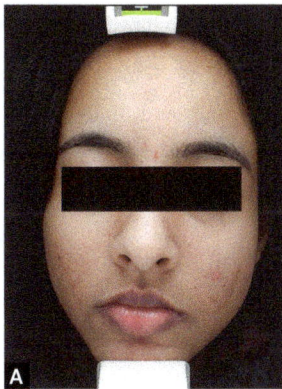 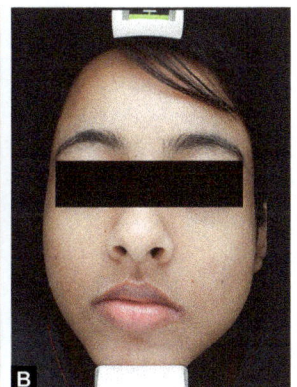

FIG. 5: **A,** Before; **B,** After one session of ferulac peel.

POSTPEEL CARE

After approximately 12 hours, the patient can wash the area with a mild cleansing gel. Patients should not expose treated skin to the sun or high temperatures for 3–7 days after the treatment. The procedure can be done every 15 days, and series of 6–12 treatments typically produce the best results.

COMPLICATIONS[28,29]

Complications are rare after Ferulac peel. There may be mild discomfort or excessive dryness after the peel.

PRACTICAL TIPS

If the patient is on topical or oral retinoids, the number of coats should be reduced to two, the time between peeling treatments should be extended to 15–30 days, and sealing with retinol should be avoided to prevent increased dryness.

Ferulac peel can be used in sequential peel with other superficial peels, such as glycolic, lactic and arginine, once they are neutralized.

CONCLUSION

Ferulac peel system is a safe peel system. Ferulac peel is one of the peel which can be

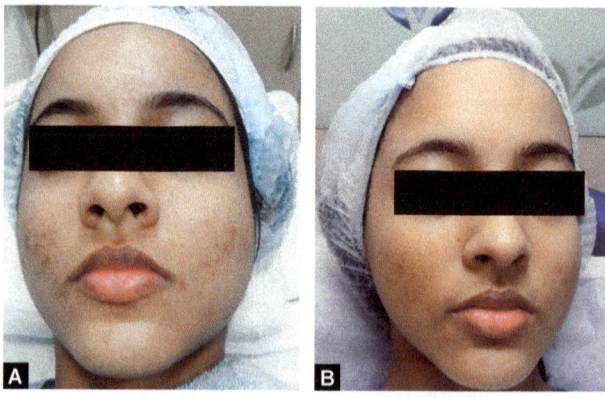

FIG. 6: **A,** Before; **B,** After one session of ferulac peel.

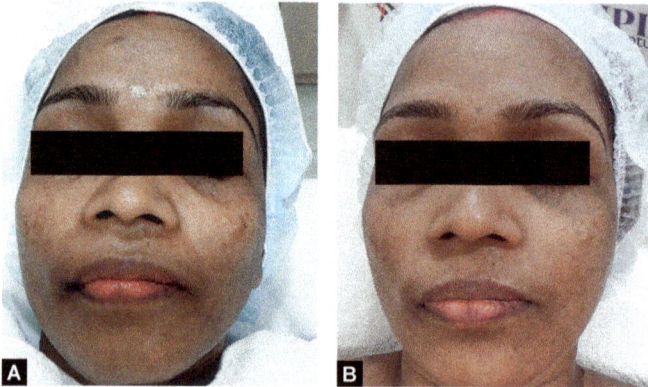

FIG. 7: **A,** Before; **B,** After one session of ferulac peel.

used in all seasons and with all skin types and races. Even with the first treatment, patients report that their skin feels smoother and looks lighter with a glow. Ferulac is a safe peel which does not produce burning or itching during application. The markedly noticeable results in the skin color improvement, make this peel one of the most valuable and beneficial products.

TAKE HOME POINTS

- Ferulac peel is a safe peel with no risk of hyperpigmentation for any Fitzpatrick skin type
- Ferulic acid has anti-inflammatory properties and enhances the antioxidant properties of vitamin C and E
- It can be used as a sequential peel.

REFERENCES

1. Monheit GD. Chemical peels. Skin Therapy Lett. 2004;9(2):6-11.
2. Guo T, Sun Y, Sui Y, et al. Determination of ferulic acid and adenosine in Angelicae Radix by micellar electrokinetic chromatography. Anal Bioanal Chem. 2003;375(6):840-3.
3. Bourne LC, Rice-Evans C. Bioavailability of ferulic acid. Biochem Biophys Res Commun. 1998;253(2):222-7.
4. Mattila P, Hellstrom J. Phenolic acids in potatoes, vegetables, and some of their products. Journal of Food Composition and Analysis. 2007;20:152-60.

5. Mattila P, Hellstrom J, Torronen R. Phenolic acids in berries, fruits, and beverages. J Agric Food Chem. 2006;54(19):7193-9.
6. Mattila P, Pihlava JM, Hellstrom J. Contents of phenolic acids, alkyl-and alkenylresorcinols, and avenanthramides in commercial grain products. J Agric Food Chem. 2005;53(21):8290-5.
7. Srinivasan M, Sudheer AR, Menon VP. Ferulic acid: Therapeutic potential through its antioxidant property. J Clin Biochem Nutr. 2007;40(2):92-100.
8. Sudheer AR, Muthukumaran S, Kalpana C, et al. Protective effect of ferulic acid on nicotine-induced DNA damage and cellular changes in cultured rat peripheral blood lymphocytes: a comparison with N-acetylcysteine. Toxicol In Vitro. 2007;21(4):576-85.
9. Tilay A, Bule M, Kishenkumar J, et al. Preparation of ferulic acid from agricultural wastes: Its improved extraction and purification. J Agric Food Chem. 2008;56:7644-8.
10. Wong DW, Chan VJ, Batt SB, Sarath G, Liao H. Engineering Saccharomyces cerevisiae to produce feruloyl esterase for the release of ferulic acid from switchgrass. J Ind Microbiol Biotechnol. 2011;38(12):1961-7.
11. Harris PJ, Hartley RD. Phenolic constituents of the cell walls of monocotyledons. Biochemical Systematics and Ecology. 1980;8(2):153-60.
12. Hartley RD, Harris PJ. Phenolic constituents of the cell walls of dicotyledons. Biochemical Systematics and Ecology. 1981;9:189-203.
13. Carpita NC. Structure and biogenesis of the cell walls of grasses. Annu Rev Plant Physiol Plant Mol Biol. 1996;47:445-76.
14. Graf E. Antioxidant potential of ferulic acid. Free Radic Biol Med. 1992;13(4):435-48.
15. Saija A, Tomaino A, Trombetta D, et al. In vitro and in vivo evaluation of caffeic and ferulic acids as topical photoprotective agents. Int J Pharm. 2000;199(1):39-47.
16. Barreca D, Bellocco E, Laganà G, et al. Biochemical and antimicrobial activity of phloretin and its glycosilated derivatives present in apple and kumquat. Food Chem. 2014;160:292 7.
17. Crespy V, Aprikian O, Morand C, et al. Biovailability of phloretin and phloridzin in rats. J Nutr. 2001;131(12):3227-30.
18. Crespy V, Morand C, Besson C, et al. Comparision of the intestinal absorption of quercetin, phloretin and their glucosides in rats. J Nutr. 2001;131(8):2109-14.
19. Rezk BM, Haenen GR, van der Vijgh WJ, et al. The antioxidant activity of phloretin: The disclosure of a new antioxidant pharmacophore in flavonoids. Biochem Biophys Res Commun. 2002;295(1):9-13.
20. Grimes PE. Salicylic acid. In: Antonella T, Grimes PE, De Padova MP (editors). Color Atlas of Chemical Peels. 2nd edition. Springer; 2012. p. 49-57.
21. Kinsley M, Metelitsa AI, Somani AK. Chemical peels. In: Wolverton SE, editor. Comprehensive Dermatologic Drug Therapy. 3rd edn. New York, NY, USA: Elsevier Saunders; 2013.
22. Small R, O'Hanlon K. Chemical peels. In: P fenniger U, Small S. Dermatologic and cosmetic proedures in office practice, Saunders: 2012. p. 259-73.
23. Small R. Aesthetic procedures in office practice. Am Fam Physician. 2009;80(11):1231-7.
24. Baumann L, Saghari S. Chemical peels. In: Baumann L. Cosmetic Dermatology: Principles and Practice. 2nd edition. McGraw Hill; 2009. p. 148-62.
25. Paula E, Angela J. Chemexfoliation and superficial skin resurfacing. In: Burgress CM. Cosmetic Dermatology. Springer; 2005. p. 63-82.
26. Monheit GD, Chastian MA. Chemical and mechanical skin resurfacing. In: Bolognia JL, Jorizzo JL, Rapini RP, editors. Dermatology. Philadelphia, PA, USA: Mosby; 2003.
27. Khunger N. Standard guidelines of care for chemical peels. Indian J Dermatol Venereol Leprol. 2008;74,Suppl S1:5-12.
28. Nikalji N, Godse K, Sakhiya J, et al. Complications of medium depth and deep chemical peels. J Cutan Aesthet Surg. 2012;5(4):254-60.
29. Anitha B. Prevention of complications in chemical peeling. J Cutan Aesthet Surg. 2010;3(3):186-8.

25

Combination Peels

Rashmi Sarkar, Zubin K Mandlewala

INTRODUCTION

A combination peel is a single formulation comprising of relatively lower concentrations of multiple chemical agents acting synergistically so as to increase the overall efficacy of the peel and further reducing the chances of overt side effects. The principle of skin peeling is to produce a controlled chemical destruction of the skin at indication-dependent depths so as to cause favorable resurfacing or rejuvenation of the skin. With a wide range of action, favorable safety profile and ease of application, combination peels have cemented their place in every dermatologist's office.

SPECIAL CONSIDERATIONS

- Depending on the Fitzpatrick skin type and hydration patterns, the treatment protocol can accordingly be modified with regards to exposure times with a particular combination peel
- Dark-skinned patients (Fitzpatrick skin types IV–VI) are more at a risk of pigmentary changes with applications of combination peels with higher concentrations of individual agents than are light-skinned patients
- If patients present with a poor skin condition, such as low hydration, transepidermal water loss (TEWL), pigmentary problems and damaged blood vessels, then avoid most peels, but use creams for boosting skin structure, repair processes, priming and preparation, regardless of skin type. Then, an appropriate sequence of peels may be considered, interspersed with creams and serums to boost their response but also to limit complication development, such as postinflammatory hyperpigmentation[1]
- Water is essential for movement through the skin; therefore, skin with poor hydration is more likely to react to the acid component of the peel (hydrogen ions). Thus, the localized damage to the surface is more irritating and more likely to lead to complications. This is because poor hydration causes less mobility for the hydrogen ions[2]
- The periorbital skin is much thinner than the rest of the face; hence, this needs to be taken into consideration. The type of agent used can be similar to other facial areas, but the strength and surface activity needs to be lower. Phenols and high strength trichloroacetic acids (TCAs) or pyruvic acid would not be appropriate. Lower concentrations of glycolic-based combination peels (e.g., also containing lactic acid, arbutin,

kojic and arginine) may be desired in such areas. The number of layers used would vary depending on the patient's skin type and sensitivity.[1] The peels in the periorbital area are likely to settle in the wrinkle furrows; hence, it is prudent to have an assistant stretch the skin throughout the procedure
- Most combination peels are relatively safe in nonfacial areas (e.g., arms, axillae, back, etc.), as they contain lower concentrations of individual agents. Yet caution must be exercised, as applying peels to a larger body surface area is not totally devoid to systemic effects (e.g., higher concentration of phenol-based combinations)
- Even the technique of application (e.g., rubbing vs. painting), peel base (e.g., gel vs. solution) and vigorous degreasing are all thought to affect penetration patterns of combination peels.

COMMON FORMULATIONS

Combination peels have multiple agents with wide range of actions; hence, each constituent should be assessed in terms of its properties and end effects (Table 1). Some common formulations include:
- 14% salicylic acid, 14% lactic acid and 14% resorcinol (Jessner's peel)
  - Indications: Acne, dyschromias, seborrhea, fine lines and wrinkles, dilated pores and hyperkeratotic conditions
- 20% salicylic acid and 10% mandelic acid (Vedasol SM gel peel, Cipla)
  - Indications: Inflammatory and non-inflammatory acne, postinflammatory and postacne hyperpigmentation, melasma
- 33% glycolic acid, 9% lactic acid, 7% kojic acid, 5% citric acid and 3% salicylic acid (Sesglicopeel K gel peel, Sesderma)
  - Indications: Inflammatory and non-inflammatory acne, acne scars, rosacea, postinflammatory or postacne hyperpigmentation, melasma
- 18% salicylic acid, 15% azelaic acid and 10% mandelic acid (Azelac M peel, Sesderma)
  - Indications: Inflammatory and non-inflammatory acne, hyperpigmentary conditions, rosacea and photoaging
- Salicylic acid, black acetic acid, potassium iodide and jasmonic acid (Black peel, Aakaar)
  - Indications: All types of acne (especially nodulocystic), acne scars
- 20% lactic acid, 20% arginine, 5% kojic acid, 5% urea, 2% citric acid and 2% arbutin (Claze gel peel, Cipla)
  - Indications: A mild peel suggested for periorbital hypermelanosis and lip hyperpigmentation
- 20% azelaic acid, 10% resorcinol and 6% phytic acid (Melanostop peel, Mesoestetic)
  - Indications: All types of acne, rosacea and hyperpigmentary conditions
- 40% pyruvic acid and 10% lactic acid (Piruvex peel, Mesoestetic)
  - Indications: Acne, actinic and fine seborrheic keratosis, fine and deep wrinkles
- 4% retinol, 1% retinyl propionate- sachet with 10% ascorbyl glucoside and 5% niacinamide–ampoule (Retises CT yellow peel, Sesderma)
  - Indications: Acne, superficial acne scars, photoaging and hyperpigmentary conditions
- 15% TCA, 8% phenol, glycolic acid, ascorbic acid, salicylic acid, mandelic acid and retinoic acid (Nomelan fenol light peel, Sesderma)
  - Indications: All types of acne, acne scars, hyperpigmentary conditions and photoaging.

TABLE 1: Active ingredients used in peels with their properties and effects

Active ingredients	Properties	Effects
Salicylic acid	• Keratolytic • Loosens horny layer increasing penetration of other peels • Comedolytic • Anti-inflammatory • Antimicrobial	• Unblocks comedones • Reduces inflammatory acne • Reduces epidermal pigmentation • Removes excess oil • Softer, thinner skin
Gylcolic acid	• Keratolytic • Anti-inflammatory • Antioxidant	• Acne reduction • Pigment lightening • Textural changes
Mandelic acid	• Keratolytic • Antimicrobial • Sebum-regulating • Bacteriostatic • Depigmenting	• Acne, folliculitis, and rosacea reduction • Pigment lightening
Lactic acid	• Keratolytic • Attracts water to stratum corneum • Stimulates collagen and ceramide synthesis • Inhibits tyrosinase • Sebostatic • Bacteriostatic • Antioxidant	• Natural moisturizing effect • Strengthens skin barrier • Pigment lightening • Improves skin turgor, smoothens skin texture, and reduces fine lines and small wrinkles
Citric acid	• Antioxidant	• Pigment lightening
Azelaic acid	• Comedolytic • Antimicrobial • Anti-inflammatory • Antioxidant • Inhibits tyrosinase	• Acne, folliculitis, and rosacea reduction • Pigment lightening
Pyruvic acid	• Keratolytic • Antimicrobial • Sebostatic • Stimulates collagen synthesis • Converted to lactic acid in the skin	• Acne reduction • Pigment lightening • Scar reduction
Phytic acid	• Antioxidant • Inhibits tyrosinase	• Pigment lightening
Kojic acid	• Inhibits tyrosinase	• Pigment lightening
Retinoic acid	• Keratolytic • Sebostatic • Anti-inflammatory • Stimulates collagen synthesis • Normalizes melanocyte activity	• Acne reduction • Pigment lightening • Correction of photodamage • Reduction of wrinkles • Textural changes

Continued

Continued

Active ingredients	Properties	Effects
Trichloroacetic acid	• Coagulation of epidermal proteins • Keratolytic • Comedolytic • Increases production of collagen and elastin • Antioxidant • Bacteriostatic and bactericidal	• Epidermal destruction • Acne scar reduction • Firms and smoothens skin • Wrinkle reduction • Pigment lightening • Reduces dilated pores
Phenol	• Keratolytic • Anesthetic • Antiseptic	• Acne reduction • Pigment lightening • Correction of photodamage • Wrinkle reduction

COMBINATION PEELS IN ACNE

Patients with acne routinely consult dermatologists to seek treatment with chemical peels, which dictates the increased awareness to such procedures. Combination peels play a major role in comedonal and active inflammatory acne. Furthermore, they are also utilized for postacne hyperpigmentation and erythematous acne scars. Early and judicious use of such peels can really aid in prevention of sequelae such as scarring. 20% salicylic acid with 10% mandelic acid in a gel base (Vedasol-SM peel, Cipla) is a safe combination peel for comedonal and active acne, the end point of which may be very slight erythema (Fig. 1). A second coat can be applied if it is tolerable and such sessions should be repeated every 2-3 weeks till adequate reduction in acne is obtained. Salicylic acid, a beta-hydroxy acid (BHA), is a worthy peeling agent in comedonal acne due to its keratolytic properties and likewise in active acne due to its anti-inflammatory effects. On the other hand, mandelic acid is a safe, mild alpha-hydroxy acid (AHA) that is prepared by the hydrolysis of bitter almond extract. Mandelic acid can be utilized in active acne for its bacteriostatic properties and anti-inflammatory effects. Garg VK, S Sinha and Sarkar R compared the therapeutic efficacy and tolerability of 35% glycolic acid and 20% salicylic + 10% mandelic acid peels in active acne and postacne scarring and hyperpigmentation. In this study, salicylic-mandelic acid combination peels (SMPs) were seen to be significantly better than glycolic acid peels in the treatment of noninflammatory lesions and hypersecretion of sebum. This is because of the unique lipophilic and anti-inflammatory properties of both acids.[2] 15% azelaic acid + 18% salicylic acid + 10% mandelic acid (Azelac M peel, Sesderma) is a suitable option in cases of active acne and erythematous acne scars (Fig. 2).[3] Azelaic acid is a saturated dicarboxylic acid that is naturally found in wheat, rye and barley. It has potent antimicrobial effects against *Propionibacterium acnes*, *Staphylococcus aureus* and *Staphylococcus epidermidis* and has keratolytic and comedolytic properties. It is suggested to be used in postinflammatory hyperpigmentation due to its ability to reduce melanin production by inhibiting tyrosinase. Usually, one coat applied on the full face or spot application on the macular hyperpigmented areas is sufficient; the endpoint being mild erythema, after which a slight pseudofrost is likely to develop. Similarly, the yellow peel (Retises CT yellow

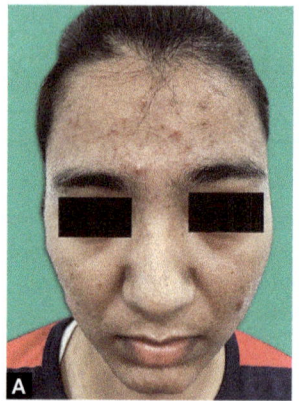
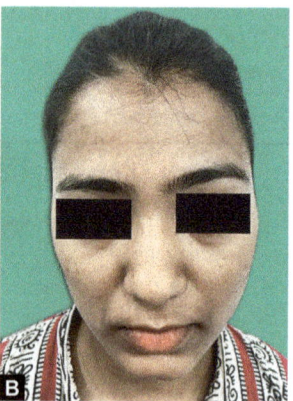

FIG. 1: Inflammatory acne treated with salicylic mandelic acid combination peel (Vedasol-SM peel). **A,** Before treatment; **B,** After 6 sessions done every 2 weeks.

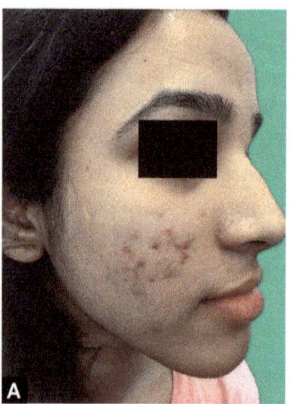
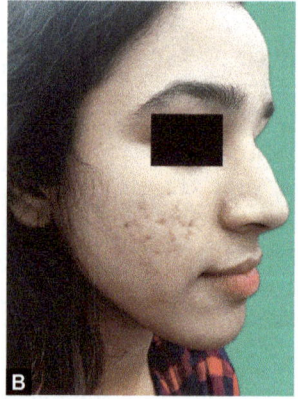
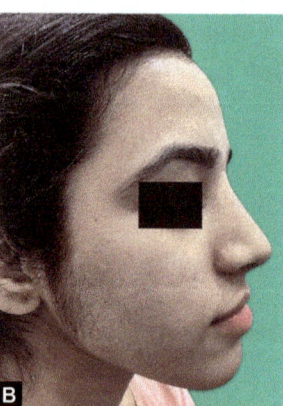

FIG. 2: Erythematous acne scars treated with a combination peel containing azelaic acid, salicylic acid, and mandelic acid (Azelac M peel). **A,** Before treatment; **B,** Reduction of erythema within acne scars after 2 sessions 3 weeks apart; **C,** After a total of 6 sessions.

peel, Sesderma) has had a tremendous fan following by both the patient as well as the dermatologist as it produces good results in inflammatory and comedonal acne along with postacne hyperpigmentation. An ampoule containing 10% ascorbyl glucoside and 5% niacinamide is applied on the full face and/or neck and left for about 5 minutes. Thereafter, a sachet containing 4% retinol and 1% retinyl propionate is adequately massaged on the face and/or neck till a thin transparent layer is visible, without the need to neutralize (Fig. 3). The yellow peel is kept on for about 8 hours (avoiding sun exposure by using sunscreens and physical sun protection) after which it can be washed. The patient is informed that some degree of exfoliation will occur for up to a week starting from the second day post peel.

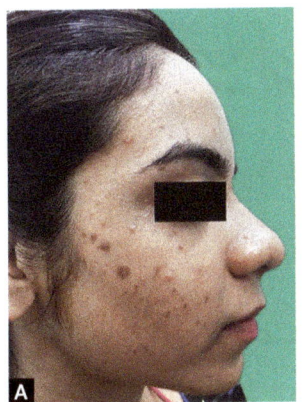
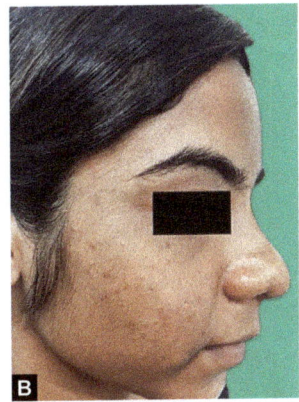

FIG. 3: Inflammatory and comedonal acne with postacne hyperpigmentation treated with yellow peel (Retises CT yellow peel). **A,** Before treatment; **B,** Pigmentary as well as textural changes noted after 3 sessions done at 3-week intervals.

COMBINATION PEELS IN MELASMA

Melasma, an entity considered stubborn by many due to evident recurrences, has also necessitated the application of chemical peels for its concerned hosts. Furthermore, apart from sunlight exacerbation as a plausible cause, other etiopathogenetic factors are complex and difficult to address (e.g., genetic). Considering that out of the two variants (epidermal and dermal or mixed melasma), the dermal or mixed element predominates; it becomes increasingly difficult to devoid the skin of such pigmentation with routine topical therapies. Even the utility of pigment lasers is controversial in melasma and hence, efficacious treatment options are limited. Due to the increasing availability of combination chemical peels, melasma patients are certainly given a ray of hope. The basic mechanism of the action of chemical peels in melasma is the removal of unwanted melanin by causing a controlled chemical burn to the skin.[4] Triple combination creams, if utilized, should be used for only 3–4 weeks at the initiation of therapy after which a combination peel can be done. The authors have used even triple combination therapy in between peels for about 6 weeks or so. After that, preference of non-hydroquinone skin lightening topical therapies must be advocated in between peels to prevent any likelihood of exogenous ochronosis, which is likely with prolonged hydroquinone-based therapies. A combination peel containing 33% glycolic acid, 9% lactic acid, 7% kojic acid, 5% citric acid and 3% salicylic acid (Sesglicopeel K gel, Sesderma) can be utilized every 2–3 weeks for about 6 sessions for melasma (more effective in the epidermal variant); the endpoint of each session being a faint erythema (Fig. 4). As the concentration of glycolic acid in the aforementioned combination peel is 33%, it will act superficially and visible results would be seen over a period of time especially in epidermal melasma. Such a combination is not only safe, but also gives a free hand to use multiple agents at lower concentrations for a better therapeutic effect. Similarly, a combination containing two known tyrosinase inhibitors, namely 20% azelaic acid and 6% phytic acid, along with a carbolic acid—10% resorcinol (Melanostop peel by Mesoestetic) has proven to be effective in reducing epidermal melasma (Fig. 5). Resorcinol, a phenol derivative with relative reduced toxicity,

Chemical Peels: A Global Perspective

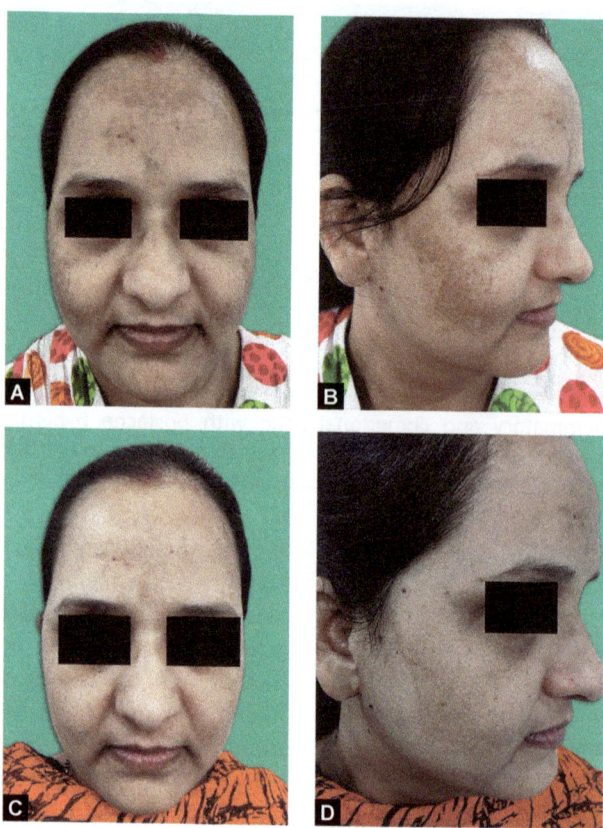

FIG. 4: Centrofacial melasma treated with a combination peel consisting of glycolic acid, lactic acid, kojic acid, citric acid, and salicylic acid (Sesglicopeel K gel). **A,** and **B,** Before treatment; **C** and **D,** Pigment reduction after a total of 6 sessions done at 3-week intervals.

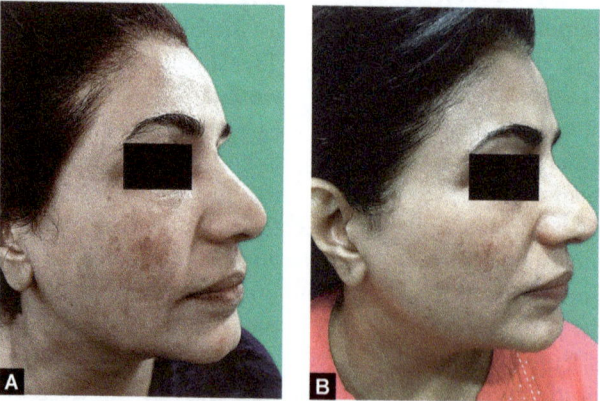

FIG. 5: Malar melasma treated with a combination of azelaic acid, resorcinol, and phytic acid (Melanostop peel). **A,** Before treatment; **B,** Malar pigment reduction and improvement of overall skin tone and texture noted after a total of 3 sessions done at 3-week intervals.

is known to improve skin texture and reduce hyperpigmentation. Melanostop peel should be done roughly every 3 weeks for a total of 6 sessions; the endpoint of each session being a mild erythema.

In a study of twenty female patients with melasma by Safoury et al.,[5] a combination of modified Jessner's solution with 15% TCA was compared with only 15% TCA, and it was found that the result was better on the side of the combination peel. Appropriate care should be taken in skin of color as darker skin is more prone to developing postinflammatory hyperpigmentation, thus aggravating an already dark melasma patch. Priming is important and the choice of the agent(s) varies, but essentially a regular and routine use of SPF 30 and above sunscreen must be advocated.

COMBINATION PEELS IN NONFACIAL AREAS

Conventionally, chemical peels are routinely performed on the face possibly due to its superior cosmetic value. With the availability of safe combination peels having multiple agents, areas such as the arms, back, chest and neck to name a few, are routinely opted for. It must be kept in mind that the density of pilosebaceous glands in the aforementioned body areas is quite less as compared to the face, hence, healing is often delayed thereby increasing the risk of complications. The common indications for which peels are performed in nonfacial areas include: postacne hyperpigmentation, postinflammatory hyperpigmentation, tanning, photoaging, acanthosis nigricans, cutaneous macular amyloidosis and keratosis pilaris. Commonly, patients who recently return from a vacation (e.g., beach-side destinations) wherein increased amount of sun-basking had taken place, present to the dermatologists' requesting treatment for tanned skin, specifically on the arms and forearms. For such tanned skin and also for large areas of postinflammatory hyperpigmentation, a combination peel consisting of: 15% TCA, 8% phenol, glycolic acid, ascorbic acid, salicylic acid, mandelic acid, phytic acid and retinoic acid (Nomelan fenol light peel, Sesderma) has shown to be quite effective (Figs. 6 and 7). As the concentration of phenol is very less in the

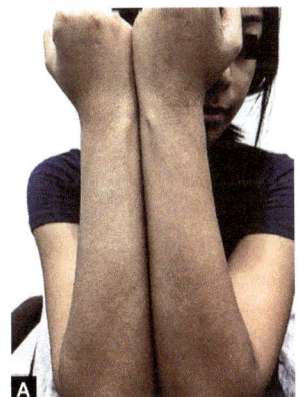 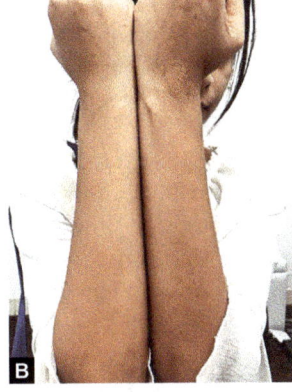

FIG. 6: Sun-tanned skin on forearms treated with a combination peel comprising trichloroacetic acid, phenol, glycolic acid, ascorbic acid, salicylic acid, mandelic acid, phytic acid, and retinoic acid (Nomelan fenol light peel). **A,** Before treatment; **B,** Evident pigment reduction after 3 sessions done at 3-week intervals.

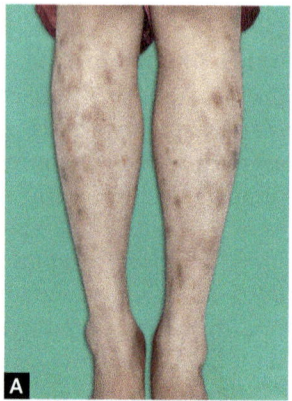 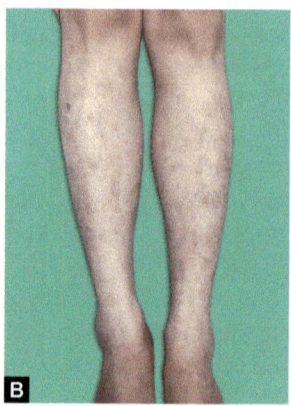

FIG. 7: Postinflammatory hyperpigmentation on legs treated with a combination peel comprising trichloroacetic acid, phenol, glycolic acid, ascorbic acid, salicylic acid, mandelic acid, phytic acid, and retinoic acid (Nomelan fenol light peel). **A,** Before treatment; **B,** Evident pigment reduction after 6 sessions done at 3-week intervals.

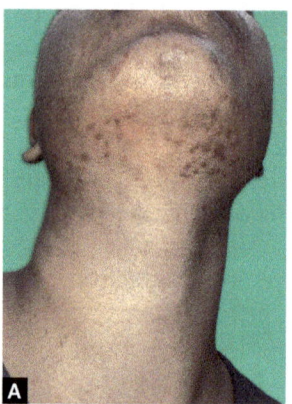 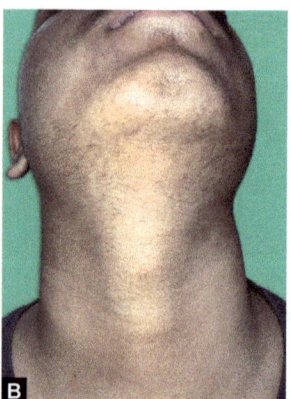

FIG. 8: Folliculitis with postinflammatory hyperpigmentation on the upper neck treated with a combination peel consisting of azelaic acid and salicylic acid (Azelan peel). **A,** Before treatment; **B,** Reduction of folliculitis, acne, and postinflammatory hyperpigmentation after 6 session done at 2-week intervals.

combination, the peel can be done safely for nonfacial areas, although, it should be avoided in patients with dry and sensitive skin. The endpoint of the nomelan fenol light peel is slight erythema with speckled frosting. The same peel can be utilized for cutaneous macular amyloidosis. In a case of folliculitis or inflammatory and comedonal acne with postinflammatory hyperpigmentation at a site like the neck, a combination of 20% azelaic acid with 20% salicylic acid (Azelan peel, Mesoestetic) done every 2–3 weeks for a total of roughly 6 sessions produces desirable results, the end point being mild-to-moderate erythema with slight pseudo frosting (Fig. 8).

PREPEEL PREPARATION

Prior to commencement of any peeling procedure, it is important to take a detailed history and to examine the skin of all patients. In the history, it is of paramount importance to mention occupation, amount of sun exposure and methods used to prevent it, past herpes simplex infection, medication history, immunocompromised states, smoking habit and history of any systemic diseases. Parameters of assessment such as skin type (Fitzpatrick's classification), tone, texture, sebaceous activity, degree of photodamage (Glogau classification) and other signs of aging, preexisting infection or inflammation, and presence of scarring or keloid formation are to be noted precisely. After a thorough examination, it is equally important to gauge and thereby address the patient's concerns, expectations, and likely outcomes of the peeling procedure to be performed. The treating dermatologist should thereafter discuss the procedure in detail by mentioning the merits, duration and the number of sittings, the cost of therapy as well as the potential risks involved. As a combination peel would be advised, due thought and consideration must be given in regards to the effect or side effect profile of individual agents in the preparation. After a mutual agreement, it is important for the treating dermatologist to initiate the therapy by priming the patient, which is typically application of a few topical agents regularly for 2-4 weeks prior in order to prepare the skin for a positive outcome of the peel procedure. Although the choice of the priming agent is governed by the skin condition for which a peel is to be done, in general, some of the more common priming agents include: broad-spectrum sunscreens (SPF >30), topical retinoids (e.g., tretinoin 0.025%), AHAs (e.g., glycolic acid 6% or 12%, lactic acid, mandelic acid), skin lightening agents (e.g., hydroquinone 2% or 4%, kojic acid, arbutin, licorice, etc.) and/or a bland soap-free cleanser for sensitive skin. Benefits of the priming process such as enhanced penetration of the peel, reduction of potential side effects and reduced wound healing time should all be conveyed to the patient. Equally important is for the patient to avoid excessive sun exposure and smoking. Emphasis should also be laid on avoidance of facials, "clean-ups", scrubs, bleaching, oil massages, steam, sauna, certain cosmetics, mechanical trauma, waxing, hair reduction laser and other procedures on the to-be-treated area during the vital priming phase. On an average, 2 days prior to the date of the peel procedure, the patient should be directed to stop the priming agent. Dermatologists are urged to take baseline, postpriming and postpeel photographs in both full-face frontal and lateral views without flash mode. For those patients who have suffered from herpetic infections in the recent past, it is advisable to start oral acyclovir a day prior to the procedure and to continue for about 7-10 days. The dermatologist must re-check that all the materials or equipment are in place and properly working, so as to avoid last minute catastrophes. It is also advisable to do a test patch of the peel in the posterior auricular region about 10 days prior to the procedure (especially for TCA-based combination peels). On the day of the peeling procedure, the skin is again examined thoroughly to view the changes after the priming phase. This is a stage when the initial choice of a particular preparation may be replaced with a more suitable one due to various changes in the skin encountered thereof (e.g., if a patient with baseline oily skin has become extremely dry post priming, then it is better to defer the initial choice of peels containing combinations of glycolic acid, salicylic acid, TCA and/or phenol). The patient prior to the therapy must sign an informed consent.

POSTPEELING CARE

Legible written instructions must be handed over to the patient following the peel procedure. With most combination peels, erythema and desquamation are common postpeel events which are encountered and which may last up to 10 days. The advice given varies with regard to the individual agents in the formulation. For example, if one of the agents in the formulation contains TCA (15%), the patient is informed that some amount of redness, burning and swelling may be experienced and the skin may become very dry and "flaky" and may even feel tight and stretchy. Bland moisturizers along with routine and regular use of broad-spectrum sunscreens (SPF >30) must be advocated in order to avoid any sun-based inflammation. In some instances, wherein there is significant erythema and edema, topical corticosteroids (e.g., Desonide 1% cream) can be prescribed for a few days. Although a neglected option by many, an umbrella and/or a wide-brimmed hat ideally should be used as a means of physical sun protection. Bathing bars should ideally be avoided for the first 48 hours post peel. Furthermore, as mentioned previously, smoking, facials, "clean-ups", scrubs, bleaching, oil massages, steam, sauna, certain cosmetics, mechanical trauma, waxing and other procedures are to be strictly avoided in the postpeel period. Once the expected degree of exfoliation has completed, the patient can resume use of topical skin care formulations, including the initial priming agents. Apart from dryness, there is a chance of development of postinflammatory hyperpigmentation. However, any hyperpigmentation remaining after the peeling procedure responds to topical hydroquinone and frequent use of sunscreens.

CONCLUSION

Combination peels by their mere synergistic and versatile nature have given dermatologists a free hand to use multiple agents at lower concentrations for a variety of indications, thereby minimizing adverse events.

TAKE HOME POINTS

- Combination peels give leverage to utilize multiple agents; hence, wider range of indications is covered
- The various agents in the peel act synergistically and gel formulations are relatively the safest to use on the face
- Reduced occurrence of adverse events as compared to higher concentration of mono peels
- Salicylic mandelic acid combination peels are preferred for inflammatory and noninflammatory acne and postacne hyperpigmentation also
- Azelaic acid based combinations play a great role in reducing erythematous acne scars and can also be utilized in epidermal melasma
- A combination of alpha (e.g., glycolic and citric acids) and BHAs (e.g., salicylic acid) along with skin lightening agents (e.g., kojic acid) in various concentrations has shown desirable results in melasma
- Trichloroacetic acid and phenol (low concentration)-based combinations are effective in tanned skin and cutaneous macular amyloidosis in nonfacial areas.

REFERENCES

1. Roberts P. Aesthetics [Internet]. Chemical Peeling; 2017 Feb 13 [cited 2017 April]. Available from: https://aestheticsjournal.com/feature/chemical-peeling.
2. Chemistry LibreTexts [Internet]. The Hydonium Ion; 2017 Oct 9 [cited 2018 July 12]. Available from: http://chem.libretexts.org/Core/Physical_and_Theoretical_Chemistry/Acids_and_Bases/Aqueous_Solutions/The_Hydronium_Ion
3. Wójcik A, Kubiak M, Rotsztejn H. Influence of azelaic and mandelic acid peels on sebum secretion in ageing women. Postepy Dermatol Alergol. 2013;30(3): 140-5.
4. Sarkar R, Bansal S, Garg VK. Chemical Peels for Melasma in Dark-Skinned Patients. J Cut Aesth Surg. 2012;5(4):247-53.
5. Safoury OS, Zaki NM, El Nabarawy EA, et al. A study comparing chemical peeling using modified Jessner's solution and 15% trichloroacetic Acid versus 15% trichloroacetic acid in the treatment of melasma. Indian J Dermatol. 2009;54:41-5.

26 CHAPTER

Proprietary Peels

Mukta Sachdev, Rachana Shilpakar

INTRODUCTION[1]

Chemical peeling is the application of a chemical agent to the skin which causes controlled destruction of a part of or the entire epidermis, with or without the dermis, leading to exfoliation, and removal of superficial lesions, followed by regeneration of new epidermal and dermal tissues. This is one of the commonest office procedures carried out in a dermatological office practice. The broad indications for a chemical peeling include pigmentary disorders, acne and superficial acne scars, aesthetic purposes, and benign epidermal skin growths. Various peeling agents are available in different formulations and compositions to achieve the maximum benefits without any side effects, while the lists of the agents are increasing with each day.

CLASSIFICATION OF PEELING AGENTS[1,2]

Histological Classification of Peels (Table 1)[1-3]

- The higher the concentration, the greater is the depth of penetration
- The concentration of the peeling agent can vary between various brands and formulations, although the label indicates the same concentration
- The pKa of solution, the pH at which half is in acid form, is the more accurate determinant of strength of the peeling agent
- The more the skin contact time of agent, the greater is the depth of penetration of the peel in alpha-hydroxy acid (AHA) peels
- Rubbing the peel into the skin achieves a greater depth than painting it with a brush
- The more the coat application in Jessner's solution, the greater the depth achieved
- The degree of frosting in salicylic acid indicates the depth of the peel reached.

Based on Ingredients[1,2]

- *Alpha-hydroxy acids and monocarboxylic acids:* Glycolic acid 35–70%, lactic acid 10–90%, mandelic acid 30–50%, tartaric acid, malic acid and phytic acid
- *Beta-hydroxy acids:* Salicylic acid 20–50%, citric acid 20–70%
- Trichloroacetic acid (TCA) 10–35%
- *Alpha ketoacids*: Pyruvic acid 40–70%
- Retinoic acid 1–5%, retinol
- Resorcinol
- Phenol 88%

Proprietary Peels

TABLE 1: Histological classification of peels and their agents

Types of peel	Histological level	Agents
Very superficial light peels	Necrosis up to the level of stratum corneum	• TCA 10% • GA 30–50% • Salicylic acid 20–30% • Jessner's solution 1–3 coats • Tretinoin 1–5%
Superficial light peels	Necrosis through the entire epidermis up to basal layer	• TCA 10–30% • GA 50–70% • Jessner's solution 4–7 coats
Medium-depth peels	Necrosis upto papillary dermis	• TCA 35–50% • GA 70% plus TCA 35% • 88% phenol unoccluded • Jessner's solution plus TCA 35% • Solid CO_2 plus TCA 35%
Deep peels	Necrosis up to mid-reticular dermis	• Baker–Gordon phenol peel • Phenol 88%

TCA, trichloroacetic acid; GA, glycolic acid.

- Combination peels like:
  - Jessner's solution (Lactic acid 14 g, salicylic acid 14 g and resorcinol 14 g)
  - Modified Jessner's solutions
  - Brody's peel (Solid CO_2 combined with 35% TCA)
  - Coleman's peel (Glycolic acid 70% with TCA 35%)
  - Monheit's peel (Jessner's solution with 35% TCA).

NEWER PEELS

The newer peels are introduced to achieve better outcome with no downtime and with minimal side effects. These agents are gentler, with lower concentrations, available singly as well as in combinations. Many have added antioxidants and humectants to make them potent, with improved tolerance and less-irritant potential. The list of the newer peeling agents used regularly in dermatological aesthetic practice is given in box 1.

BOX 1 Newer peeling agents[4]

- Lactic acid
- Mandelic acid
- Azelaic acid
- Pyruvic acid
- Ferulic acid
- Phytic acid
- Arginine
- Retinoic acid
- Polyhydroxy acid
- Citric acid
- Enzyme peels
- Obagi blue peels
- Black peels
- Dermamelan peel
- Cosmelan peel
- Milk peel
- Mela peel
- Mela peel forte
- Cosmo peel
- Mask peel
- Bio C

Indications of Chemical Peels[1]

Pigmentary Disorders

- Melasma
- Postinflammatory hyperpigmentation
- Freckles
- Lentigines
- Facial melanosis.

Acne
- Superficial acne scars
- Postacne pigmentation
- Comedonal acne
- Acne excoriee
- Mild-to-moderate acne vulgaris.

Aesthetic
- Photoaging
- Fine superficial lines
- Dilated pores
- Superficial scars.

Epidermal Growths
- Seborrheic keratoses
- Actinic keratoses
- Xanthelasma
- Warts
- Milia
- Sebaceous hyperplasia
- Dermatoses papulosa nigra.

Contraindications of Peels
- Active bacterial, viral (herpetic) and fungal infection
- Open wound
- Pre-existing active inflammatory dermatoses like atopic dermatitis, psoriasis
- History of drugs with photosensitizing potential
- Patient with unrealistic expectation, body dysmorphic disorder
- History of hypertrophic scars, keloidal tendency, atrophic skin, isotretinoin use in last 6 months for medium-depth and deep peels.

Prepeel Preparation (Priming)
- Priming of skin should be started 2–4 weeks prior to the procedure
- Priming helps to accelerate healing, assist in uniform application of the peel, enhance penetration and reduce risk of complications. It also decreases the incidence of postinflammatory hyperpigmentation (PIH) in dark skins
- It reinforces compliance of the patient in sun protection and application of topical agents to maintain results of the peel
- A standardized priming regimen helps to maintain and compare results
- Priming agents are
  - Broad-spectrum sunscreen
  - Tretinoin 0.025–0.05%, adapalene 1%, glycolic acid 6–12%, kojic acid, azelaic acid, arbutin, licorice and hydroquinone 2–4%.
- Priming agents should be stopped at least 3 days prior to procedure
- Avoid laser hair removal, electrolysis, waxing and the use of depilatory creams for 5–7 days prior to peel
- Avoid having the peel until skin has completely healed from any procedures, such as intense pulsed light (IPL), laser or microdermabrasion.

Peel Procedure in General[1]
- The patient lies on the bed or the procedure chair preferably with head elevated at 45° and eyes closed
- The hair is secured with the hairband and ear with the cotton
- The skin is cleaned with alcohol and then degreased with acetone
- The sensitive areas—inner and outer canthi of eyes, nasolabial folds, and around lip margins—are protected with Vaseline
- The suitable peeling agent is taken in a cup and applied with the brush or cotton-tipped applicator or gauze
- The peel is quickly applied as cosmetic units on the entire face—the forehead, right cheek, nose, left cheek and chin. Perioral,

lower and upper eyelids, if required, are treated last. Feathering strokes are applied at the edges to blend with the surrounding skin and prevent demarcation lines
- Neutralization is done for glycolic acid peel after around 3 minutes or immediately if erythema, epidermolysis occurs using 10–15% sodium bicarbonate. For TCA peels, neutralization is done with a neutralizing agent or cold water after frosting appears. For salicylic acid peel, it is washed with cold water after a pseudofrost appears
- The skin is then cleansed with wet cotton or gauze until irritation disappears
- The skin can be soothened with spring water spray, applied the hydrating mask (optional)
- Then a moisturizer and sunscreen is applied.

Postpeel Care

- A good postpeel care prevents or minimizes complications and ensures early recovery
- Mild soap or a nonsoap cleanser may be used daily for cleansing
- Regular use of moisturizer and sunscreen should be emphasized
- Scratching, scrubbing and use of products with active ingredients should be avoided for couple of days post peeling.

PROPRIETARY PEELS

Obagi Blue Peel[4]

It consists of a fixed concentration of TCA with the a company-designed proprietary blue peel base (containing glycerin, saponins and a nonionic blue color base) which gives a bluish tint to the skin after the procedure is complete and remains on the skin for 12–24 hours. The blue base causes a reduction in the surface tension of TCA ensuring a slow and more uniform penetration of TCA.

Obagi ZE et al. in their study have noted an unexpected benefit of appearance of skin tightening and a reduction of skin laxity in many cases.[5] Hong P et al. have observed a significant improvement in melasma lesions after 4 weeks of therapy with no difference between 1550-nm fractional erbium laser and Obagi blue peel treated sides.[6]

ZO® Medical 3-Step Peel™ (By ZO Skin Health, Inc.)

- Multifunction treatment designed to provide long-lasting results
- *Improves*:
  - Acne
  - Melasma
  - Sun damage
  - Fine lines
  - Rough or dull texture
  - Large pores.
- Suitable for any skin type or color
- Quick and easy to perform
- Usage studies show remarkable safety with minimal burning and stinging
- Minimal or no downtime
- Can be repeated every 3–4 weeks.

Three Steps Designed

Step 1: Peel Solution

To remove the outermost layers of skin (Table 2).

TABLE 2: Functions of different peeling ingredients

Ingredients	Function
17% SA, 10% TCA, 5% LA	Exfoliating, peeling agents
Glycerin	Hydrator, moisture replenisher
Saponins	Anti-irritant

TCA, trichloroacetic acid; SA, salicylic acid; LA, lactic acid.

Step 2: Retinol Crème

To stimulate deeper skin layers for more profound benefits, increasing cellular function
- 6% retinol for collagen regulation, firming and wrinkle reduction
- CoQ10 for cellular renewal stimulation
- Marrubium vulgare and Leontopodium alpinum meristem cell culture for antioxidant and ant-irritant benefits
- Beta-glucan for DNA protection and antioxidant benefits
- *Myristoyl tripeptide-4:* A collagen-boosting peptide for firming and wrinkle reduction.

Step 3: Calming Crème— Postprocedure Skin Relief

To suppress skin inflammation that can be caused by peels, sun, hormones and pollution postprocedure.
- Hydrolyzed sericin works as biomimetic stimulant and upregulates hyaluronan (HA) and collagen
- Buddleja Davidii meristem cell culture is a powerful antioxidant with outstanding anti-irritant properties
- Ceramide 2 works to replenish natural skin moisture and improves the barrier function
- Myristoyl tripeptide-4 is a collagen-boosting peptide used for firming and wrinkle reduction
- Cholecalciferol is an immune function "booster"—vitamin D3 precursor.

Professional Protocol Given by Company

Peeling at Office

Step 1: Peeling

Peel solution: Shake well before use. Apply peel solution evenly using the provided nonwoven pads. You may see some frosting in certain areas. Apply gradually with gentle painting action, avoid dripping and avoid the eye area. The peeling step is complete when the entire solution (8 mL) is applied.

Step 2: Stimulation—Part 1

Retinol Crème: Tear the two packets apart. Apply 1 packet of the Retinol Crème to the treated area. Give the patient the second retinol crème packet to take home and apply no sooner than 5 hours postpeel procedure.

Step 3: Hydrating and anti-inflammation—Part 1

Calming Crème postprocedure skin relief: Apply a thin layer of the Calming Crème after the first application of the Retinol Crème. Give the patient the remainder of the product to take home. The patient should avoid washing their face for at least 5 hours, preferably, the next morning postpeel procedure.

Postpeel Care

The day after the peel:

Step 1: Cleanse face or treated area with cleanser from your ZO® daily skin care program. Rinse and pat dry.

Step 2: Stimulation (Part 2): Retinol Crème— Apply the second packet (2.5 g) of Retinol Crème. Massage into skin.

Step 3: Hydrating and anti-inflammation (Part 2): Calming Crème postprocedure skin relief—Apply a thin layer of the Calming Crème postprocedure skin relief after applying the Retinol Crème. Apply on the peeled area up to 3 times daily.
- Redness, stinging, itching, mild swelling, flaking and peeling are all normal signs after the peel and vary based on patient responses
- Exfoliation generally starts 2–3 days after treatment and ends by day 5
- Avoid rubbing, peeling skin with fingers and scratching while healing

- Broad-spectrum sunscreen SPF 50 can be used as needed
- Avoid direct sun exposure for at least 7–10 days following the peel
- Do not use AHAs, beta-hydroxy acids, benzoyl peroxide, retinoids and other irritating products until the skin is healed
- Avoid procedures, such as facials, hair removal, microdermabrasion and laser until skin is fully healed
- After skin is healed, return to your daily skin health program.

MILK PEEL TREATMENT (DERMACEUTIC LABORATOIRE)

Ingredients

Gycolic acid, lactic acid and salicylic acid.

Indications

Skin exfoliant, chemical removal keratinized structures of the epidermis; in preparation for skin treatments with lasers.

Milk Peel Treatment Protocol

- Cleanse using 4 pumps of Foamer 15, rinse and dry
- Pour 2.5 mL of milk peel into a cup and apply on the entire face with a brush starting from forehead, then T-zone followed by cheeks
- Leave on for indicated time as in table 3 below. A light erythema will appear
- Rinse abundantly with water and dry
- Apply Hyal Ceutic to calm and hydrate the skin after treatment.

Milk peel may be used up to 4 times in total at 2 weeks intervals.

Recommended Home Care Treatment

- Hyal Ceutic to restore
- Sun Ceutic 50 to protect
- Light Ceutic or turnover to stimulate.

Recommended Time for Leave on of Milk Peel

The recommended time for leave on of milk peel as per phototype skin is mentioned in table 4.

MELA PEEL TREATMENT

Indications

- Epidermal melasma
- Pigment spots
- Postinflammatory pigmentation.

Three Combined Actions for Optimal Effect

- *Activa peel:* Prepares and exfoliates the skin for Mela peel application. Fastens the active ingredients penetration
- *Mela peel:* Inhibits melanin production and exfoliates skin to decrease the appearance of pigmentation
- *Mela cream:* Regulates pigment production in the long-term and boosts Mela peel treatment's depigmenting action.

TABLE 3: Recommended time for leave on of milk peel as per phototype skin

	Oily or acne prone skin	Mild-to-moderate skin aging	Advanced skin aging
Phototype I	30 s	30 s	1 min
Phototype II	30 s	1 min	1 min 30 s
Phototype III	1 min	1 min	1 min 30 s
Phototype IV–VI	30 s	1 min	1 min

Chemical Peels: A Global Perspective

TABLE 4: Ingredients of Mela peel procedure

Activa peel	Mela peel	Mela cream
Azelaic, salicylic, ferulic, and phytic acids	Lactic, salicylic, phytic, and kojic acids. Retinol and arbutin	Salicylic, phytic, mandelic, and kojic acids. Niacinamide, retinol, arbutin, licorice extract, and exonolone

Ingredients

Ingredients of Mela peel procedure are given in table 4.

Mela Peel Treatment Protocol

- *Foamer 15:* To cleanse the face—using four pumps.
- *Activa peel:* To be applied to the whole face—2–3 layers—using two cotton buds. Leave on skin for 2–3 minutes after the last application and remove excess with humid cotton pads
- *Mela peel:* To be massaged on the entire face—4 pumps. Reapply 3 pumps on pigment spots
- Patient goes home and rinses it off with water after 2–6 hours
- *Mela cream:* To be applied every morning and/or evening following protocol adapted to skin sensitivity.

Two to three in-clinic sessions for optimal results.

MELA PEEL FORTE

It is a medium chemical peel which is used for removal of pigmentation with visible skin desquamation. It follows 2-step Jessner-power formula (Salicylic and lactic acids, resorcinol). It can be used up to 2 times at 1-month interval.

Indications

- Reduced melasma and pigment spots, homogenous complexion
- Improved skin radiance and brightness.

Ingredients

Mela Peel Forte

- *5% citric acid*: Antiseptic and anti-inflammatory effect
- *5% resorcinol*: Antibacterial and whitening effect
- *10% lactic acid*: Hydrating and whitening effect
- Kojic acid, phytic acid, arbutin and retinol.

Activa Peel Forte

- 20% salicylic acid
- 5% citric acid
- 20% azelaic acid and 5% phytic acid
- 10% ferulic acid.

Mechanism of Action

- Decreases the cohesion between corneocytes and provides intense flaking.

Dermaceutic Solution—2-step Jessner's Formula

Step 1: Activa Peel Forte

- Apply one layer (1.5 mL) of Activa peel forte to the face using cotton buds
- Apply a second layer on the pigment spots
- Wait a couple of minutes and ventilate in between each layer.

Step 2: Mela Peel Forte

- Apply and massage 4 pumps of Mela peel forte
- Apply a second layer on stubborn pigment spots.

COSMO PEEL

Indications

- Reduces wrinkles
- Improves skin texture, smoker's complexion
- Reduces pigment spots and acne.

Ingredients

- *Foamer 15 cleanser:* Glycolic acid 15%, enoxolone
- *Cosmo peel:* TCA 12–15% superficial peel, 18–20% medium peel
- *Cosmo peel cream:* Lactic acid, salicylic acid, citric acid, retinyl palmitate, ascorbic acid, selenomethionine and alpha-tocopherol.

Cosmo Peel Treatment Protocol

- Cleanse with Foamer 15 cleanser
- Take 1.5 mL of TCA and apply using two cotton buds held together to whole face starting from forehead, then T-zone followed by cheeks. Apply two layers successively over each area, both vertically and horizontally
- Ventilate and allow to dry between two layers. Do not rinse
- Apply and massage six pumps of cosmo peel cream to the area being treated with gloved fingers. The patient goes home with the cream on and rinses off with water after 12 hours
  - The higher the concentration and number of layers applied, the more destructive the effect
  - The more concentrated the TCA, the more acidic it will be and the deeper it will penetrate into the skin seeking water to be neutralized
  - Much stronger than glycolic acid pH close to 0.

MASK PEEL

Indication

- Regulates oily skin, dilated pores and excessive sebum
- Brightens dull complexion.

Ingredients

Glycolic acid, salicylic acid and bentonite.

Mask Peel Treatment Protocol

- Cleanse the face using 4 pumps of Foamer 15, rinse and dry
- Apply a small amount of mask peel on the face. Always start by applying the product on the T-zone, followed by the jawline and mouth, and finish with the cheeks
- Leave for 1.5–2.5 minutes on the face (for body protocol, leave up to 10 minutes). A light erythema will appear
- Rinse abundantly with water and dry the face
- Apply Hyal Ceutic to calm and hydrate the skin after treatment.

Advanced protocol: Increase application's duration up to 5 minutes.

BLACK PEEL

Black peel is a new chemical peel solution based on black vinegar (black acetic acid). As a natural organic acid, the black acetic acid of Theraderm® Black Peel is made through the fermentation of black rice. It contains large amounts of organic materials, minerals and especially high concentrations of essential amino acids.

Ingredients

Tetra-hydro-jasmonic acid and salicylic acid: Plays an important role in the pathogen defense response, have anti-inflammatory effect as well as exfoliating property.

Potassium iodide: Empirically used for deep fungal infection and has wound recovery effect.

Black acetic acid: Contains large amount of organic materials, minerals and especially high concentrations of essential amino acids. It has anticancer properties as well as antioxidant activity.

Indications

- *Acne*: Pustules, nodules—black peel clear and black peel spot
- Improves PIH
- Skin resurfacing, cell renewal, antioxidant—black peel resurfacing.

Black Peel Procedure

Step 1: Preparation—cleanser and toner .

Step 2: Comedones extraction.

Step 3: Application of black peel clear—Apply this solution starting from the outside edges of the face, leaving the sensitive areas of the face until the last moment. Apply the solution two times or more on the oozing or bleeding acne lesions opened by extraction. Wait approximately 10 minutes to calm down the redness and warming sensation. Cleanse with the soft sponge soaked in cold water.

Step 4: Sebo Hydra Infused Mask—Apply mask on the face to calm down and hydrate the irritated skin. For deeper penetration, use Sonophoresis for 5–10 minutes and leave it for another 10 minutes. Do not rinse after taking it off, instead, massage gently the residue to be absorbed completely.

Step 5: Sunscreen.

Black Peel Protocol

Day 0: Black peel application at office.

Day 1-5: Peeling occurs postpeel.

Day 6-13: Black peel acne spot (home care)
- Contains black acetic acid, bio sulfur (comedolytic), potassium iodide, jasmonic acid, salicylic acid and lactic acid
- Patient applies at home over black and white heads, nodules, cysts and pores several times for maximum penetration and leaves overnight.

Day 14-20: Time for healing and skin repair.

Day 21: Black peel.

Four to six sessions are recommended depending on acne severity.

NEOSTRATA PROSYSTEM RETINOL PEEL

It consists of 3% retinol plus retinol boosting complex. It is a superficial peel suitable for most to exfoliate and improve the appearance of fine lines and wrinkles, laxity, mottled pigmentation, pore size, and to enhance clarity and radiance.

Peel Procedure Guidelines

- After priming the skin for 2–4 weeks, prepare patient for the peel procedure as usual
- Remove one unit-dose vial from the carton and break open. Pour entire contents of retinol peel into a cup
- Apply carefully the solution uniformly to the skin using a disposable fan brush. Apply one layer for a lighter peeling effect and multiple layers for a stronger peeling effect
- For approximately 10 minutes, observe for signs of erythema and inquire patient about discomfort
- If skin experiences uncomfortable erythema and/or other signs of discomfort, wash off the peel
- After 10 minutes, if the peel is tolerated well, gently rub in any remaining peel that

may be left on skin. Neutralization is not required
- Instruct patient to wash off any remaining peel after 8 hours or overnight and avoid sun exposure. For a lighter peeling effect or sensitive skin, instruct patient to wash off peel after 3 hours
- Apply moisturizer and sunscreen after wash.

Patient can get visible peeling beginning approximately 2-3 days postpeel and may continue for approximately 1 week.

Subsequent peels can be performed at 6-8 week intervals if the skin has fully healed.

DERMAMELAN PEEL

Dermamelan depigmentation treatment is a very versatile, dynamic process which is easily adapted to the needs of each individual patient. The mechanism is based on the inhibition of tyrosinase, a basic enzyme in the melanin formation process. Several of the substances present in the Dermamelan formula act by blocking this enzyme, or even by inverting the metabolic process of the transformation chain.

Indication

- Improves melasma, PIH, pigment spots and blotchy skin
- Increases luminosity and smoothness
- Effective for pigmentation failed to resolve by traditional lightening agents, superficial chemical peels
- Prevents postlaser and postpeel hyperpigmentation.

Ingredients

Dermamelan 1: Mask
Azelaic acid, kojic acid, phytic acid, ascorbic acid, arbutin and titanium dioxide.

Dermamelan 2: Maintenance Cream (30 g)
Titanium dioxide, kojic acid, phytic acid and ascorbic acid.

Mesoestetic® Hydra Vital Factor K Cream (50 mL)

Hydro nutritional cream for face and neck. Contains Hydroviton, vitamin K, vitamin E, amniotic fluid, glycerin and silicone oil.

Dermamelan Peel Procedure

- Apply Dermamelan 1 at office after cleansing the face at the hyperpigmented spots
- Wait for couple of minutes. If no irritation, apply moisturizer and sunscreen
- Patient washes face after 4-6 hours
- Patient will start applying Dermamelan 2 at spots at night for 3-4 weeks along with the skin care.

COSMELAN PEEL

This is similar to Dermamelan peel; however, the ingredients are 20% lower in concentration.

Cosmelan 1: Mask
Azelaic acid, kojic acid, phytic acid, ascorbic acid, arbutine and titanium dioxide.

Cosmelan 2: Maintenance Cream (30 g)
Titanium dioxide, kojic acid, phytic acid and ascorbic acid.

Mesoestetic Hydra Vital Factor K Cream (50 mL)

Hydro nutritional cream for face and neck. Contains Hydroviton, vitamin K, vitamin E, amniotic fluid, glycerin and silicone oil.

The indications, mechanism of action and peel procedure are similar to Dermamelan peel.

BIO C (PARTY PEEL)

It is an antiaging and brightening peel by Coherent Medical Systems. The combination of gentle peeling acids with hyaluronic acid and vitamin C ensures maximum tolerance of this antiaging peel.

Indications

- Premature skin aging, toning and brightening
- Maintaining results of previous peels.

Ingredients

- *Solution 1:* Lactobionic acid 25%, mandelic acid 10%, lactic acid 10% and glycolic acid 10%
- *Solution 2:* Ascorbic acid 15%, hyaluronic acid 10% and vitamin A 1%.

Application Technique

- Clean and degrease the face with cleanser
- Take 2 mL of Inno-Exfo Bio C in a bowl
- Apply solution with brush and leave for 5–10 minutes
- Push the button and mix vitamin C
- Do not wipe off the product solution after application
- Apply sunscreen and post-treatment care products
- Recovery time 2–3 days. Recommended 6–8 sessions.

CONCLUSION

Chemical peeling is a simple, safe and common dermatological procedure. The proper peel selection and adequate preparation of the skin prior to peeling are mandatory to achieve maximum benefit. The nuances of proprietary chemical peels aid in dealing with resistant cases, achieve maximum desired effect and minimal or no side effects.

TAKE HOME POINTS

- Proper medical history including herpes infection and keloidal tendency is mandatory
- Adequate counseling and recognize patients with body dismorphic disorders and unrealistic expectation
- Adequate priming of the skin for maximum benefit and to avoid side effects
- Document written informed consent, photographic consent and images prior to peel
- Choose the right peel. Always check label of peel
- Apply peel following cosmetic unit, secure sensitive areas with Vaseline
- Emphasize on postpeel care
- Detect complications early, if present
- Be extra careful in ethnic skin due to high chances of postinflammatory hyperpigmentation
- Combine low strength peels, mix and match peels segmentally and sequentially for optimized results
- Repeat peels at intervals. Emphasize on maintenance with topical skin care regimen
- Proprietary peels exist for resistant cases and sensitive skin.

REFERENCES

1. Khunger N. Standard guidelines of care for chemical peels. Indian J Dermatol Venereol Leprol. 2008;74: S5-12.
2. Khunger N. Types of peels. In: Khunger N (Ed.). Step-by-Step Chemical Peels, 2nd Edition. New Delhi: Jaypee Brothers Medical Publishers (P) Ltd.; 2014. pp. 17-26.
3. Savant SS. Superficial and medium depth chemical peeling. In: Savant SS (Ed.). Textbook of Dermatosurgery and Cosmetology, 2nd Edition. Mumbai: ASCAD; 2005. pp. 177-95.
4. Talwar A, Talwar K. Newer superficial peels. In: Mysore V (Ed.). ACS(I) Textbook of Cutaneous & Aesthetic Surgery, 2nd Edition. New Delhi: Jaypee Brothers Medical Publishers (P) Ltd; 2017. pp. 749-58.
5. Obagi ZE, Obagi S, Alaiti S, et al. TCA-based blue peel: a standardized procedure with depth control. Dermatol Surg. 1999;25(10):773-80.
6. Hong SP, Han SS, Choi SJ, et al. Split-face comparative study of 1550 nm fractional photothermolysis and tricholoacetic acid 15% chemical peeling for facial melasma in Asian skin. J Cosmet Laser Ther. 2012;14:81-6.

27
CHAPTER

Combination Therapy: Chemical Peels with Other Technologies

Mukta Sachdev, Rachana Shilpakar

INTRODUCTION

Chemical peel is a very popular and old dermatological outdoor procedure. Chemical peels are versatile and varied in their composition. With the increasing demand of youthful, radiant skin all over the world with minimal side effects, newer chemical peels are being added up at a faster pace. Chemical peeling procedure is expanding the horizon of its indications from the clinical dermatological conditions such as acne, postinflammatory hyperpigmentation, postacne marks, acne scars and pigmentary disorders like melasma to aesthetic conditions like resurfacing and rejuvenation of skin. With the advent of fast-growing aesthetic world, a plethora of resurfacing technologies, such as nonablative and ablative lasers, fractional lasers of various wavelengths, to meet the specific demands have been developed.

Currently, combining the chemical peel procedure with the different procedure at the same setting is gaining the popularity. The combination approach leads to an increased efficacy with reduced risk of complications. However, the choice of the combination should be individualized depending on the indication and site to achieve better outcome.

LIST OF COMBINATION THERAPIES[1]

Chemical peels can be combined with—
- Microdermabrasion
- Dermasanding
- Dermabrasion
- Lasers—various types with different wavelengths
- Botulinum toxin
- Fillers
- Microneedling
- Subcision.

INDICATIONS

Combination treatment can be done for various dermatological and aesthetic conditions such as:
- Acne
- Acne scars
- Pigmentary disorders
  - Melasma
  - Postinflammatory hyperpigmentation of any cause
  - Age spots.
- Rejuvenation
- Photoaging.

PRETREATMENT PROCEDURE

- The proper detailed history and general examination is mandatory
- The patient expectation has to be considered and the probable outcome of the combined technique has to be explained properly
- The procedure has to be explained in detail; the number of sessions, the downtime, if any, and side effects have to be discussed
- Serial photographs are mandatory and written informed consent is must
- It is advisable to prepare the skin 2-4 weeks prior with tretinoin, retinaldehyde, glycolic acid or lightening agent including moisturizer and sunscreen for better outcome
- The patient should be advised to stop the priming agents 2-4 days prior to the procedure.

THE PROCEDURE

- The patient is once again explained about the procedure in detail
- The treated area is cleansed with a cleanser and degreased
- The sensitive areas are secured properly.

Chemical Peels with Lasers

Chemical peeling can be combined with lasers for acne scars and facial rejuvenation. Both the procedures are done simultaneously on the same setting to optimize the results.

Acne and Acne Scars

Treatment of acne scars is challenging as the outcome is with marginal success. Taylor MB et al. have described a combination of a superficial chemical peel, subcision and fractional carbon dioxide laser resurfacing in a single-treatment session as a novel treatment approach for rolling acne scars.[2] The authors have concluded that the combination of a trichloroacetic acid (TCA) 20% chemical peel, subcision and fractional CO_2 laser resurfacing combined with tumescent anesthesia is both safe and effective in the treatment of rolling acne scars.

Lekakh O et al. have conducted a study to evaluate the safety and efficacy of concurrent use of salicylic acid peels with pulsed dye laser versus salicylic acid alone in the treatment of moderate-to-severe acne vulgaris.[3] It was a randomized split-face designed study wherein patients were treated with pulsed dye laser (595 nm) at laser settings of 7 mm spot size, energy 10 Joules, 10 millisecond pulse duration, cooling setting 2 (only on one half of face). Finally, two coats of a 30% salicylic acid peeling solution with large cotton-tipped applicators were applied to the subject's entire face and remained in place for 3-5 minutes. Once a white crystallization appeared, cool washcloths were applied for subject comfort, and the face was wiped clean with water. Triamcinolone acetonide (0.1%) was then applied to the entire face. Subjects received a total of three treatments at 3-week intervals and assessment done at 0-9 weeks. The patients experienced greater benefit from pulsed dye laser treatment used in conjunction with salicylic acid peels. Hence, the authors concluded that adjunctive utilization of pulsed dye laser to salicylic acid peel therapy can lead to better outcomes in acne management.

Pigmentary Disorders

Lee GY et al. have carried out the study to demonstrate the effect of combination treatment of the recalcitrant pigmentary disorders with pigmented laser and chemical peeling.[4] The studies was carried out in 24 patients with recalcitrant facial pigmentary disorders and was treated with Q-switched alexandrite laser at fluences of 7-8 J/cm^2 or pigmented lesion dye laser at fluences of 2–2.5 J/cm^2, and the same session, 15–25% TCA with or without Jessner's solution were used for the chemical peeling. Both the patients and clinicians rated good response without significant complications. Hence, the combination treatment with pigmented laser and chemical peeling is effective, safe, and relatively inexpensive treatment modalities in the recalcitrant pigmentary disorders.

Lee MC et al. had conducted study wherein the patients with melasma were treated with the 1064 nm Q-switched neodymium-doped yttrium aluminum garnet (Nd:YAG) laser for 4 sessions with various parameters at 1-month intervals.[5] Ice packs were applied for 5 minutes followed by ultrasonic application of vitamin C over melasma on right side of face while the other side received only a moisturizing lotion. The patients were followed up 3 months post four laser treatments. The improvement was more pronounced during second to fourth sessions. There was no rebound or postinflammatory hyperpigmentation detected during the 3-month follow up period.

Chemical Peel with Microdermabrasion

Microdermabrasion can be combined with superficial chemical peel to enhance outcome. Hexsel D et al. had conducted the study to evaluate photoaging, in which one group patients underwent three sessions of microdermabrasion followed by 5% retinoid acid (RA) application at 7–10 days interval while the second group underwent only 5% RA application.[6] The author concluded that the combination of microdermabrasion followed by a 5% RA peel showed slightly greater improvement in the histological alterations resulting from photoaging. Briden E et al. had concluded that superficial GA peels can be combined with microdermabrasion to maximize treatment results and patient satisfaction.[7] The authors carried out two methods. The first method included alternating GA peels and microdermabrasion treatments every 2 weeks, enabling the patient to receive both a peel and microdermabrasion in the same month. With the second method, microdermabrasion may be used prior to the superficial GA peel to increase the exfoliation and antiaging effects of both treatments within the same visit. This second method is considered to be a more aggressive approach and usually is reserved for patients with a history of procedures. Hence, combining treatments can be used to maintain a patient's skin after the initial treatment stage, usually performed every other month or seasonally, depending on the patient.

Chemical Peel with Dermasanding[1]

Dermasanding is a procedure wherein sterile sandpaper is used to abrade the skin up to papillary dermis level. While combining chemical peel with dermasanding, a greater depth of peeling is possible without increasing the concentration of the peeling agent followed by faster re-epithelialization reducing downtime. The combination is usually used for acne scars and striae treatment.

Fulton JE et al. had adopted the step-by-step methodology for neck rejuvenation wherein the patients preconditioned their face and neck skin with vitamin A or glycolic skin conditioning lotions for 6–8 weeks prior to surgery.[8] Following this, the chest and neck area was treated with the Jessner–trichloroacetic acid peel. Then, the middle section of the neck was sanded with one hundred fifty grit sandscreen. Finally, the central area was resurfaced with the UltraPulse CO_2 laser using reduced power settings. Usually two passes were adequate to shrink the skin of this central section of the neck. A petrolatum-based ointment was applied during the initial 7-day postoperative period. After re-epithelialization, a sunscreen-moisturizer was used during the day and hydrocortisone moisturizer was applied at night. The study showed that the blending from the décolleté area to the hairline produced rejuvenation without a line of demarcation and an improved texture of the neck developed without visible scarring.

Adatto MA et al. had treated striae at various sites with sand abrasion followed by combination peel (carboxylic acid, L ascorbic acid, citric acid, excipients and 15% TCA) application, following which patented-cream application under plastic occlusion for 6–24 hours.[9] The study has resulted around 70% improvement after 1–8 sessions in all types of striae.

Chemical Peel with Dermabrasion

Whang KK et al. had conducted a three-staged operation in acne scar surgery.[10] A focal chemical peeling was performed on all patients and then two laser, scar excision and punch grafts were used for deep scars. Finally, dermabrasion was done for the remaining scars. The degree of improvement increased as the follow-up periods and number of focal chemical peeling procedures increased and as the 3-staged operation progressed. Thus, a 3-staged operation is effective in the treatment of patients with various types of acne scars.

Chemical Peel with Microneedling

Microneedling can be combined with chemical peel for acne scars and skin rejuvenation. Microneedling will help to improve atrophic scars while the chemical peel improves textures and hyperpigmentation. Kontochristopoulos G et al.[11] has concluded in their study that combination of microneedling followed by 10% TCA constitute an innovative combination treatment for infraorbital hyperchromia with encouraging results and minor side effects. Sharad J had carried out the study in Indian population with acne scars in which the author conducted comparative study between microneedling alone versus sequential microneedling followed by 35% GA peeling.[12] Five sessions were done once in 6 weeks and concluded that the combined sequential treatment with GA peel caused a significant improvement in the acne scars along with improvement in skin texture and reduction in postacne pigmentation, without increasing morbidity in Indian skin in combination group.

Chemical Peel with Subcision

Chemical peel can follow subcision in the same setting in treatment of acne scars. Taylor MB et al. have described a combination of a superficial chemical peel, subcision and fractional carbon dioxide laser resurfacing in a single-treatment session in acne scars.[2]

Chemical Peel with Botulinum Toxin[1]

The scientific basis for combining botulinum toxin and chemical peeling is that the toxin relaxes the muscles thereby provides better remodeling during new collagen formation following chemical peeling. Landau M had shown in the study that by combining chemical peels with fillers and botulinum toxin injections synergistic beneficial effect is achieved.[13] These rejuvenating procedures significantly increase the satisfaction rate of patients. Bosniak S et al. had concluded in their study that combined technologies provide results superior to the use of individual therapy lone in oculofacial rejuvenation.[14]

Chemical Peel with Fillers[1,13,14]

Chemical peeling is done first and superficial temporary fillers are used after inflammation subsides and healing occurs completely. The chemical peels aids in improving superficial signs of photoaging, textures, age spots while fillers helps to increase volume, and helps in depressed scars and wrinkles optimizing the benefits to the patients. However, semi-permanent and permanent fillers are used 4–8 weeks prior to the chemical peel procedure.

POSTPROCEDURE CARE

All the patients should be advised to use moisturizer and sunscreen liberally and avoid direct and prolonged exposure to sunlight. Instruction should be given clearly not to pick the scales and scabs, if any.

COMPLICATIONS

The common complications of combined procedures are:
- Persistent erythema
- Hypopigmentation
- Hyperpigmentation
- Lines of demarcation
- Scarring.

CONCLUSION

Chemical peels can be combined with other existing and emerging technologies to achieve optimized results in the shortest possible time, with minimal downtime and lesser side effects for various clinical and aesthetic indications. The combination modality should be individualized for better outcome.

TAKE HOME POINTS

- Chemical peeling can be combined with various other technologies to optimize the result
- The concentration of the peeling agent can be lowered due to combination technology
- Proper medical history including herpes infection and keloidal tendency is mandatory
- Adequate counseling and recognize patients with body dysmorphic disorders and unrealistic expectation
- Adequate priming of the skin for maximum benefits and avoids side effects
- Document written informed consent, photographic consent, and images prior to procedure
- Choose the right combination. Always check label of peel. The combination should be individualized
- Emphasize on postprocedure care
- Educate the patient on downtime, if any
- Detect complications early, if present
- Be extra careful in ethnic skin due to high chances of postinflammatory hyperpigmentation
- Repeat combination procedure at intervals if required. Emphasize on maintenance with topical skin care regimen
- As with all combination treatments, safety precautions and monitoring the patient's skin throughout treatment are crucial to success.

REFERENCES

1. Khunger N. Combination therapies. In: Khunger N (Ed.). Step-by-Step Chemical Peels, 2nd Edition. New Delhi: Jaypee Brothers Medical Publishers (P) Ltd.; 2014. pp. 195-205.
2. Taylor MB, Zaleski-Larsen L, McGraw TA. Single session treatment of rolling acne scars using tumescent anesthesia, 20% trichloroacetic acid extensive subcision, and fractional CO2 laser. Dermatol Surg. 2017;43 Suppl:S70-4.
3. Lekakh O, Mahoney AM, Novice K, et al. Treatment of acne vulgaris with salicylic acid chemical peel and pulsed dye laser: A split face, rater-blinded, randomized controlled trial. J Lasers Med Sci. 2015;6(4):167-70.
4. Lee GY, Kim HJ, Whang KK. The effect of combination treatment of the recalcitrant pigmentary disorders with pigmented laser and chemical peeling. Dermatol Surg. 2002;28(12):1120-3.

5. Lee MC, Chang CS, Huang YL, et al. Treatment of melasma with mixed parameters of 1064nm Q-switched Nd: YAG laser toning and an enhanced effect of ultrasonic application of vitamin C: a split-face study. Lasers Med Sci. 2015;30(1):159-63.
6. Hexsel D, Mazzuco R, Dal'Forno T, et al. Microdermabrasion followed by a 5% retinoid acid chemical peel vs. a 5% retinoid acid chemical peel for the treatment of photoaging—a pilot study. J Cosmet Dermatol. 2005;4(2):111-6.
7. Briden E, Jacobsen E, Johnson C. Combining superficial glycolic acid (alpha-hydroxy acid) peels with microdermabrasion to maximize treatment results and patient satisfaction. Cutis. 2007;79(1 Suppl Combining):13-6.
8. Fulton JE, Rahimi AD, Helton P, et al. Neck rejuvenation by combining Jessner/TCA peel, dermasanding, and CO2 laser resurfacing. Dermatol Surg. 1999;25(10):745-50.
9. Adattoo MA, Deprez P. Striae treated by a novel combination treatment – sandabrasion and a patent mixtue containing 15% trichloroacetic acid followed by 6-24 hours of a patent cream under plastic occlusion. J Cosmet Dermatol. 2003;2(2):61-7.
10. Whang KK1, Lee M. The principle of a three-staged operation in the surgery of acne scars. J Am Acad Dermatol. 1999;40(1):95-7.
11. Kontochristopoulos G, Kouris A, Platsidaki E, et al. Combination of microneedling and 10% trichloroacetic acid peels in the management of infraorbital dark circles. J Cosmet Laser Ther. 2016;18(5):289-92.
12. Sharad J. Combination of microneedling and glycolic acid peels for the treatment of acne scars in dark skin. J Cosmet Dermatol. 2011;10(4):317-23.
13. Landau M. Combination of chemical peelings with botulinum toxin injections and dermal fillers. J Cosmet Dermatol. 2006;5(2):121-6.
14. Bosniak S, Cantisano-Zilkha M, Purewal BK, et al. Combination therapies in oculofacial rejuvenation. Orbit. 2006;25(4):319-26.

28

Chemical Peels in Melasma

Sahar MF Ghannam, Zubin K Mandlewala, Rashmi Sarkar

INTRODUCTION

Melasma is a common, distressing, chronic and recurrent disorder of hyperpigmentation, with a female preponderance. It is characterized by the development of light to dark brown macules and patches distributed relatively symmetrically over sun-exposed areas such as the face. On the basis of location, melasma can be classified as centrofacial, malar and/or mandibular. It can also be classified histologically as epidermal, dermal or mixed melasma.[1] Such a classification is essential as it guides in choice of treatment modalities. Fitzpatrick skin types IV through VI, living in areas of intense ultraviolet (UV) light exposure, are mostly affected. Some common risk factors incriminated in the initiation of melasma include: Genetic, UV exposure, pregnancy, oral contraceptive pills and thyroid disease. Likewise, cosmetic products and some photosensitive medications may also be implicated as plausible factors in causation.[2,3] The Melasma Quality of Life Scale (MELASQOL) has shown that this disorder may have a significant effect on patient's quality of life.[4,5] The use of oral and topical medications for melasma has very rarely given substantial clinical improvement and hence modalities such as chemical peels are warranted to supplement ongoing therapy.

PATIENT PREPARATION

It is important to speak to the patient about the nature and course of the disease and the treatment options that can be offered. An initial assessment by Wood's lamp can aid in delineating the level of pigmentation (epidermal vs. dermal). This can be substantiated with dermatoscopy. Similarly, a detailed history regarding occupation, onset during pregnancy, development of thyroid disorder and/or use of any medication that may have contributed to the causation of melasma have to be noted. Primarily, the amount and continuous/regular use of a sunscreen having a sun protection factor-30 or above has to be advocated in the therapeutic protocol. The patient should also be told about the effectiveness of physical measures such as wide-brimmed hats, umbrellas, shades, etc. when out in the sun, as the goal is not only to clear but also to prevent further pigmentation. After meticulous assessment of the skin over the affected areas, a proper peeling program can be formulated. About 2-4 weeks prior to the initiation of the peel procedure, it is very important to prepare the patient's skin with certain topical medications, known as priming agents. Such agents are known to enhance the effect of the peeling agent by virtue of their action on the skin in the transitory period before the peel. Common priming agents include: Topical retinoids (e.g., tretinoin 0.025%), α-hydroxy acids [e.g., glycolic acid (GA) 6% or 12%, lactic acid, mandelic acid], skin lightening agents (e.g., hydroquinone 2% or 4%, kojic acid, arbutin, licorice, etc.) and/or a bland soap-free cleanser for sensitive skin. In a study by Garg et al,[6] they studied 80 Indian patients with melasma who were randomly allocated into three groups, one group receiving GA peel only, the other groups GA primed with 0.025% tretinoin and 2% hydroquinone respectively. The fall in Melasma Area Severity Index (MASI) score was highest in the group receiving 2% hydroquinone as a priming agent with minimum relapse and postinflammatory hyperpigmentation (PIH). After verbal consent, a baseline photograph should be taken.

CHEMICAL PEEL FORMULATIONS

Chemical peels form an important tool in a dermatologist's armamentarium when treating melasma. Peels act by causing a controlled chemical burn to the skin and thereby removal of unwanted melanin.[7] After the priming process, some amount of exfoliation and xerosis maybe experienced and if it becomes very troublesome, the use of peels may be deferred to a future date. If the above issues are not present on the day of the procedure, peels may be started after written consent and photographic documentation. Peels may be selected according to the depth of penetration and generally deeper peels are to be avoided in darker skin types (Table 1).

Alpha-hydroxy Acid Peels

Glycolic Acid Peels

Glycolic acid is an alpha-hydroxy acid derived from sugar cane that thins the stratum

TABLE 1: Chemical peels for melasma

Depth	Histological location	Peels
Very superficial	Epidermis: Stratum corneum	• TCA 10–20% • GA 20–50% • SA 20% • MA 10–20% • Jessner's (single coat)
Superficial	Epidermis: Stratum granulosum to stratum basale	• TCA 25–30% • GA 50–70% • SA 30% • Jessner's (>1 coat)
Medium	Epidermis till papillary dermis	• TCA 35–50% • TCA 35% + GA 70% • TCA 35% + Jessner's • TCA 35% + Solid CO_2
Deep	Epidermis till mid-reticular dermis	Avoid in melasma and dark skin

TCA, trichloroacetic acid; GA, glycolic acid; SA, salicylic acid; MA, mandelic acid.

corneum, disperses melanin in the epidermis and improves the distribution of other drugs in the skin making it a useful adjunct to other topical hypopigmenting agents.[8] Glycolic acid peels act in melasma by accelerating desquamation and its additive inhibitory effect on melanin synthesis resulting in quick pigment dispersion. For the treatment of melasma, GA peels ranging from 20–70% have been utilized routinely (Fig. 1). Many clinical studies have been undertaken demonstrating the utility and thereby effectiveness of GA peels in melasma. Javaheri et al. carried out a study in 25 Indian female patients who were primed with 10% GA lotion and sunscreen followed later by monthly 50% GA facial peels for 3 months. An improvement in melasma (reduction in MASI score) was observed

Chemical Peels in Melasma

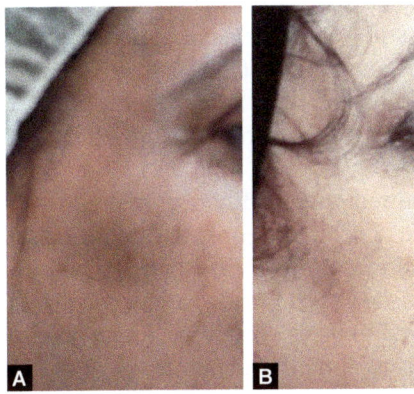

FIG. 1: **A,** Malar melasma in type III Fitzpatrick skin before applying 35% glycolic acid peels; **B,** Malar melasma in Type III Fitzpatrick skin after applying six serial 35% glycolic acid peels.

in 91% of patients (p <0.01).[9] Grover et al. formulated a study wherein 15 patients of melasma were initially primed with tretinoin cream (0.025%) followed by serial glycolic acid peels (10–30%) at fortnightly intervals. A good to fair improvement was noted at the end of the study period.[10] Sarkar et al. published a comparative study wherein 40 Indian melasma patients were divided into two groups of 20 each. One group received serial GA peels (30% for the first three sittings and 40% for the next three sittings) combined with the modified Kligman's formula. The other received only the modified Kligman's formula. A significant decrease in the MASI score from baseline to 21 weeks was observed in both groups (p <0.001). However, the group receiving the GA peels showed more rapid and greater improvement, with statistically significant results (p <0.001).[11] Dayal et al. published a study wherein 60 patients of epidermal melasma were enrolled for 24 weeks. Patients were divided into two groups: (1) study group received serial GA peel every 3 weeks with twice daily 20% azelaic acid cream; (2) control group received only 20% azelaic acid cream.[12] Clinical improvement was assessed objectively using MASI. The improvement in MASI score and percentage decrease in MASI scoring were statistically significant 12 weeks onward in the study group as compared to control group. There was also a significant reduction in MELASQOL scores in the study group as compared to the control group after treatment. Hence, it was concluded that GA peels enhance the therapeutic efficacy of topical azelaic acid cream in melasma. Garg et al. did a single-blind study in which 60 patients of melasma were randomly assigned into three groups of 20 each. Group I received only GA peels while Groups II and III were primed with 0.025% tretinoin and 2% hydroquinone creams, respectively, for 2 weeks before peeling.[13] The patients received serial GA peels fortnightly for the first 3 months and then monthly for the next 3 months and were then followed up for the next 3 months after the peeling was stopped. The result of their study was an overall decrease in MASI score from baseline to 6 months in all three groups but it was highly significant between group I and III (p <0.001) at 6 and 9 months and significant between groups II and III (p <0.01) at 9 months, thus highlighting the importance of hydroquinone along with GA peels in the treatment protocol of melasma. In general, GA peels should be used with much caution especially in skin of color as they can cause burns and thereby PIH.

Salient Points about Glycolic Acid Peels

- Glycolic acid is a time-dependent peel; hence, the treating dermatologist must stay in the room at all times (with timer on) to observe the peeling end point
- It must be mentioned to the patient that they may experience a slight stinging/tingling/burning sensation during the procedure and ideally a portable fan can be used to cool the area

- As it is preferable to treat the epidermal variant of melasma, lower concentrations of GA (20–50%) should be applied ideally as a single coat for up to 3 minutes before neutralizing
- The peeling end-point is usually mild to moderate erythema
- The GA peel should be neutralized preferably with a base such as 10–15% sodium bicarbonate or cold water
- Patients may experience slight redness and xerosis in the postpeel period, which may last up to a week and thus importance lies in the regular use of sunscreens and moisturizers
- Skin types V and VI are more prone to develop PIH with GA peels and thus topical skin lightening agents (e.g., hydroquinone, kojic acid, azelaic acid, etc.) may be initiated along with the continuance of other priming agents if the need arises.

Other Alpha-hydroxy Acid Peels

Other α-hydroxy acids such as mandelic and lactic acid can also be tried for patients with melasma. Mandelic acid, which is derived from bitter almond, has large molecular size and thus uniformly penetrates the epidermis very slowly making it a favorable option in patients with dark, sensitive skin. Lactic acid, which is derived from sour milk, has catered a bit of attention recently for its relative safety profile especially in skin of color. Lactic acid reduces the thickness of the stratum corneum by reducing corneocyte cohesion, and should be the treatment option for patients with dry skin.[14] Sharquie et al. published a study wherein 92% lactic acid peels were applied on 20 patients every 3 weeks up to a maximum of six sessions, after which an assessment was done on the 6th month.[14] All patients who completed the study showed a marked improvement (statistically significant) in MASI score. Sharquie et al. published a split-face study on 24 melasma patients comparing lactic acid peels (full strength 92%) with Jessener's solution.[15] Lactic acid and Jessner's peel were applied on respective halves of the face every 3 weeks until desired results were obtained and follow-up assessment was done at 6th month post-treatment cessation. Patients showed marked improvement (statistically significant) and lactic acid peels proved to be as effective as Jessner's solution in the treatment of melasma.

Beta-hydroxy Acid Peels

Salicylic acid (SA), which is a lipid soluble agent derived from the bark of willow tree, is the chief β-hydroxy acid. Although it is more commonly used for acne, it has similarly found its place in peel formulations for melasma (Fig. 2). Salicylic acid based peels work by way of its anti-inflammatory property thereby reducing PIH and also produce a diffuse "whitening effect".[16] Grimes et al. had published a pilot study on efficacy of SA peels on dark skinned individuals (Fitzpatrick skin types V and VI) with various skin conditions such as acne, PIH and melasma. Patients were primed for two weeks with 4% hydroquinone after which two 20% then three 30% SA peels were performed sequentially at 2 week intervals for a total of five sessions.[17] They noted that four out of the six patients (66%) of melasma had moderate to significant improvement at the end of the study. More commonly, 20% SA is used in combination with 10% mandelic acid (α-hydroxy acid), as a safe and effective option in patients of melasma. The SA component penetrates the epidermis quickly and also enhances the further absorption of mandelic acid, which is larger in size and disperses slowly. Sarkar et al. had published a study wherein 90 patients diagnosed with melasma were randomly allocated into three groups of 30 patients

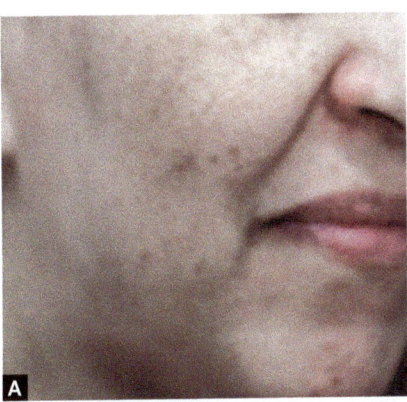 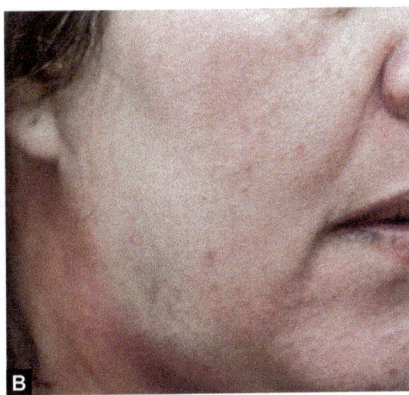

FIG. 2: **A,** Melasma at baseline; **B,** Melasma after six 20% salicylic acid peels.

each. Group A received 35% GA peel, Group B received 20% SA + 10% mandelic acid combination peel (SM peel) and Group C received phytic combination peels. Each group was primed with 4% hydroquinone and 0.05% tretinoin cream 4 weeks prior to the peels.[18] Chemical peeling was done after every 2 weeks in all groups until 12 weeks. Clinical evaluation using MASI score and photography was recorded at every visit and follow-up was done until 20 weeks. It was concluded that SM peels were as safe and effective as the GA peel and had a better tolerability profile as compared to the others.

Salient Points about Salicylic Acid Peels

- One coat of SA peel can be applied for anywhere between 2-10 minutes depending on tolerability
- Mild burning and stinging sensations may be experienced
- The patient may experience anesthesia of the face within 1-3 minutes due to anesthetic properties of SA
- Within one minute a dry white precipitate may be noticed referred to as "pseudofrost" which occurs due to crystallization of SA (excessive pseudofrosting should be avoided in melasma)
- Neutralizing the peel is not required
- Bland cleansers and moisturizers should be continued for 48 hours postpeel.[19]

Trichloroacetic Acid Peels

Tricholoroacetic acid (TCA) is available as anhydrous hygroscopic white crystals dissolved in distilled water. It is considered as a versatile peel due to its varied depth-guided concentrations (mainly superficial and medium depth) for use in a host of skin conditions. TCA peels have also found a place in the treatment of melasma, (Fig. 3) but must be used with extreme caution especially in skin of color because overzealous use can lead to the development of PIH and scarring. Tricholoroacetic acid works by denaturing epidermal proteins thereby causing exfoliation. Kalla et al. compared 55-75% GA versus 10-15% TCA peels in 100 patients with recalcitrant melasma.[20] They reported that both the time to response and degree of response were more favorable with TCA compared with GA. Soliman et al. reported that 20% TCA peels plus topical 5% ascorbic acid was superior to TCA peeling alone in 30 women with epidermal melasma.[21]

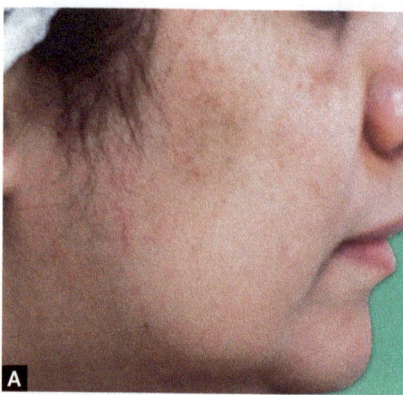 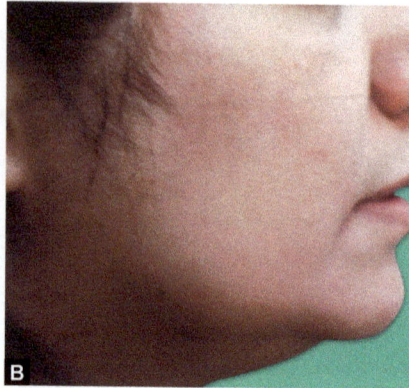

FIG. 3: **A,** Melasma at baseline; **B,** Lightening of melasma after six 20% trichloroacetic acid peels.

Salient Points about Trichloroacetic Acid Peels

- Results are coat-dependent, and hence application of one coat is enough as the epidermal variant of melasma should ideally be the only indication to be treated
- After dipping the brush in the solution, excess solution should be wiped off against the side of the bowl
- A superficial depth based TCA peel concentration (ideally 10–20%) is preferred; the end point of which would be mild erythema and scattered frosting (not uniform)
- Frosting is due to precipitation of skin proteins and once frosting occurs, cold water should be applied via gauze at specific frosted sites
- The patient is instructed to wash the face with cold water a few times without a cleanser and without rubbing the skin, after which the skin can be patted dry with a dry gauze
- Postpeel sunscreen should be applied and should be continued even after cessation of desquamation
- Moisturizers are equally important and should be applied as frequently as possible till the desquamation subsides
- The patient should be informed that dark, dry and stretchy patches may develop in a few/all areas and he/she shouldn't pick nor peel off these areas
- All salon based procedures such as facials and clean-ups or even other topical therapies that aren't recommended by the dermatologist should be avoided at all costs.

Jessner's Solution

Jessner's solution is a combination of resorcinol, salicylic acid, lactic acid and ethanol used as a superficial peeling agent. As resorcinol tends to cause burning and other side effects, it is often replaced by an α-hydroxy acid namely, citric acid; the combination being labeled as "modified Jessner's solution". It is routinely used for conditions like acne, photodamaged skin, keratosis pilaris, etc. It has also been tried in melasma with varying results (Fig. 4). Safoury et al. published a comparative study wherein 20 female patients with melasma had undergone full-face 15% TCA peel with the exception of the left malar area, to which a combination of 15% TCA and modified Jessner's solution were applied.[22] The results showed that the side where the combination peel (left malar area) was applied

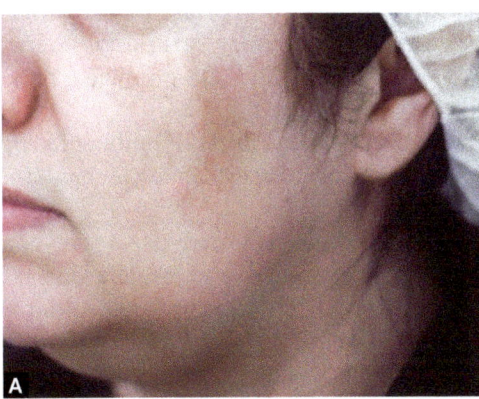 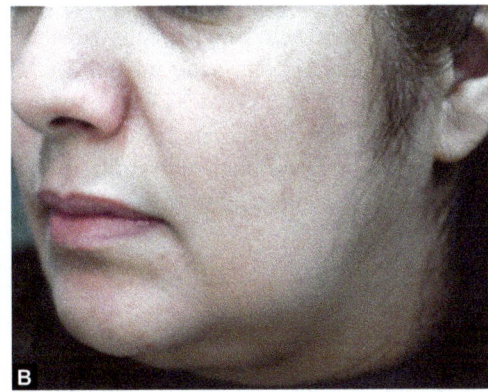

FIG. 4: **A,** Melasma at baseline; **B,** Lightening of melasma after six modified Jessner's peels.

produced a much better outcome (statistically highly significant) when compared to other areas of the face.

Salient Points about Jessner's Solution

- The resorcinol component is known to cause a lot of burning
- One coat is sufficient when treating epidermal variant of melasma
- Mild to moderate erythema may be noted followed by a powdery whitening of the skin after application of the peel
- If the peel reaches a little deeper (due to application of more than one coat), a brownish discoloration can be seen for up to 2 days postpeel which is further followed by peeling
- Patients are instructed that some amount of exfoliation may occur in the postpeel period, for which an emollient can be used along with routine and regular use of sunscreens
- If erythema, burning and stinging are experienced in the postpeel period a mild topical corticosteroid cream (e.g., 0.05% desonide) may be applied twice a day for up to 3 days
- Jessener's solution should be avoided over large body areas due to potential systemic toxicity (due to the salicylic acid and resorcinol components).

Other Peels

- Khunger et al. published a pilot study in which serial 1% tretinoin peels were found to be as effective a therapy for melasma in dark skinned individuals as 70% GA in a sample size of 10 female patients[23]
- Pyruvic acid, an α-keto acid having keratolytic, sebostatic and antimicrobial properties, penetrates very rapidly and deeply. It has been tried in melasma, the limiting factor being the intense burning and possible postpeel crusting experienced by patients. Berardesca et al. conducted a study wherein 50% pyruvic acid peel was applied on 20 subjects for a total of four sessions performed every 2 weeks.[24] Instrumental evaluation revealed a significant pigment reduction in melasma patients
- The phytic acid peel, an α-hydroxy acid, allays the need for neutralizing and thereby lessens the likelihood of any adverse effects in the event of overpeeling[25]
- Combination peels are composed of two or more agents within a single formulation. Such peels are beneficial because they reduce the burden of using higher concentrations of a single agent and thus reducing the risk of side effects in dark skin. Common formulation includes

33% glycolic acid, 9% lactic acid, 7% kojic acid, 5% citric acid and 3% salicylic acid (Sesglicopeel K gel, Sesderma) and can be utilized every 2-3 weeks for about six sessions for melasma (more effective in the epidermal variant); the endpoint of each session being a faint erythema.

CONCLUSION

Although, numerous therapeutic modalities exist for melasma, we are yet to see a definitive cure for this disorder stereotypically known for its frequent recurrences. As systemic and topical therapies provide modest improvements in reduction of pigmentation, a variety of peels with varying characteristics certainly can be implemented in day-to-day practice. Ideally, the epidermal variant responds exceptionally well to the judicious use of chemical peels. Yet, Kligman's formula with its modifications (for a limited duration), other skin lightening topical agents and sunscreens continue to be the cornerstone of melasma treatment.

TAKE HOME POINTS

- Melasma is a stubborn disorder with frequent relapses and thus apart from topical/systemic therapies, peels work as formidable adjuvants
- Epidermal variant of melasma responds best to peels; dermal variant has to be tackled very cautiously as darker skin types may end up with PIH
- Broad spectrum sunscreens and other topical therapies work as priming agents cum definitive therapeutic modalities which have to be utilized during, before and even after cessation of peels
- Glycolic acid peels are time-dependent peels that are used most commonly either as a solo formulation or as a part of combination peels
- Salicylic acid peels work by way of their anti-inflammatory property thereby reducing PIH and also produce a diffuse "whitening effect"
- Salicylic + Mandelic acid combination peel is a safe and effective option for epidermal melasma
- Tricholoroacetic acid peels are coat-dependent peels and usually one coat suffices in the treatment of epidermal melasma
- Modified Jessner's solution, 1% tretinoin, 50% pyruvic acid and phytic acid have been utilized with varying results in melasma
- Many now consider combination peels the cornerstone and preferred choice in melasma because it gives the leverage to use a single formulation containing multiple agents at lower concentrations for a variety of indications without compromising safety, tolerability and efficacy.

REFERENCES

1. Sanchez NP, Pathak MA, Sato S, et al. Melasma: A clinical, light microscopic, ultrastructural, and immunofluorescence study. J Am Acad Dermatol. 1981;4:698-710.
2. Grimes PE. Melasma. Etiologic and therapeutic considerations. Arch Dermatol 1995;131:1453-7.
3. Victor FC, Gelber J, Rao B. Melasma: A review. J Cutan Med Surg. 2004;8:97-102.
4. Freitag FM, Cestari TF, Leopoldo LR, et al. Effect of melasma on quality of life in a sample of women living in southern Brazil. J Eur Acad Dermatol Venereol. 2008;22:655-62.
5. Pandya A, Berneburg M, Ortonne JP, et al. Guidelines for clinical trials in melasma. Pigmentation Disorders Academy. Br J Dermatol. 2006;156:21-8.
6. Garg VK, Sarkar R, Agarwal R. Comparative evaluation of beneficiary effects of priming agents (2% hydroquinone and 0.025% retinoic acid) in the treatment of melasma with glycolic acid peels. Dermatol Surg. 2008;34:1032-40.
7. Sheth VM, Pandya AG. Melasma: A comprehensive update: Part II. J Am Acad Dermatol. 2011;65:699-714.
8. Ball Arefiev KL, Hantash BM. Advances in the treatment of melasma: A review of the recent literature. Dermatol Surg. 2012;38:971-84.

9. Javaheri SM, Handa S, Kaur I, et al. Safety and efficacy of glycolic acid facial peel in Indian women with melasma. Int J Dermatol. 2001;40:354-7.
10. Grover C, Reddu BS. The therapeutic value of glycolic acid peels in dermatology. Indian J Dermatol Venereol Leprol. 2003;69:148-50.
11. Sarkar R, Kaur C, Bhalla M, et al. The combination of glycolic acid peels with a topical regimen in the treatment of melasma in dark-skinned patients: A comparative study. Dermatol Surg. 2002;28:828-32; discussion 832.
12. Dayal S, Sahu P, Dua R. Combination of glycolic acid peel and topical 20% azelaic acid cream in melasma patients: Efficacy and improvement in quality of life. J Cosmet Dermatol. 2017;16:35-42.
13. Garg VK, Sarkar R, Agarwal R. Comparative evaluation of beneficiary effects of priming agents (2% hydroquinone and 0.025% retinoic acid) in the treatment of melasma with glycolic acid peels. Dermatol Surg. 2008;34:1032-9; discussion 1340.
14. Sharquie KE, Al-Tikreety MM, Al-Mashhadani SA. Lactic acid as a new therapeutic peeling agent in melasma. Dermatol Surg. 2005;31:149-54.
15. Sharquie KE, Al-Tikreety MM, Al-Mashhadani SA. Lactic acid chemical peels as a new therapeutic modality in melasma in comparison to Jessner's solution chemical peels. Dermatol Surg. 2006;32:1429-36.
16. Sarkar R, Bansal S, Garg VK. Chemical peels for melasma in dark-skinned patients. J Cutan Aesthet Surg. 2012;5(4):247-53.
17. Grimes PE. The safety and efficacy of salicylic acid chemical peels in darker racial-ethnic groups. Dermatol Surg. 1999;25:18-22.
18. Sarkar R, Garg V, Bansal S, et al. Comparative evaluation of efficacy and tolerability of glycolic acid, salicylic mandelic acid, and phytic acid combination peels in melasma. Dermatol Surg. 2016;42(3):384-91.
19. Arif T. Salicylic acid as a peeling agent: A comprehensive review. Clin Cosmet Investig Dermatol. 2015;8:455-61.
20. Kalla G, Garg A, Kachhawa D. Chemical peeling--glycolic acid versus trichloroacetic acid in melasma. Indian J Dermatol Venereol Leprol. 2001;67:82-4.
21. Soliman MM, Ramadan SA, Bassiouny DA, et al. Combined trichloroacetic acid peel and topical ascorbic acid versus trichloroacetic acid peel alone in the treatment of melasma: A comparative study. J Cosmet Dermatol. 2007;6:89-94.
22. Safoury OS, Zaki NM, El Nabarawy EA, et al. A study comparing chemical peeling using modified Jessner's solution and 15% trichloroacetic acid versus 15% trichloroacetic acid in the treatment of melasma. Indian J Dermatol. 2009;54:41-5.
23. Khunger N, Sarkar R, Jain RK. Tretinoin peels versus glycolic acid peels in the treatment of melasma in dark-skinned patients. Dermatol Surg. 2004;30:756-60; discussion 760.
24. Berardesca E, Cameli N, Primavera G, et al. Clinical and instrumental evaluation of skin improvement after treatment with a new 50% pyruvic acid peel. Dermatol Surg. 2006;32:526-31.
25. Deprez P. Easy phytic solution: A new alpha hydroxy acid peel with slow release and without neutralization. Int J Cosm Surg Aesth Derm. 2003;5:45-51.

Chemical Peels for the Treatment of Postinflammatory Hyperpigmentation

Nisha V Parmar, Rashmi Sarkar

INTRODUCTION

Postinflammatory hyperpigmentation (PIH) refers to an acquired excess of pigment deposition at the sites of prior inflammatory dermatoses or on procedural sites. It occurs more commonly in persons with Fitzpatrick skin types III–VI.

EPIDEMIOLOGY

Epidemiologic data on PIH is scarce; a study by Halder et al. in 1983 revealed PIH to be the third most common dermatosis amongst African Americans.[1] A Singaporean study in 1992 on 74,589 patients reported the prevalence of PIH to be 12.2% in Indians (n = 7,384.3) and 11.3% in Malays (n = 4,176.98).[2] PIH is the most common complication of laser treatments in individuals with darker skin. The incidence of PIH post laser treatment varies from 11.2% to 92% depending on the depth and type of lasers used.[3-5] PIH occurred in as high as 92% of patients with Fitzpatrick skin type IV after ablative fractional carbon dioxide laser procedures in comparison to 32% of patients with skin types I to III undergoing the same procedures.[3,4]

ETIOPATHOGENESIS OF POSTINFLAMMATORY HYPERPIGMENTATION

The "individual chromatic tendency" theory suggests that every person's ability to heal with either hypopigmentation or hyperpigmentation is determined genetically.[6] As a result of cutaneous inflammation, cytokines including prostaglandins and eicosanoids are released. Leukotrienes B_4, C_4, D_4, E_4 and prostaglandins E_2 and D_2 stimulate melanocyte proliferation and leukotriene C_4 has been found to stimulate tyrosinase activity.[7]

CLASSIFICATION OF POSTINFLAMMATORY HYPERPIGMENTATION

Classification of PIH is based on the depth of pigment deposition in the skin. PIH is thus classified as epidermal, dermal, or mixed. Epidermal PIH manifests as tan brown to dark brown pigmentation, which may fade away spontaneously within months without treatment. Dermal PIH manifests as blue-gray macules, which may persist indefinitely. Mixed PIH consists of both epidermal and dermal components. It is important to classify PIH before planning management as treatment outcomes depend upon the type of PIH. Noninvasive investigatory tools such as Wood's lamp examination, colorimetry and dermoscopic evaluation can be used to accurately assess the depth of pigmentation prior to treatment initiation.

TREATMENT OF POSTINFLAMMATORY HYPERPIGMENTATION

Postinflammatory hyperpigmentation can have great impact on the quality of life of affected individuals. Treatment is sought often with high expectations regarding clearance of pigmentation and restoration of normal skin color as fast as possible. Each individual patient needs to be carefully counseled regarding treatment options and outcomes, and the need for patience during the treatment period.

CHEMICAL PEELS FOR POSTINFLAMMATORY HYPERPIGMENTATION

Treatment is based on the type of PIH in the individual patient. Chemical peels are currently used for the management of epidermal and mixed PIH and form the second-line treatment option. Chemicals peels should be used with caution and only by experienced dermatologists due to the possibility of subsequent treatment related side effects.

Superficial peels are the peels of choice for the treatment of PIH. They act by exfoliating the epidermis and upper papillary dermis and include glycolic acid (GA) in a concentration of 20-50%, salicylic acid in concentrations of 20-30%, trichloroacetic acid in concentrations of 10-35%, tretinoin peel and Jessner's solution (salicylic acid, lactic acid and resorcinol).

Prior to peeling, the following regime has to be advised to the patients:[8]

- Use of a broad-spectrum sunscreen lotion with a sun protection factor of 30 to be used on the sun-exposed areas at intervals of 3 hours during the daytime
- Use of a priming agent at bedtime to the areas where peeling is to be done. Priming agents include hydroquinone 2-4% in a cream base, tretinoin 0.025-0.05% in a cream base, or GA 6-12% in a cream base. The aim of priming is to ensure uniform penetration of peel during the procedure and to prevent subsequent post-treatment related PIH. Application of the priming agent should be done for preferably 4 weeks prior to the peeling and should be stopped 2 days before the peeling
- Avoidance of the use of scrubs, loofahs and exfoliators before, during and after the whole treatment duration. This is to avoid any irritation to the treatment sites which could lead to subsequent PIH
- Use of gentle cleansers with a pH of 5.5 (normal pH of skin) for cleaning the areas to be treated.

Peeling Procedure

The first peel is performed 2-4 weeks after priming, and subsequent peels performed every 2-3 weeks thereafter. The contact time of peel depends on the peeling agent used and increases during subsequent sessions:

- *Glycolic acid*: 2 minutes to start with and sequentially increased to a maximum of 5 minutes
- *Salicylic acid*: 3 minutes to start with, increased to 5 minutes subsequently.
- *Trichloroacetic acid*: 10-30% applied as one coat; endpoint is frosting
- *Tretinoin peel*: leave on peel washed after 4-6 hours.

Postpeel Care

The goal of postpeel care is to ensure faster recovery of the skin with minimal complications. Redness, minimal edema and exfoliation are expected to occur within 1-3 days of peeling using superficial peels.

Post peel care includes use of broad-spectrum sunscreen, adequate moisturization using bland nonscented moisturizers, complete avoidance of manually peeling or rubbing the peeling sites, and use of gentle facial cleansers.

Instructions for postpeel care should be preferably handed to patients in a printed manner and explained carefully to avoid complications.

Application of priming agents can be resumed 5-7 days after a superficial peel.

Current Evidence on the Use of Chemical Peels for Postinflammatory Hyperpigmentation

Burns et al. first studied the role of GA in the treatment of PIH in combination of a topical regimen.[9] Nineteen patients were randomized into two groups, one receiving only the topical regimen consisting of hydroquinone 2%, GA 10% and tretinoin 0.05%, and the other group receiving the topical regimen combined with six serial GA peels from 50% to 68% concentrations. Statistically significant results were obtained in the peels group as assessed by colorimetry and hyperpigmentation area severity score.

Grimes studied the use of salicylic acid peels in ethnic skin in a pilot study including 25 patients; five of these had PIH. The peels were performed using 20% and 30% salicylic acid every 2 weeks for a total of five peels per patient. Assessment was done using serial photographic evaluation. Four out of five patients with PIH had significant improvement (>75%) at the end of the study and one patient had moderate improvement (51-75%).[10]

Joshi et al. conducted a randomized spilt face study on the use of salicylic acid peels for treatment of PIH in 10 dark-skinned patients.[11] Three peels of 20% salicylic acid followed by three peels of 30% salicylic acid were used on one side of the face whereas the other half remained untreated. Results were assessed using the visual analog scale, dermatology life quality index (DLQI) and a patient structured treatment quality questionnaire. Improvement on the treated side (as assessed by individual raters), as well as DLQI were not statistically significant. However, subjects' visual analog scale (VAS) scores suggested significant improvement on treated side.

More recently, Sarkar et al. evaluated the use of GA 30-50% in combination with modified Kligman's formula consisting of hydrocortisone 1%, hydroquinone 2% and tretinoin 0.05% in 30 patients, 15 of which received both peels and topical regimen, and 15 topical regimen alone.[12] Results were established using the hyperpigmentation area and severity index (HASI) score and clinical photography, and revealed statistical significance difference between the peel group and topical regimen alone group, favoring the peels group.

Current Recommendations on the Use of Chemical Peels for Postinflammatory Hyperpigmentation[13]

Current recommendations place chemical peels as second line in the treatment of epidermal and mixed PIH. The peels recommended are:

- Glycolic acid peels starting with 50% and performed every 3 weeks (Level of evidence: A) (Fig. 1). Start with lower concentrations in darker skin types

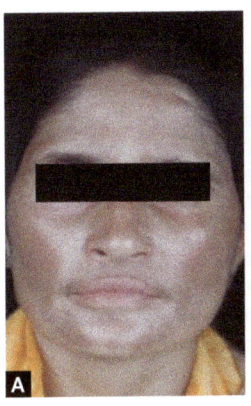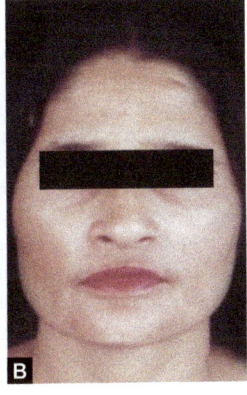

FIG. 1: Treatment of postinflammatory hyperpigmentation with glycolic acid (GA) peels. **A,** Pretreatment; **B,** After six peels, three with 25% GA, three with 35% GA.

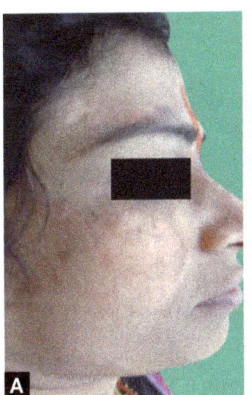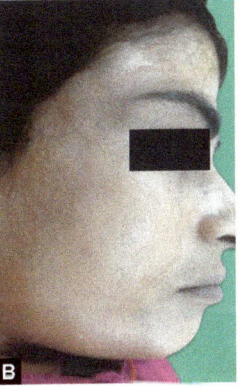

FIG. 2: Treatment of postinflammatory hyperpigmentation with salicylic acid (SA). **A,** Pretreatment; **B,** After six peels, three with 20% SA, three with 30% SA.

- Salicylic acid peels starting with 20-30% scheduled every 2 weeks (Level of evidence: B) (Fig. 2).

CONCLUSION

Chemical peels are reserved for treatment of epidermal and mixed PIH that is refractory to topical treatment modalities. Optimal results are achieved when peels are used in combination with topical treatments in the intervening periods. Only a handful of studies are available on the use of chemical peels in PIH and these support the use of superficial chemical peels glycolic acid and salicylic acid.

TAKE HOME POINTS

- Postinflammatory hyperpigmentation is a common acquired disorder of pigmentation in individuals with Fitzpatrick's skin types III-VI
- Postinflammatory hyperpigmentation is classified as epidermal, dermal and mixed depending on the depth of pigment deposition
- Management of PIH should be carefully planned as procedural modalities such as chemical peels bear the risks of subsequent treatment-related PIH
- Superficial chemical peels are the peels of choice and reserved for second line in the treatment algorithm
- Data on the use of chemical peels for PIH is limited to two peels: Glycolic acid 30-68% and salicylic acid 20-30%.

REFERENCES

1. Halder RN, Grimes PE, Mc Laurin Cl, et al. Incidence of common dermatoses in a predominantly black dermatologic practice. Cutis. 1983;32:388-90.
2. Chuah-Ty G, Goh CL, Koh SL. Pattern of skin diseases at the national skin center (Singapore) from 1989-1990. Int J Dermatol. 1992;31:555-9.
3. Chan HH, Manstein D, Yu CS, et al. The prevalence and risk factors of postinflammatory hyperpigmentation after fractional resurfacing in Asians. Lasers Sur Med. 2007;39:381-5.
4. Manuskiatti W, Triwongwaranat D, Varothai S, et al. Efficacy and safety of a carbon-dioxide ablative fractional resurfacing device for treatment of atrophic acne scars in Asians. J Am Acad Dermatol. 2010;63:274-83.
5. Chapas AM, Brightman L, Sukal S, et al. Successful treatment of acneiform scarring with CO2 ablative fractional resurfacing. Lasers Surg Med. 2008;40:381-6.

6. Ruiz-Maldonado R, Orozco-Covarrubius ML. Postinflammatory hypopigmentation and hyperpigmentation. Semin Cutan Med Surg. 1997;16:36-43.
7. Tomita Y, Maeda K, Tagami H. Melanocyte stimulating properties of arachidonic acid metabolites: possible role in postinflammatory hyperpigmentation. Pigment Cell Res. 1992;5:357-61.
8. Khunger N. Standard guidelines of care for chemical peels. Indian J Dermatol Venereol Leprol. 2008;74:S5-12.
9. Burns RL, Prevost-Blank PL, Laury MA, et al. Glycolic acid peels for postinflammatory hyperpigmenatation in black patients: a comparative study. Dermatol Surg. 1997;23:171-4.
10. Grimes PE. The safety and efficacy of salicylic acid chemical peels in darker racial ethnic groups. Dermatol Surg. 1999;25:18-22.
11. Joshi SS, Boone SL, Alam M, et al. Effectiveness, safety and effect on quality of life of topical Salicylic acid peels for treatment of postinflammatory hyperpigmentation in dark skin. Dermatol Surg. 2009;35:638-44.
12. Sarkar R, Parmar NV, Kapoor S. Treatment of postinflammatory hyperpigmentation with a combination of glycolic acid peels and a topical regimen in dark-skinned patients: a comparative study. Dermatol Surg. 2017;43(4):566-73.
13. Postinflammatory hyperpigmentation: a comprehensive review-treatment options and prevention. J Am Acad Dermatol. 2017;77:607-21.

CHAPTER 30

Chemical Peels for Acne and Acne Scars in Dark Skin

Monica B Dassi

INTRODUCTION

Acne and its complications including postinflammatory hyperpigmentation (PIH) and scarring constitute one of the most common dermatological problems. The erstwhile "physiological self-resolving teenage disorder" has now attained a new dimension, that of persistence beyond teenage, especially in women stemming from a rising incidence of polycystic ovarian syndrome. Some being temporary like hyperpigmented or erythematous macular scar or permanent scarring both atrophic and hypertrophic. The etiological factors of acne including hormonal imbalance, eventuate into the tetrad of follicular hyperkeratinization, excess sebum production, bacterial proliferation and generation of proinflammatory mediators; the local skin alterations that produce the lesions of acne.

The general properties, effects and mechanism of action of chemical peels have been discussed in great detail in the initial chapters of this book. In this chapter, we shall concentrate on the role of chemical peels in general, role of specific peels and optimizing their use in improving acne and associated scarring.

Oral isotretinoin is perhaps the only molecule that targets the entire tetrad of acne pathogenesis. However, chemical peels also possess acne-reduction properties and when used in combination, can reduce follicular hyperkeratinization, control sebum levels, exert antibacterial effect and control inflammation. Additionally, their depigmenting and resurfacing effects also halt the ongoing PIH and scarring and with judicious use of select peels, the established PIH and scarring can be reversed to a significant extent, with or without additional physical interventions. Though topical and oral treatments work well for acne vulgaris, conventionally peels have been considered a great adjuvant therapy for resistant or recalcitrant acne. However, the changing trend and the author's personal experience favors early introduction of chemical peels in majority of patients, along with the medical therapy, since the overall cosmetic outcome seems to be much better with this approach.

GENERAL DETERMINANTS

General determinants defining the benefit of adding on peels for acne and selection of the peel:

- Grade of acne
- Severity and grading of established PIH and scarring
- Possibility of impending PIH and scarring
- The duration, nature and response to medical therapy
- Concomitant use of oral isotretinoin
- Patient's expectations, compliance and commitment to meticulous postpeel care
- Skin sensitivity
- Costing and patient affordability
- Need for additional physical procedures.

COMMON PEELS USED FOR ACNE

- Salicylic acid (SA) peel
- Jessner's solution (JS)
- Glycolic acid (GA) peel
- Trichloroacetic acid (TCA) peel
- Mandelic acid (MA) peel
- Pyruvic acid (PA) peel
- Lactic acid (LA) peel
- Retinoic acid peel
- Newer peels or combination peels like black peel.

SALICYLIC ACID PEEL

Salicylic acid has been used in various skin conditions for over 2,000 years. Chemically, SA is 2-hydroxybenzoic acid or orthobenzoic acid. It is found in nature in willow barks, winter green leaves and sweet birch. It was labelled as beta-hydroxy acid (BHA) by Kingman, but Yu and Van classified it as a phenolic aromatic acid.[1] SA has aromatic benzene ring to which are attached the carboxyl (-COOH) and hydroxyl (-OH) groups directly. In case of true BHA, there is an aliphatic carbon atom chain. It has a pKa value of three.

Salicylic acid ability to work on acne is due to its lipid-soluble properties and penetrates into the pilosebaceous units. The acne formation started from the excessive keratinization in the mid portion of the follicular canal. This leads to the comedones formation. Lipophilicity leads to the penetration of salicylic acid in the pilosebaceous unit and comedolysis. It is easily miscible with epidermal lipids and sebaceous gland lipids, reduces sebum secretions and has sebumetric effects which adds to the therapeutic benefit. It has keratolytic and comedolytic properties. Being a lipophilic agent, SA removes intercellular lipids, which are linked covalently to the cornified envelop surrounding the surface epithelial cells, decreases corneocyte adhesion, loosens these cells and subsequently causes detachment. SA is considered a desmolytic agent rather a keratolytic agent since it extracts desmosomal protein including desmoglein, disrupting cellular junction rather than lysing intercellular keratin filaments.[3] This causes loosening of the epidermal cell and exfoliation. Being a salicylate, SA also has anti-inflammatory properties, rapidly reduces the postpeel erythema and erythematous macular scars. It also has an anesthetic effect, making the peel more acceptable to the patient. It has antimicrobial and antifungal properties. Whitfield's ointment which contains benzoic acid and SA has antifungal properties.

Various formulations of SA are used for peeling purpose. SA is prepared in ethyl alcohol containing 10-50% SA (w/v) or as newer formulation 20-30% SA in polyethylene glycol. The risk of salicylism in intact skin with this formulation is low. It has also been found to reduce ultraviolet B-induced skin cancers in hairless mice.[4] The properties of SA change with the concentration of SA. 20-30% are usually used for the acne as superficial peeling agents. Pearl et al. in his study on ethnic skin observed moderate to significant improvement in papules, comedones and microcomedones, and mild reduction in pustular and cystic acne.[5] There was rapid reduction in microcomedones and textural improvement in rough oily skin and open pores. Combination of 4% hydroquinone with regular SA peel reduced the postacne hyperpigmentation faster than would occur with conventional treatment. Side effect profile with SA is low. Lee et al. noticed reduction in both inflammatory and noninflammatory acne with significant reduction in the total facial lesion count.

Indications in Acne

Salicylic peel works very well in grade I and II acne causing significant reduction in microcomedones. Indications are listed below:
- Reduction in microcomedones, comedones and inflammatory acne (Fig. 1)
- Reduction rapidly in erythematous acne scars and postinflammatory hyperpigmentation
- Seborrhea
- Open pores
- Uneven skin tone with rough skin
- Pigmentation in a sensitive skin type.

Contraindications

- Allergy to salicylates, aspirin
- Pregnancy or lactation; SA is a category C drug
- Very dry skin

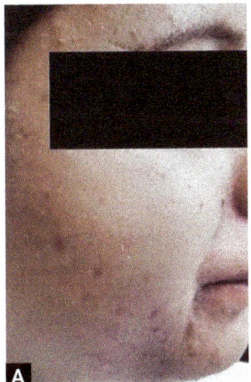 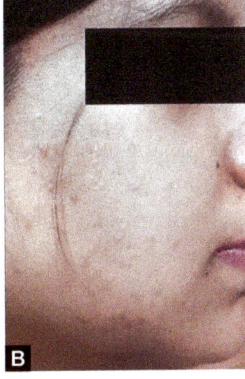

FIG. 1: **A,** 30-year-old female with jawline comedonal acne and **B,** after 3 sessions of 20% salicylic peel with serial comedone extraction after each session.

- Unrealistic expectation or patient not willing to continue 4–6 sessions of the peel.

Complications

They are rare. Commonly associated with dryness and burning sensation. Lee et al. observed persistent erythema in few patients lasting for 2 days in 8.8% of the cases.[6] Incidence of superficial crusting in the periorbital area was observed especially in first session but no permanent pigmentation or scarring seen.

For application on face, salicylism is not known. Systemic toxicity due to cutaneous absorption can cause salicylism. It is very rare but of serious concern. It is characterized by tinnitus, dizziness, abdominal cramps, deafness, psychosis stupor, coma and death. It occurs when the blood concentration of salicylate exceeds 35 mg/dL. Salicylate toxicity is reported when 20% SA is applied to 50% body surface area. Fung et al. concluded that facial peeling with 30% SA formulation do not pose risk of systemic toxicity.[6]

Salicylic acid is a weak contact sensitizer, and rare contact dermatitis with SA or other components of the preparation may be noticed.

Key Points about Salicylic Peel

- Salicylic peels are ideal peels for young adults or teenagers with acne
- It can be concomitantly used with oral isotretinoin and has a cumulative benefit
- Grade I acne warrants for removal of comedones prior to the peel dual benefit of faster clearance of lesions and prevention of postpeel flare up. It can also prove beneficial in difficult to treat topical steroid damaged/dependent face (TSDF) with monomorphic grade I acne
- Peel should be poured seconds before the application as it precipitates fast

- Within few minutes of peel application, it leaves behind a white precipitate of SA or pseudofrost. Penetration is arrested once the vehicle has volatilized. This is unlike the frosting, which occurs in medium-depth peels due to coagulation of surface proteins
- Drinking large amount of water before or after the peel prevents incidence of salicylism
- Salicylic acid is self neutralizing.

JESSNER'S PEELS

Jessner's solution is a combination of alpha-hydroxy acid (AHA), SA along with phenol derivative resorcinol in combination of 14% SA, 14% resorcinol or citric acid and 14% LA in 95% ethanol. Resorcinol also known as resorcin, it is slightly more acidic than phenol and is used as a component of the superficial peel. Though, it belongs to the phenol group but is less toxic than phenol. In modified Jessner's peel, resorcinol is replaced with citric acid. Citric acid produces reduction of open pores, which is often associated with oily skin type. By eliminating resorcinol, side effects and toxicity is reduced and efficacy is increased. Many modified versions of JS containing kojic acid, hydroquinone etc. are also available.

Indications in Acne

It has antiseptic, antipruritic and keratolytic properties. The weak hydrogen links of keratin are broken by its proteolytic power even at lower concentrations. At higher concentration, it can precipitate skin proteins and become a protein coagulant. The efficacy of JS varies with skin thickness, sensitivity, skin preparation, force of application, type of applicator, number of coats used, quality and type of prepared solution. Jessner's peel does not cause systemic effects like dizziness, tinnitus or faintness as described with resorcinol paste. But, in case resorcinol peel is applied on larger surface area, one must be aware of the absorption that may occur and salicylism is described.

Degreasing with acetone and alcohol is recommended. Jessner's is applied slowly, second coat only when the first coat is dry. The number of coats describes the strength of the peel. Depth also depends on the force of application. First coat causes erythema, pinpoint frosting and some pseudofrosting. Unlike true frosting which is due to protein coagulation, pseudo frosting can be brushed away. Skin should be allowed to dry for 4–5 minutes in between two subsequent coats. Second and third coats are associated with more pronounced erythema and cloudy-white frosting. Flaking occurs after 4–5 days. More than three coats are not recommended. It eliminates comedones, improves dyschromia and relieves folliculitis.

Studies comparing Jessner's peel with SA by Dayal et al. and Bae et al. clearly concluded that salicylic peel achieved clearance of noninflammatory comedones faster within 6 weeks of start of therapy which was not possible for Jessner's peel even after 12 weeks.[8,9] In inflammatory acne, papules showed earlier clearance as fast as 1 week with SA peel while with JS, the clearance was slower. Though at the end of 12 weeks of study, both achieved similar results. Pustular lesion reduced similarly over 4 weeks and the difference in lesion count was statistically insignificant. Side effects like prolonged erythema were more common with JS as compared to SA. Incidence of postinflammatory hyperpigmentation was also higher with Jessner's peel. Overall improvement in acne was 85% with SA than 20% with JS.[8]

Jessner's solution can be done before a deeper peel like TCA as a skin preparatory peel, for example Monheit technique.

Monheit technique: Jessner's peel is applied first resulting in a uniform erythema. Once dry, TCA is applied over it resulting in increased penetration and more efficacy.

It works best in people with thick, acne-prone and oily skin. This technique can be used before an AHA known as the Moy technique. But, the limitation of this technique is that AHA when applied on the erythematous skin post JS, may cause frosting. This is because the endpoint of AHA is also erythema which may not be appreciated on the erythematous skin.

Contraindications

It is best avoided in patient with hepatic and renal insufficiency, patients with arrhythmia, and pregnant and breastfeeding women. Jessner's solution is known to be absorbed into capillaries due to its small molecular size. Methemoglobinemia has been described after application on leg ulcer but never with peels. Salicylism has been described only on application to large body parts. Surface, body weight and the hydration are important for salicylism.

Pigmentation is also common post Jessner's peel. Effective sun protection is important.

Key Points in Jessner's Peel

- Jessner's is an effective peel in active inflammatory acne
- Additional benefit in case of thick oily skin or actinically damaged skin
- Complication are rare, though PIH is known to happen after Jessner's peel
- Allergy to resorcinol manifests as generalized pruritic, erythema and disproportionate edema
- Systemic toxicity can occur with both resorcinol and SA, when they are applied on large surface areas.

GLYCOLIC ACID

Glycolic acid is the most popular AHA for peeling. GA is the smallest AHA with the chemical nomenclature aliphatic: alpha-hydroxy acetic acid.

Unlike SA, it is highly hydrophilic solution and has multiple mode of action. Various concentration ranging from 20% to 70% are used. Its activity is determined by the pH of the solution. At a low concentration and acidic pH, it causes lysis of the desmosomes, removes the stratum corneum, unroofs the papules and pustules, scatters basal melanocytes and stimulates epidermolysis.[10] It behaves as a moisturizer at higher pH. The absorption of GA in human skin depends on the pH, concentration of the GA, skin type and the time and site of application. Since it does not cause any coagulation of the protein like TCA peel, the endpoint is erythema and not frosting.

Indication in Acne

Usually all grades of acne respond to glycolic peel, though effect increases with number of session. Noninflammatory lesion responds faster, though the response of inflammatory lesion like papules is also significant. It not only improves the lesion count but also improves postinflammatory hyperpigmentation, macular scars and overall skin texture. It has an antibacterial effect as shown by Takenaka and colleagues and can also help in combating the ever-increasing antibiotic resistance to *Propionibacterium acnes*.[11] No or minimal response was seen in nodulocystic acne. Exfoliation and stimulating growth in the basal layer in the epidermis also causes melanocyte stimulation and sensitization of the skin and can cause postinflammatory hyperpigmentation.

Glycolic acid peels have been studied both in comparison and as combination with other peels. Seventy percent GA was found to be equally effective as Jessner's peel, though the response with glycolic peel was initially less dramatic and Jessner's peel was associated

Chemical Peels: A Global Perspective

with more exfoliation.[12] As compared to salicylic–mandelic acid combination peel (SMP), active acne- and postacne scarring responded better to SMP than glycolic peel.[13] For facial acne, concentration of 50% or less is most effective with contact time of 1–3 minutes. Unexpected frosting with higher concentration and prolonged contact time delays the healing process and also makes the patient susceptible to postpeel complications. For back acne, higher concentration of 50% or 70% for 4–10 minutes can be used. Frosting on the back is a sign of greater effectiveness. Inflamed acne responds best to AHA. Figure 2 shows the improvement in inflammatory acne and the skin tone and complexion after three sessions of GA peel 35% and 50%.

Complications

Usual side effect of glycolic peel includes erythema, burning, irritation and postinflammatory pigmentation.

Contraindications

- Contact dermatitis and glycolate hypersensitivity
- It is category B drug and may be used in pregnancy in lower concentrations.

Key Points of Glycolic Peel

- Priming before the peel significantly improves the results of the peel and reduces the complications too
- Glycolic acid is the smallest of all AHAs, followed by lactic, pyruvic, malic, tartaric

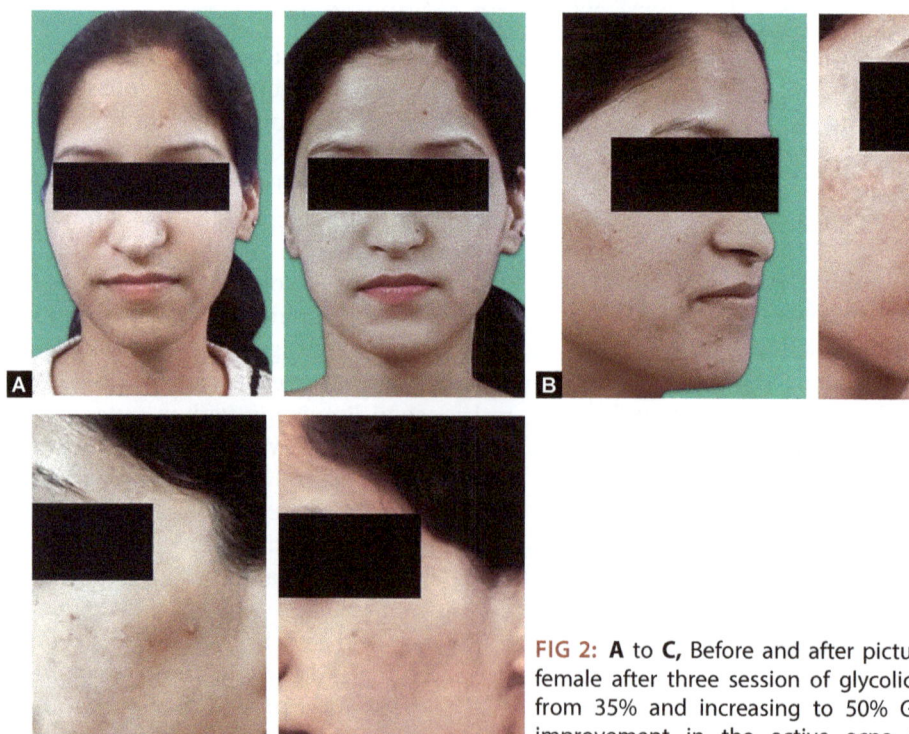

FIG 2: **A** to **C,** Before and after pictures of a young female after three session of glycolic peels starting from 35% and increasing to 50% GA. Apart from improvement in the active acne lesions, visible improvement is also noticed in the skin texture, complexion and PIH.

and citric acids. The bioavailability of the AHAs increases as pH decreases
- The peel is time dependent and need neutralization with sodium bicarbonate
- pH and the contact time of the peel both are important in the acidifying power and depth of the peel
- Glycolic acid works well both for grade II acne and PIH secondary to acne. It gives an overall rejuvenated look
- Ideal for patients with acne and pigmentation
- One should watch out for acneiform eruption as a postpeel complication and in such cases, it is best to stop the glycolic peel.

TRICHLOROACETIC ACID PEEL

Trichloroacetic acid is classified as haloacetic acid, which are derivatives of acetic acid in which one or more hydrogen atoms on the alpha carbon are replaced by halogens. TCA is a chlorine derivative of the acetic acid. It is a strong acid with pKa 0.26. It comes as a white or colorless crystal with a distinct pungent smell. The TCA crystals are hydrophilic and readily dissolve on exposure to atmospheric humidity. TCA is unstable in water and its concentration becomes more and more dilute and therefore less effective over time. TCA in simple aqueous solution (TCA-SAS) is prepared by simply dissolving TCA crystal in water, are unstable and can give unpredictable outcome and severe complication. It is, therefore, safer to not use crystals but TCA in the solution form which do not have the capacity to hydrate by themselves. Various adjuvants are added like glyceryl monooleate and propylene glycol to stabilize it. TCA peel is a tricky peel; different methods of preparing the peel can give different results with the same concentration of the peel. Depth of destruction also depends on the concentration of the peel. TCA is a self-neutralizing peel.

Indications in Acne

Trichloroacetic acid is a caustic and causes coagulation of the skin protein which appears as frosting. Fig. 3 illustrates the frosting observed with TCA peel which cannot be rubbed off as the pseudofrost of SA. The intensity of frosting gives a rough measure of the depth of the peel. Penetration of TCA depends on its concentration and on the thickness of the skin. Prepeel priming with tretinoin and degreasing with acetone causes membrane lipid modification and increases penetration. TCA causes destruction of the living cells of the epidermis and part or whole of dermis depending on its concentration. Surrounding surviving cells cause regeneration of new cells. Subsequently new collagen is also formed. 10%, 15% and 25% are the various strengths used. It behaves as a superficial peel at 10%, 15% and 25% and as medium-depth peel at 35%.

Due to its keratolytic properties, it is useful in comedonal acne and also in active acne. Coagulation of the skin proteins and reepithelialization causes reduction in comedonal and active acne, and also acne-induced PIH and superficial scarring. TCA can be done for all types of acne. Severe

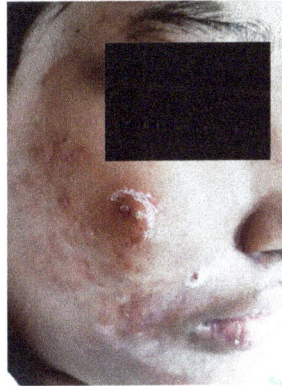

FIG. 3: Frosting seen with 15% trichloroacetic acid peel.

acne should be treated medically first and controlled before undergoing a peel. Medium-depth concentration till the basal layer are effective for all acne lesions like comedonal, microcystic, papular or papulopustular. Deeper peel in active acne increases the risk of infection. It is an ideal peel for active acne with postinflammatory hyperpigmentation. To obtain better results and to prevent postpeel flare of acne, we can remove the comedones and microcysts immediately before the peel. This intervention gives faster and better results. Seborrhea is reduced, pigmented acne scars become better, and shallow acne scar softens though there is no improvement of ice-pick scars. Endpoint of the TCA peel is the erythema signaling epidermal depth and pinpoint or cloudy-white frosting signaling deeper penetration.

Trichloroacetic acid has an added benefit for treatment of superficial acne scars and also ice-pick scars which are otherwise difficult to treat with chemical reconstruction of skin scars (CROSS) technique.

Complications

To avoid complications, care needs to be exercised during application of the peel and postpeel. Burns and irritation on contact with skin, eyes and mucosa are known. The complication of TCA peel includes skin atrophy, scarring and hypopigmentation invariably with higher concentration of TCA peels where there is appendageal damage and reepithelialization is hampered. This can also result in hypopigmentation and depigmentation due to necrosis of the melanocyte reserve along with keratinocytes, which results in scarring. There are reported incidence of infection, persistent erythema, hypopigmentation and hyperpigmentation, scarring, milia and textural changes.[14]

Contraindications

- Keloidal tendency
- Recent facial surgical procedure or flaps, which may have compromised circulation
- Immunocompromised patient
- Non-compliant patients who cannot adhere to thorough post care regimen.

Key Points of Trichloroacetic Acid

- Endpoint of the TCA peel is frosting
- Intensity of erythema and levels of frosting are important indicators of the penetration of the peel
- Self-neutralizing, not absorbed systemically even at higher concentration
- Penetration of TCA may be uneven due to no apparent reason. These are known as hot spot. One should be vigilant for these hot spots during application of the peel.

MANDELIC ACID PEEL

Mandelic acid is an AHA obtained from amygdalin, a glycoside found in peaches, bitter almonds and apricots. It has a phenyl group as a side chain substitute. MA has a pKa value of 3.41 at 25°C and is therefore stronger acid that GA which had pKa of 3.83. But, it has a high molecular weight, therefore a larger size and hence the penetration is low.

It works similar to other AHA. The phenolic group as a side chain renders it more lipophilic as compared to other AHA and can be used for acne-prone and oily skin. It has an antibacterial activity and is also used as antibiotic in urinary tract infections. Due to its antimicrobial action, it is used in active acne especially in people with sensitive skin.

Indications in Acne

Mandelic peel is ideal for use in infected acne, sensitive skin and darker skin type. Large molecular weight and low penetration of MA is advantageous in cases of people with sensitive skin with acne and pigmentation but has also been a disadvantage of not being assessed as a peeling agent. The endpoint in mandelic peel is difficult to appreciate and due to absence of visible peeling, patient satisfaction may be low. It is also a good peel option in case of apprehensive patient worried about stinging in peeling process. It can be used as a stand-alone peel at the concentration of 20–50% or in combination with other superficial peel, the most popular being SA peel with SA 20% and MA 10%.[13] Mandelic peel 40% is also used in combination with azelaic acid 20% for postinflammatory pigmentation and acne. MA can improve both the lesion count in type II and III grade acne but also lightens, rejuvenates the skin with lightening of the macular scars due to its ability to inhibit melanogenesis. As a combination, it improves the erythema associated with acne. Its antibacterial properties are useful for preventing gram-negative folliculitis post laser resurfacing or due to prolonged use of antibiotics in acne. MA can be applied as a leave on peel also depending on the patient's skin type. Fig. 4 shows the significant improvement in the pustules and the erythema after two sessions of salicylic mandelic peel.

Complications

Complications are rare.

Key Points of Mandelic Acid Peel

- Ideal use in patient of acne with sensitive skin who are unable to tolerate glycolic or trichloroacetic acid peels
- Can be used sequentially or as combination peels. The most popular combination being with SA
- There is no specific endpoint.

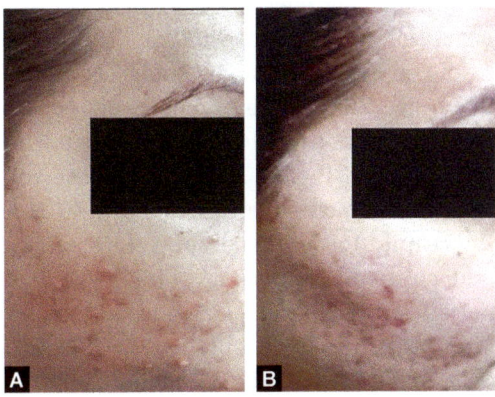

FIG. 4: **A,** Young female with grade II acne vulgaris; **B,** after 3 session of sequential peels with 20% SA and mandalic acid sequential peels with marked reduction in the inflammatory acne and the erythematous macules.

PYRUVIC ACID PEEL

Pyruvic acid is an alpha-keto acid which has a carboxylic acid having a keto group at alpha position of the aliphatic carbon atom. It is converted partly to LA by lactate dehydrogenase and is physiologically in equilibrium with LA. It is a potent acid with pKa of 2.39 and a small molecular size facilitating deeper penetration. Presence of LA makes it a well-tolerated peel.

Indications in Acne

Pyruvic acid has a lipophilic nature like SA and has keratolytic, antimicrobial and sebostatic activities. LA is a humectant. It causes keratolysis in the epidermis but also causes collagen induction in the dermis. Sebostatic nature makes it ideally suited for oily skin. There is no coagulation of protein so no frosting. Endpoint is blanching and mild erythema. Forty percent PA in a well-balanced proportion with water and ethanol is used for superficial peeling.

Comedolytic effect and lipophilic nature is beneficial in grade I acne and seborrhea; also helpful in open pores and superficial scarring due to its effect on dermal collagen, elastin and glycoproteins. Gel form formulation with stabilized 40% PA and 5% LA treats acne and seborrhea. Cotellessa et al. study with 40–50% PA in mild-to-moderate acne, 40% patient had complete remission, while 50% had partial remission, and 10% had no effect.[15] Similar results were obtained by Pacifico et al. and Tosson et al.[16,17] Patient with mild acne revealed better response as compared to severe acne. Stinging, persistent erythema and mild scaling are the common side effects. Application of sodium bicarbonate 10% rapidly relieved the burning. However, it is good option for peeling in patient with photodamaged dull skin with acne.

Complications

Since its molecular size is small, PA penetrates rapidly to the dermis. The side effect of the pyruvic peel is the intense stinging sensation on application and post peel erythema which may last for 15–30 minutes. One needs to be careful especially while treating thin sensitive skin for fear of scarring.

Contraindications

Individuals with thin skin.

Key Points of Pyruvic Peel

- Deeper penetration, excess burning and stinging sensation but well tolerated due to presence of LA
- Superficial thin desquamation for 7–10 days
- Blanching suggestive of the depth of penetration but may be difficult to appreciate in darker skin type.

LACTIC ACID

Lactic acid is a weak AHA derived from sour milk or bilberries. It has a pH of 3.5 at 90% concentration. It is also used as combination peel in Jessner's peel and other rejuvenating or party peels. Full strength LA peel 92% can be safely used in skin of color. It reduces the thickness of stratum corneum by reducing intracorneocyte adhesion. It is a humectant and has moisturizing properties. It can improve skin texture, pigmentation and general appearance of the skin. It has a comparatively larger size so it penetrates slowly and therefore is not associated with inflammation and complications.

Indications in Acne

Alpha-hydroxy acids give good to excellent results in acne. Keratinocyte cohesion is reduced in the follicles, and prevents follicle canal clogging. It has antimicrobial and anti-inflammatory properties. Since it is a humectant, it improves skin texture. It can be used mostly in inflammatory acne and postinflammatory pigmentation or dull skin. A study by Sachdeva with 90% LA in Indian skin for acne scar and acne showed greater than 75% clearance in four sessions fortnightly apart in 42.84% of the patients.[18]

Complications

- Mild erythema or frosting in very sensitive or dry dehydrated skin
- Used with caution in patients with lactose intolerance.

Contraindication

None.

Key Points of Lactic Acid Peel

- Used in patients with rosacea and sensitive skin

- Moisturizing agent and humectant so can be used in dry skin.

TRETINOIN PEELS OR YELLOW PEEL

These are the vitamin A-derivative peels usually retinoic acid or retinaldehyde 0.3% solution with ethanol alcohol. Retinoids cause regulation of cellular turnover and keratinization process. It also inhibits melanogenesis, discourages hyperkeratinization and stimulates collagen production. Tretinoin peels are yellow peels that are left on for 4–5 hours and then washed away.

Indications in Acne

It is rarely used alone. It is used as a sealing agent with combination peels or TCA peels. It increases exfoliation, reduces follicular plugging and hyperkeratinization, and inhibits melanogenesis. All these factors are important for pathogenesis of acne and acne scars.[19]

Complications

- Postinflammatory hyperpigmentation
- Acneiform eruptions
- Bronzing effect
- Excessive peeling and dermatitis.

NEWER PEELS

Acetic Acid Peel or Black Peel

Combination of black acetic acid, SA, jasmonic acid and potassium iodide. Acetic acid also known as ethanoic acid has a pKa of 4.76 and a low molecular weight. It is formed by distilling vinegar. Potassium iodide induces fast wound healing. Jasmonic acid has anti-inflammatory properties.

It works in all types of acne and also on postinflammatory hyperpigmentation.

Nomelan Peel

Combination of 8% phenol with TCA 15%. It works well in post acne PIH or erythematous scars.

Enzyme Peel

An enzyme peel contains natural fruit ingredients to gently remove top layers of skin and expedite cell turnover. Conditions treatable by the method include, but are not limited to, age-related conditions such as lines and wrinkles, infections, pigmentary disorders, follicular disorders such as acne and hyperkeratotic disorders such as warts.[20]

Some of the commonly used enzyme peels include:
- Papain and bromelain, proteolytic enzymes that are isolated from unripe papaya fruit and pineapple, respectively, have been used in various types of topical formulations
- *Pomegranate enzyme:* Pomegranate is a powerful antioxidant that brightens the skin. It contains 11% LA, 4% alpha-arbutin and 2% SA. It promotes deep hydration, reduced oiliness and lightens the skin from irregular pigmentation.

POTENTIAL PROBLEMS DURING ACNE TREATMENT WITH PEELS

Peels may not always give the desired results.

It is often prudent to reevaluate the patient in such case. Sometimes simple measures like addition of a topical retinoid or oral antibiotic may be required or we may often need to change the peel. Table 1 enumerates various problems encountered during treating acne with peels.

TABLE 1: Problems encountered during treatment of acne with peels and their solutions

Problem	Solution
Temporary aggravation of the acne	Immediately put on oral antibiotics
Recurrence	Do maintenance peels
Ineffectiveness	Relook at the etiology and suitable treatment
Comedones difficult to extract	Do a TCA/SP first, this causes keratolysis and softening of the comedones and extraction to be done in the next session
Too many comedones	Phasic extraction before each session of the peel
Patient on isotretinoin therapy	Do not go beyond pinpoint frosting
Postinflammatory hyperpigmentation	Priming the skin with hydroquinone or tretinoin
Folliculitis barbae	Oral antibiotics
	Opening the comedones and applying the peel

TCA, trichloroacetic acid.

ROLE OF PEELS IN ACNE SCARS

With the advancement of technology, better lasers like fractional CO_2, erbium glass and fractionated microneedling radiofrequency, role of peels in the improvement of acne scars may look insignificant. The improvement with lasers is much more visible and appreciated than with peels. But peels also do have a role in improvement of atrophic, erythematous and macular acne scar. More importantly, early intervention with peels help in reducing the probability of scar formation and improving the general skin texture.

Glycolic acid peels are also known to cause neocollagenesis by increasing secretions of interleukin-6.[12] Glycolic acid increases dermal and epidermal glycosaminoglycans (GAG). GAG has an immense ability to bind with water, about 1,000 times their weight in water though their dry weight is 0.1–0.3% the weight of dermis. Therefore, a small increase in dermal GAG improves epidermal and dermal hydration, skin quality and texture substantially. This further provides for a more stable and permanent matrix for collagen formation. In combination with other procedures like microneedling, the improvement in atrophic acne scars was significant.[22]

Pyruvic peel, which is an important peel for antiaging in view of its deeper penetration due to its small molecular weight, and subsequent collagen and elastin formation also plays a role in superficial acne scars. Similar results are also observed with 90% LA peels and 15–25% TCA peels. Macular erythematous scars respond to azelaic, salicylic and MA peels.

One of the most important techniques which is very important in acne scar improvement is the CROSS technique, first described by Lee et al. for the treatment of ice-pick scar.[23] Ice-pick scars are narrow, less than 2 mm, but deep scars. They respond poorly to EBD and CROSS technique provides a simple and effective technique for their improvement. High concentration of TCA like 50–100% are applied in the depth of the scar with a sharpened wooden applicator. Frosting subsequent to coagulation of protein self-neutralizes the peels. There is controlled inflammation and wound healing causing neocollagenesis. Healing is prompt due to sparing of the surrounding normal tissue and the adnexal tissue. The process needs repetition at an interval of 12 weeks. Care should be taken about the contact time with the wooden applicator as in case of wider area of necrosis, it can worsen the scar and make it wider, delay healing and cause scarring. Transient hypopigmentation is common and distressing complication in the skin of color.

CONCOMITANT USE OF ORAL ISOTRETINOIN AND PEELS

The initial apprehension about use of concomitant oral isotretinoin and peels due to reports of hypertrophic scarring are more or less put to rest. Though not all, but superficial peels can safely be done along with low dose isotretinoin. Study by BR Kar et al. documented that the inflammatory and comedonal acne cleared faster and the scarring as a sequel to acne was less obvious in patients on concomitant therapy.[24] Twenty percent salicylic peel being superficial peel has no direct effect on collagen remodeling. The deeper peels have a direct influence on collagen remodeling and can adversely affect the outcome by keloid formation. Patient who are prone to develop hypertrophic scars in acne or have a keloidal tendency should not be subjected to concomitant therapy.

Report of scarring and hyperpigmentation are reported with use of low dose isotretinoin 10 mg alternate day with glycolic peels.

The exact mechanism of atypical reepithelialization and scarring due to isotretinoin is still unclear. It is postulated to be due to stimulation of angiogenesis or production of collagenase inhibitors resulting in hypertrophic scars or keloids.[25]

But the systemic review of literature by Spring et al. confirmed that superficial chemical peels can be concomitantly done in patients on low dose isotretinoin though mechanical dermabrasion, ablative lasers and deeper collagen modulating peels should be avoided.[26]

FINDING THE RIGHT PEEL

It may be often difficult to decide the best peel for the patient. Salient characteristics of the peels often help us to decide which peel would give predictable results. Table 2 enumerates various clinical situations normally encountered in our daily practice and how best we can give optimum results by selecting the right peel and the adjuvant therapy.

TABLE 2: Ready reckoner for selection of peeling agent for various grades of acne and acne scars

Grade and type of acne	Peel characteristic and depth required	Peeling agent	Combination with other procedures, EBD or medications	Special considerations and results
Grade 1 or topical steroid-induced acne	Lipophilic nature Superficial depth, up to stratum corneum	SA 20–30% Modified Jessner's peel TCA 10–15%	Serial comedone extraction in every session, or low dose isotretinoin or topical tretinoic acid as short contact	Flare up of inflammatory acne. May be reduced with oral antibiotics. In case of too much flare, reduce the dose or stop isotretinoin
Grade II	Lipophilic nature Anti-inflammatory	SA 20–30% Modified Jessner's GA 20–50%	Oral antibiotics Alternate sessions with IPL with 390 nm filter only on inflammatory acne	Sun protection mandatory To prevent postinflammatory hyperpigmentation
Acne grade II with generalized erythema or sensitive skin	Mild peels Anti-inflammatory property	SA peel 20% Mandelic acid peels	Alternate sessions with IPL filter 590 nm	Test patch with peel recommended

Continued...

Chemical Peels: A Global Perspective

Continued ...

Grade and type of acne	Peel characteristic and depth required	Peeling agent	Combination with other procedures, EBD or medications	Special considerations and results
Acne any grade with darker skin type, higher possibility of PIH	Anti-inflammatory, inhibition of melanogenesis	SA 20%, GA 20–35%, mandelic acid 30–50%	–	–
Acne vulgaris grade III–IV without isotretinoin	Medium-depth peels Lipophilic peels Antibacterial	Acetic acid peels, glycolic peel 50% TCA 15–20% Mandelic acid 40–50%	Oral antibiotics. Weekend therapy with isotretinoin.	–
Acne vulgaris grade III–IV with isotretinoin	Superficial peels	SA 20–30%, GA 20–35%	Oral antibiotics and low dose isotretinoin	–
Acne excoriee or individuals prone to PIH, recurrent acne	Inhibition of melanogenesis and reduction of seborrhea	Salicylic and mandelic combination peels, GA 35–50%, TCA peel	Oral antihistaminic Carbon peel with Qs Nd:YAG, IPL with 590 nm filter can be combined	–
Adult acne with photodamage/fine line/uneven tone	Collagen neogenesis and remodeling	Pyruvic peel, combination peels like nomelan (TCA, salicylic and phenol) GA 50–70%	Rule out hormonal acne. Medical management accordingly	–
Acne with superficial acne scars	Collagen neogenesis remodeling	Lactic acid 90%, TCA 15–20%, GA 50–70%, Jessner's peel alone or in combination with TCA	Alternate session with microneedling (manual/RF)	–
Active acne with deeper scars	–	TCA 25% Pyruvic acid peels, GA 50–70%	To work on scars only when active acne has reduced. Use of fractional CO_2, subcision once acne reduced.	Initiation of early peels reduce the possibility of impending scarring
Acne with oily thick skin with open pores	–	Modified Jessner's solution, lactic acid 90%, GA 50%, SA 30%	Combination with microneedling/DR	–

PIH, postinflammatory hyperpigmentation; TCA, trichloroacetic acid; GA, glycolic acid; SA, salicylic acid; Nd:YAG, neodymium-doped yttrium aluminum garnet.

PRACTICAL TIPS

- Peels produce only the cosmetic effect. They do not change the pathogenic factors responsible for acne, nor do they alter the blood levels of testosterone or activity of 5-alpha reductase. So, the peels should always be accompanied by appropriate medical management
- Treatment of acne must be multifocal
- Getting early results with peels is a good sign. If the results are slow even after the second or third session, results are unlikely going to be satisfactory, may be only partial and patient may need medical management
- Patient with preexisting pigmentation, those on hormonal therapy or oral contraceptive or those who give history of postinflammatory hyperpigmentation should be primed 2 weeks prior with hydroquinone or 6–12% GA to prevent postinflammatory hyperpigmentation
- Low-strength peels should be combined to increase efficacy
- Customize treatment as per patients' skin type, sensitivity, type of acne and scarring
- Introduction of peels early in the treatment reduce possibility of postinflammatory hyperpigmentation and also impending scarring
- It improves patient compliance in view of faster results.

CONCLUSION

Chemical peels are effective adjuvant therapy in the management of acne vulgaris. With the exact etiology of acne still unclear and increase in the incidence of polycytic ovarian syndrome in young females, peels offer an effective resurfacing tool. Moreover, it works on both inflammatory and noninflammatory acne skin lesions. The sequel to acne like acne scars, pigmentation and erythema can all be addressed. Peels also prolong and maintain the effect of systemic therapy like antibiotics and isotretinoin. Newer formulations and combination peels have made it possible to deliver deeper peels with minimum side effect in the skin of color, taking care both as therapeutic and preventive management tool.

REFERENCES

1. Kligman AM. Salicylic acid: an alternative to alpha-hydroxy acids. J Geriatr Dermatol. 1997;5:128-31.
2. Yu RJ, Van Scott EJ. Salicylic acid: not a beta-hydroxy acid. Cosmet Derm. 1997;10:27.
3. Imayama S, Ueda S, Isoda M. Histologic changes in the skin of hairless mice following peeling with salicylic acid. Arch Dermatol. 2000;136:1390-5.
4. Ueda S, Mitsugi K, Ichige K, et al. New formulation of chemical peeling agent: 30% salicylic acid in polyethylene glycol. Absorption and distribution of 14C-salicylic acid in polyethylene glycol applied topically to skin of hairless mice. J Dermatol Sci. 2002;28:211-8.
5. Pearl E Grime. The safety and efficacy of salicylic acid chemical peels in darker racial-ethnic groups. Dermatol Surg. 1999;25(1):18-22.
6. Lee HS, Kim IH. Salicylic acid peels for the treatment of acne vulgaris in Asian patients. Dermatol Surg. 2003;29:1196-9.
7. Fung W, Orak D, RE TA. Relative bioavailability of salicylic acid following dermal application of 30% salicylic acid skin peel preparation. J Pharm Sci. 2008;97:1325-8.
8. Dayal S, Amrani A, Sahu P, et al. Jessner's solution vs. 30% salicylic acid peel: a comparative study of the efficacy and safety in mild-to-moderate acne vulgaris. J Cosmet Dermatol. 2017;16(1):43-51.
9. Bae BG, Park CO, Shin H, et al. Salicylic acid peel versus Jessner's solution for acne vulgaris: a comparative study. Dermatol Surg. 2013;39:248-53.
10. Rivera AE. Acne scarring: a review and current treatment modalities. J Am Acad Dermatol. 2008;59:659-76.
11. Takenaka Y, Hayashi N, Takeda M, et al. Glycolic acid chemical peeling improves inflammatory acne eruptions through its inhibitory and bactericidal effects on Propionibacterium acnes. J Dermatol. 2012;39:350-4.
12. Kim SW, Moon SE, Kim JA, et al. Glycolic acid versus Jessner's solution: which is better for facial acne patients? A randomized prospective clinical trial of split-face model therapy. Dermatol Surg.1999;25;270-3.

13. Garg VK, Sinha S, Sarkar R. Glycolic acid peels versus salicylic Mandelic acid peels in active acne vulgaris and post-acne scarring and hyperpigmentation: a comparative study. Dermatol Surg. 2009;35:59-65.
14. Deprez P. Phenol: properties and histology. In: Textbook of Chemical Peels: Superficial, Medium and Deep Peels in Cosmetic Practice. London: Informa Healthcare; 2007. p. 193-202.
15. Cotellessa C, Manunta T, Ghersetich I, et al. The use of pyruvic acid in the treatment of acne. J Eur Acad Dermatol Venereol. 2004;18:275-8.
16. Pacifico A, Fargnoli MC, Ferrari A, et al. The use of pyruvic acid in the treatment of acne. J Am Acad Dermatol. 2004;50:11.
17. Tosson Z, Attwa E, Al-Mokadem S. Pyruvic acid as a new therapeutic peeling agent in acne, melasma and warts. Egypt Dermatol Online J. 2006;2:7.
18. Sachdeva, S. Lactic acid peeling in superficial acne scarring in Indian skin. J Cosmet Dermatol. 2010;9:246-8.
19. Dreno B, Castell A, Tsankov N, et al. Interest of the association retinaldehyde/glycolic acid in adult acne. J Eur Acad Dermatol Venereol. 2009;23:529-32.
20. Fein H. Selective enzyme treatment of skin conditions. Washington: US Patent Office; 2001.
21. Treating acne. In: Deprez P. Textbook of chemical peels: Superficial, medium and deep peels in cosmetic practice. London: Informa Healthcare; 2007. p. 128.
22. Sharad J. Combination of microneedling and glycolic acid peels for treatment of acne scars in dark skin. J Cosmet Dermatol. 2011;10:317-23.
23. Lee JB, Chung WG, Kwahch H, et al. Focal treatment of acne scars with trichloroacetic acid: chemical reconstruction of skin scars method. Dermatol Surg. 2002;28:1017-21.
24. Kar BR, Tripathy S, Panda M. Comparative Study of Oral Isotretinoin Versus Oral Isotretinoin + 20% Salicylic Acid Peel in the Treatment of Active Acne Cutan Aesthet Surg. 2013;6(4):204-8.
25. Abdelmalek M, Spencer J. Retinoids and wound healing. Dermatol Surg. 2006;32:1219-30.
26. Spring LK, Krakowski AC, Alam M, et al. Isotretinoin and timing of procedural interventions: a systematic review with consensus recommendations. JAMA Dermatol. 2017;153(8):802-9.

31
CHAPTER

Special Scenario: Peels for Photoaging

Sonali Langar

INTRODUCTION

The quest to retain a youthful skin transcends all social, economic, cultural and racial barriers. Skin being the most visible of all the organs conveys aging to the utmost extent. Aging of the skin is a result of genetic (intrinsic) and environmental (extrinsic) factors. Intrinsic or chronological aging is the biological aging due to age-dependent deterioration of structures and functions of the skin. Extrinsic aging occurs in the setting of intrinsic aging and is due to the chronic and cumulative effect of environmental factors as ultraviolet radiation (UVR), infrared radiation type A (IRA), smoking and pollution-related particulate matter. Among these, long-term exposure to UVR is most important determinant of extrinsic aging, aptly a process thus called photoaging.[1]

INTRINSIC AGING VERSUS EXTRINSIC AGING

Intrinsic and extrinsic aging can be differentiated from each other on the basis of clinical, histological and molecular features. Nevertheless, it is imperative to state that they are finely intermingled as well. Intrinsic aging is the culmination of subtle changes occurring over a lifetime in an individual, whereas extrinsic aging tends to occur against the backdrop of intrinsic aging and it accelerates and exaggerates the process of biological aging. Intrinsic aging of the skin manifests as smooth, relatively atrophic, finely wrinkled, or lax skin. The color is generally homogeneous without dyspigmentation. This type of aging is also appreciable in the sun-protected areas of the body as inner aspect of arms. Histologically, the stratum corneum appears to be normal with atrophic epidermis and flattening of the dermo-epidermal junction. There is decreased density of extracellular matrix (ECM) components due to decrease in biosynthetic capacity of fibroblast with age. Extrinsic aging of skin is characterized by coarse and fine wrinkling, mottled pigmentary changes, rough texture and telangiectasias on photoexposed areas of the face, neck and forearms. Histologically, epidermal thickness may be increased or decreased corresponding to areas of hyperplasia or atrophy. There is loss of polarity of epidermal cells with keratinocyte atypia. Dermis shows elastosis, degeneration of collagen with evidence of chronic inflammatory changes. Blood vessels appear dilated and twisted (Table 1).[2,3]

TABLE 1: Various types of aging

Intrinsic or chronological aging	Extrinsic or photoaging
• Biological process	• Due to chronic or cumulative exposure to sunlight, pollution and smoke
• Age-dependent deterioration of skin's structures and functions	• Occurs in the setting of intrinsic aging accelerates and exaggerates the process of biological aging
• Manifest as smooth, relatively atrophic, finely wrinkled, or lax skin. Color of skin is generally homogeneous without dyspigmentation	• Manifest as coarse and fine wrinkling, mottled pigmentary changes, rough texture and telangiectasias on photoexposed areas

PHOTOAGING: THE CUMULATIVE ENVIRONMENTAL EFFECT

Much of the manifestations of photoaging are due to long-term exposure of UVR. Ultraviolet B (UVB) (290–320 nm) acts primarily on the epidermis damaging the DNA and facilitating the production of soluble factors including proteolytic enzymes which affect the ECM in the dermis. Erythema, sunburn, solar elastosis, hyperpigmentation, DNA damage and skin cancers have been implicated due to UVB exposure. Ultraviolet A (UVA) (320–400 nm) more abundant in the sunlight penetrates more deeply in the skin exerting direct effects on both the epidermis and dermis. However, it requires a much higher dose to induce erythema. Ultraviolet C (UVC) is mainly absorbed by ozone layer and does not affect the skin.[4]

Aging of skin is not restricted to the effects of UVRs alone. IRA (770–1,400 nm) have also been implicated in collagen breakdown contributing to the formation of coarse wrinkles.[5] Air pollution exposure, especially to particulate matter, causes pigment spots and to a lesser extent wrinkles. Smoking exposure has been attributed to cause wrinkle, elastosis and telangiectasia.[6]

PHOTOAGING: MOLECULAR MECHANISMS

Various mechanism acting at the molecular level have been implicated in causation and perpetuation of extrinsic aging.

Mitochondrial DNA Mutations

Damage to mitochondrial DNA (mtDNA) contributes significantly to the genesis of photoaging as well as chronological aging. The common deletion mutation in the mtDNA due to chronic UVR exposure is specifically taken as a marker of photoaging in an individual. This mutation, however, is not related with chronological aging.[7]

Effect on Collagen and Matrix Metalloproteinases

Ultraviolet radiation causes decreased synthesis and excessive degradation of collagen. There is failure to replace the damaged collagen and accumulation of abnormal elastin containing material in the dermis. UVR exposure also induces matrix metalloproteinases (MMPs) within hours of irradiation. MMPs are endopeptidases that degrade collagen and elastin. In the normal skin, MMPs are regulated by tissue-specific inhibitors of metalloproteinases (TIMPs), which inactivate them and regulate the breakdown of collagen and elastin. As UVR induces MMPs without affecting the expression or activity of TIMPs, increased proteolysis occurs leading to decreased resilience of skin and appearance of wrinkles.[8]

Effect on Vascularization

Damage to the cutaneous blood vessels due to ultraviolet insult range from venular wall thickening in mild photodamage to gross vessel wall thinning and reduction in the number of supporting perivascular veil cells in case of severe photodamage. Studies have demonstrated increase in skin vascularization following acute and chronic UVB irradiation. There is increased expression of vascular endothelial growth factor (VEGF) in chronic UVB damaged skin leading to endothelial cell proliferation and formation of new blood vessels.[9]

Effect on Inflammation

There is increased presence of mast cells, histiocytes and mononuclear cells in the dermis with production of soluble mediators affecting the production and degradation of collagen and elastin.[10]

Effect on Protein Oxidation

Both UVB and UVA radiation lead to an increase in reactive oxygen species (ROS) which damage cell walls, lipid membranes, mitochondria and DNA. ROS signaling blocks transforming growth factor beta (TGF-beta) leading to decreased production of collagen and promotes upregulation of collagenases through epidermal growth factor receptor pathway leading to increased collagen breakdown. Function of proteasome which degrades oxidized proteins is also diminished leading to accumulation of oxidized proteins within the cell and dermis.[11]

Infrared Radiation Effect

Infrared radiation causes increased expression of *MMP1* and decreased expression of *COL1A1* and *COL1A2*. It also decreases expression of *TIMP1* leading to increased activity of *MMP1* resulting in enhanced ECM degradation.[12]

ETHNIC VARIATIONS IN PHOTOAGING

Clear ethnic variations exist in the appearance of clinical signs of aging in individuals across the globe. Genetics plays a crucial part in determining the skin's defenses to protect itself from the deleterious effects of sun exposure. Photoaging manifest differently in lighter and darker skin types. The lighter skin types age more noticeably in comparison to their darker counterparts who age gradually because of the protective effects of melanin. Individuals with Fitzpatrick type I-III skin demonstrate increased propensity of premalignant and malignant lesions as actinic keratoses, basal cell carcinoma, squamous cell carcinoma and melanomas along with wrinkling. Individuals with Fitzpatrick type IV-VI on the other hand manifest photoaging in the form of wrinkles to a lesser extent. Textural changes and pigmentary deviations ranging from patchy involvement to diffuse hyperpigmentation predominate. There is a definite less propensity for malignant lesions.[13]

GLOGAU CLASSIFICATION OF PHOTOAGING[14]

Glogau classification is commonly used to classify the degree of photoaging through mild, moderate, advanced and severe score. Mild photoaging shows minimal to absent wrinkles, mild dyschromia and absent keratosis. Moderate photoaging manifest as wrinkles in motion, dyschromias, and early senile lentigines and actinic keratosis. Advanced photoaging is marked by wrinkles at rest, dyschromias, telangiectasias and visible keratosis. Severe photoaging shows wrinkles throughout, actinic keratosis and skin malignancies. This classification acts as a guide for the practitioner in choosing the

Chemical Peels: A Global Perspective

> **BOX 1** **Glogau classification of photoaging (Fig. 1)**
>
> *Type I: No wrinkles*
> Early photoaging
> - Mild pigmentary changes
> - No keratosis
> - Minimal wrinkles
>
> Younger patient: 20s–30s
> Minimal or no makeup
>
> *Type II: Wrinkles in motion*
> Early-to-moderate photoaging
> - Early senile lentigines visible
> - Keratosis palpable but not visible
> - Parallel smile lines beginning to appear lateral to the mouth
>
> Patient age: Late 30s or 40s
> Usually wears some foundation
>
> *Type III: Wrinkles at rest*
> Advanced photoaging
> - Obvious dyschromia
> - Visible keratoses
> - Wrinkles even when not moving
>
> Patient age: 50s or older
> Always wears heavy foundation
>
> *Type IV: Only wrinkles*
> Severe photoaging
> - Yellow gray skin color
> - Prior skin malignancies
> - Wrinkled throughout, no normal skin
>
> Patient age: 60s–70s
> Cannot wear makeup – cakes and craks

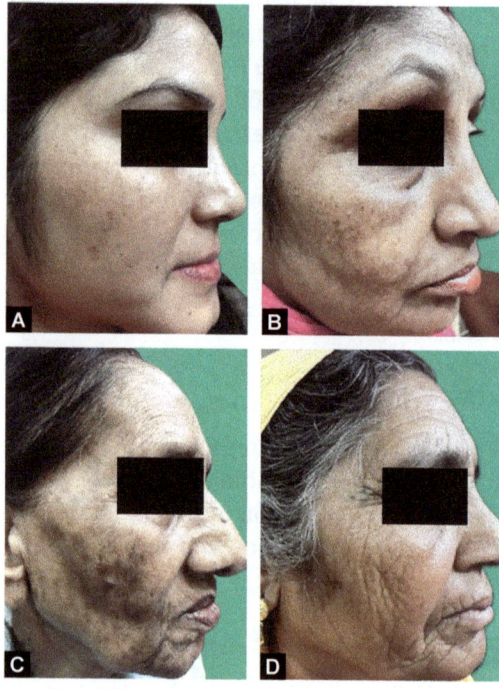

FIG. 1: Series of patients showing mild, moderate, advanced and severe photoaging according to Glogau classification.

PEELS FOR PHOTOAGING: MECHANISM OF ACTION

Peels form the first step in managing photoaging. A number of skin modifications have been reported after several weeks of peel treatment. Peeling induces controlled wounding of the skin followed by epidermal regeneration with a more uniform distribution of melanocytes and homogenous thickness of the basal membrane. Melanin grains distribute homogenously within the melanocyte.[16] Postinflammatory new subepidermal band of collagen forms with remodeling of ECM. Increased and dense rearrangement of collagen-1 or collagen-3

appropriate antiaging therapeutic modality for the patient. Mild photodamaged skin responds to topical antiaging therapies and superficial peels. Moderate to advanced photodamaged skin require medium depth to deep peeling procedures. Ablative resurfacing and face lifting techniques along with medium depth to deep peeling procedures benefit advanced photodamaged (Box 1).[15]

Special Scenario: Peels for Photoaging

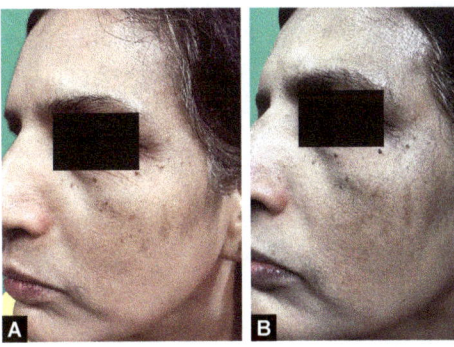

FIG. 2: Improvement in fine wrinkling following 4 sessions fortnightly of glycolic acid 50% peels.

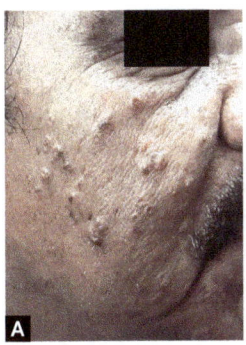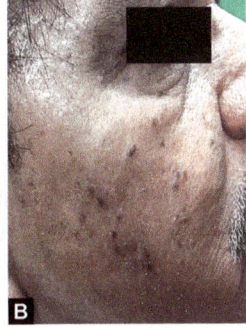

FIG. 3: Advanced photoaging. Significant improvement following 4 sessions thrice weekly of Jessner's—35% trichloroacetic acid peel (Monheit's technique).

fibers and elastic fibers occur in the dermis. Elastic fibers form network parallel to collagen.[17] There is increased evidence of epidermal and dermal hyaluronic acid with increased collagen gene expression.[18] The resultant effect is improved color, texture and fine lines (Figs. 2 and 3).

Currently, superficial, medium-depth and deep peeling agents are used for the treatment of photodamaged skin depending upon the severity of involvement and the Fitzpatrick skin type of the patient.

Superficial Peels

- Alpha-hydroxy acids (AHAs)
  - Glycolic acid 30–50%
  - Lactic acid 50–90%
  - Pyruvic acid.
- Beta-hydroxy acids
  - Salicylic acid (SA) 20–30%
  - Derivative of SA—lipohydroxy acid (LHA).
- Jessner's solution (14% lactic acid, 14% resorcinol and 14% SA)
- Trichloroacetic acid (TCA) 10–30%.

Superficial peels help to treat mild-to-moderate photodamage. Pioneering work to document the beneficial effect of AHAs in photodamaged skin was done by Van Scott and YU whose results were later reinforced by various studies.[19] These agents exfoliate epidermal layer without going beyond the basal layer. Glycolic acid is the most common AHA peel having anti-inflammatory, keratolytic and antioxidant effects. Corneosomes are targeted resulting in desquamation and increased epidermal activity of enzymes leading to epidermolysis and exfoliation. Bernstein et al. showed increased type I collagen messenger RNA and hyaluronic acid content along with dermal remodeling of the ECM in glycolic acid-treated skin. SA and lactic acid peels have shown to be effective as well. SA is lipophilic and removes intercellular lipids that are covalently linked to the cornified envelope surrounding cornified epithelioid cells. It also exerts an antihyperplastic effect on the epidermis.[20] At low concentration (<30%), lactic acid reduces sulfate and phosphate groups from the surface of corneocytes, breaking the intercellular desmosomal bonds and inducing exfoliation. At higher concentration, its effect is mainly destructive. It also appears to have dermal effects and has been shown to increase the production of mucopolysaccharides and collagen in the dermis resulting in increased skin thickness and improved skin hydration and suppleness.[21] Pyruvic acid is an alpha-keto acid which is converted physiologically to lactic acid. It is used in concentrations of 40–70% in water or ethanol solutions. Serial peels with pyruvic acid improves signs of photoaging.[22] Jessner's solution combines multiple acids (SA, lactic acid and resorcinol) each at a lower concentration to maximize the therapeutic outcome and minimizes the potential side effects of any one ingredient when used at a higher concentration. Its effect on improving the signs of photoaging is well documented.[23]

Medium-depth Peels

- Glycolic acid 70%
- TCA 35%
- Monheit's combination (Jessner's + TCA)
- Coleman's combination (Glycolic acid 70% + TCA)
- Jessner's solution with glycolic acid.

Medium-depth peels reach up to the upper reticular dermis. They cause coagulation of membrane proteins, destroy living cells of the epidermis, and depending on the concentration, the dermis. TCA is a versatile peel and chemical cauterant which causes protein coagulation when applied to the skin. TCA in strengths of 10–30% is a superficial peel and strength of 35% is a medium-depth peel. Strengths of TCA above 35% gives unpredictable results, dyschromic sequel and scarring, and its use should be reserved to cauterize isolated lesions in photodamaged skin. Alone or in combination TCA improves fine lines, elastosis, lentigines, complexion and skin tone. Monheit's and Coleman's combinations involve the use of Jessner's solution and glycolic acid solution, respectively, prior to TCA application facilitating the depth and uniform penetration of TCA.[24,25] The TCA concentration can be adjusted between 15% and 35% depending upon the patient's thickness of skin and Fitzpatrick type.

Deep Peels

- TCA more than 50%
- Phenol.

These agents penetrate up to the lower reticular dermis. Deep peels coagulate proteins and produce complete epidermolysis, restructure the basal layer and restore the dermal architecture. As stated earlier, TCA in strengths above 35% should be used to treat isolated lesions like seborrheic keratosis, actinic keratosis and lentigines in photodamaged skin. Phenol peel is the deepest of peels indicated for severe photodamage. However, due to its toxic potential, profound postpeel skin changes, and potential risk of scarring and pigmentary deviations, its use should be restricted to specifically treat those conditions which cannot be treated by other peels. Various modifications have been introduced since the original Baker-Gordon formula. Regardless of any formula used, phenol peel is only indicated for its use in Fitzpatrick skin types I–III. Wangli et al., however, demonstrated the safe use of phenol peel in light colored Asian skin.[26]

PATIENT PREPARATION

Preparation starts with prevention and correction of extrinsic modifiable factors that contribute to photoaging as avoidance of smoking, pollution and UVR. Correction of life style, nutrition and dietary habits with regular exercise is a must. A detailed history taking and clinical examination should be conducted before undertaking peeling procedure. Preparing the patients skin

24 weeks prior to the actual peel is the key to get better therapeutic results and overall efficacy of the peel. Pretreatment enhances even and increased peel penetration and minimizes chances of potential postpeel complications. The regular use of topical pretreatment medications psychologically prepares the patient for the procedure and also enforces compliance for the use of topical medications post peel. Basic priming agents, which can be used to prepare the skin, include topical retinoids, bleaching agents as azelaic acid, kojic acid, arbutin, licorice and AHAs as glycolic acid and lactic acid. A broad-spectrum UVA or UVB sunscreen with a minimum SPF 30, with regular cleansing and moisturization, should accompany any regimen. Use of topical retinoids (tretinoin cream 0.025–0.05%) for 2–4 weeks prior to peeling thins the stratum corneum enhancing the penetration of the peeling agent. These agents increase epidermal turnover, reduce the content of epidermal melanin and facilitate epidermal wound healing.[27] When treating for dyschromias, the skin should usually be prepared for 2–4 weeks with either a formulation of hydroquinone 2–4% or with any of the bleaching agents to reduce epidermal melanin.[28] The AHAs in low percentages decrease keratinocyte adhesion causing desquamation and thinning of epidermis enhancing the overall uniform penetration of peel. Topical ascorbyl glucoside has anti-inflammatory, photoprotective and skin-lightening properties, and can be used as an excellent priming agent.[29] It is worthwhile to mention that providing apt information of the procedure and advising the patient to have realistic expectations is also an important step of patient's preparation.

POSTPEEL CARE

Postpeel care includes regular use of bland moisturizers and broad-spectrum sunscreen of SPF 30 or higher. Low-to-mid potency steroid cream can be used for 2–3 days in case of pronounced erythema. Topical antibacterial ointment should be used to prevent bacterial infection in case of crusting. Analgesics though routinely not needed may be advised in case of persistent burning. The flaking should not be picked or scrubbed as fiddling can lead to scarring and pigmentary deviations. Avoid strenuous physical activity which cause excessive perspiration, use of steam rooms, saunas, or excessively hot showers in the first few days following peel as this can increase the risk of complications. Use of general skin care products, topical retinoids, emollients with 2% hyaluronic acids and bleaching agents can be resumed after peeling subsides.

PRACTICAL TIPS

- Peels being simple and inexpensive procedures hold significant position in the antiaging arsenal. They improve fine lines, texture and dyspigmentation
- Peels do not improve deep wrinkles and other established signs of aging; therefore, patients should be reinforced with acceptance of other antiaging treatment modalities
- Concomitant use of sunscreens, vitamin C, hyaluronic acid, depigmentary creams and oral antioxidants should accompany treatment protocols for enhanced outcomes
- Management of aging skin should be long term and tailored according to patients' needs.

CONCLUSION

Aging is a perpetual process undesired by all. Clear ethnic variations exist in aging pattern of skin with light skin manifesting more of wrinkles as compared to the dark skin which has more of texture and pigmentary changes. Extrinsic modifiable factors that exaggerate the aging process should be identified and rectified, such as avoidance of smoking, pollution and UVR exposure, adoption of healthy lifestyle with well-balanced diet and regular exercise. Superficial and medium-depth peels are simple, safe and inexpensive tools to minimize the unwanted signs of aging, for example, fine lines, rough texture and pigmentation. Deep peels have significant downtime with potential risk of scarring and pigmentary deviations. Their use is restricted to Fitzpatrick skin types I–III only. As aging is a continuous process, maintenance is long time along with daily use of sunscreens, moisturizers, depigmentary creams, topical vitamin C and hyaluronic acid. Peels do not improve other established signs of aging which can be dealt with other antiaging modalities.

REFERENCES

1. Krutmann J. Skin Aging. In: Krutmann J, Humbert P (Eds). Nutrition for Healthy Skin. Strategies for Clinical and Cosmetic Practice. New York: Springer, 2011. pp. 15-24.
2. Bhawan J, Andersen W, Lee J, et al. Photoaging versus intrinsic aging: a morphologic assessment of facial skin. J Cutan Pathol. 1995;22(2):154-9.
3. Lavker RM. Cutaneous aging: chronologic versus photoaging. In: Gilchrest BA (Ed). Photodamage. Cambridge: Blackwell Science; 1995. pp. 123-35.
4. Berneburg M, Plettenberg H, Krutmann J. Photoaging of human skin. Photodermatol. Photoimmunol. Photomed. 2000;16:239-44.
5. Schroeder P, Schieke S, Morita A. Premature skin aging by infrared radiation, tobacco smoke and ozone. In: Gilchrest BA, Krutmann J (Eds). Skin Aging. New York: Springer; 2006. pp. 45-54.
6. Vierkötter A, Schikowski T, Ranft U, et al. Airborne particle exposure and extrinsic skin aging. J Invest Dermatol. 2010;130(12):2719-26.
7. Koch H, Wittern KP, Bergemann J. In human keratinocytes the Common Deletion reflects donor variabilities rather than chronologic aging and can be induced by ultraviolet A irradiation. J Invest Dermatol. 2001;117:892-7.
8. Scharffetter-Kochanek K, Brenneisen P, Wenk J, et al. Photoaging of the skin: From phenotype to mechanisms. Exp Gerontol. 2000;35:307-16.
9. Yano K, Ouira H, Detmar M. Targeted over expression of the angiogenesis inhibitor thrombospondin-1 in the epidermis of transgenic mice prevents ultraviolet-B-induced angiogenesis and cutaneous photodamage. J Invest Dermatol. 2002;118:800-5.
10. Lavker RM, Kligman A. Chronic heliodermatitis: a morphologic evalauatuion of chronic actinic dermal damage with emphasis on the role of mast cells. J Invest Dermatol. 1988;90:325-30.
11. Fisher GJ, Datta SC, Talwar HS, et al. Molecular basis of sun-induced premature skin ageing and retinoid antagonism. Nature. 1996;379:335-9.
12. Buechner N, Schroeder P, Jakob S, et al. Changes of MMP-1 and collagen type I alpha 1 by UVA, UVB and IRA are differentially regulated by Trx-1. Exp Gerontol. 2008;43:633-7.
13. Grimes PE. Benign manifestations of photodamage: ethnic skin types. In: Goldberg DJ (Ed). Photodamaged skin. New York: Marcel Dekker Inc.; 2004. pp. 175-96.
14. Glogau RG. Chemical peeling and aging skin. J Geriatr Dermatol. 1994;2:30-5.
15. Fulton JE, Porumb S. Chemical peels: their place within the range of resurfacing techniques. Am J Clin Dermatol. 2004;5(3):179-87.
16. Brown AM, Kaplan LM, Brown M. Phenol-induced histological skin changes: hazards, technique, and uses. Br J Plast Surg.1960;13:158-69.
17. Vagotis FL, Brundage SR. Histologic study of dermabrasion and chemical peel in an animal model after pretreatment with Retin-A. Aesthetic Plast Surg. 1995;19:243-6.
18. Bernstein EF, Lee J, Brown DB, et al. Glycolic acid treatment increases type I collagen mRNA and hyaluronic acid content of human skin. Dermatol Surg. 2001;27(5):429-33.
19. Van Scott EJ, Yu RJ. Hyperkeratinization, corneocyte cohesion, and alpha hydroxy acids. J Am Acad Dermatol. 1984;11:867-79.
20. Kligman D, Kligman AM. Salicylic acid peels for the treatment of photoaging. Dermatol Surg. 1998;24(3):325-8.
21. Ghersetich I, Brazzini B, Peris K, et al. Pyruvic acid peels for the treatment of photoaging. Dermatol Surg. 2004;30(1):32-6.
22. Fulton JE Jr. The Progressive Peel: The Combined Jessner, TCA, Retinoid Peel. In: Tung R, Rubin MG (Eds). Chemical Peels. Philadelphia: Saunders/Elsevier; 2010. pp. 49-60.
23. Dinner MI, Artz JS. The art of the trichloroacetic acid chemical peel. Clin Plast Surg. 1998;25(1):53-62.

24. Monheit GD. The Jessner's - trichloroacetic acid peel. An enhanced medium-depth chemical peel. Dermatol Clin. 1995;13:277-83.
25. Coleman WP 3rd, Futrell JM. The glycolic acid trichloroacetic acid peel. J Dermatol Surg Oncol. 1994;20(1):76-80.
26. Phenol—Indications. In: Deprez P (Ed). Textbook of Chemical Peels. Superficial, medium and deep peels in cosmetic practice. Boca Raton: Taylor & Francis; 2017. pp. 250-63.
27. Hevia O, Nemeth AJ, Taylor JR. Tretinoin accelerates healing after trichloroacetic acid chemical peel. Arch Dermatol. 1991;127(5):678-82.
28. Garg VK, Sarkar R, Agarwal R. Comparative evaluation of beneficiary effects of priming agents (2% hydroquinone and 0.025% retinoic acid) in the treatment of melasma with glycolic acid peels. Dermatol Surg. 2008;34(8):1032-40.
29. Telang PS. Vitamin C in dermatology. Indian Dermatol Online J. 2013;(4):143-6.

32
CHAPTER

Special Scenario: Chemical Peeling in Sensitive Skin

Surabhi Sinha

INTRODUCTION

Sensitive skin can be defined as abnormal subclinical sensory responses to drugs, cosmetics and toiletries in the absence of visible signs of irritation.[1] The symptoms include burning, stinging, itching and tightness of the skin. Common triggers include cosmetics, drugs and toiletries, ultraviolet light, heat, cold and wind. There are no specific clinical signs; hence no clear consensual definition has yet been accepted. It is often a self-diagnosed condition, difficult to manage due to the lack of clear evidence-based options.

It is mostly seen or felt on the face because of its denser nervous network and its great exposure to cosmetic or physical triggering factors.[2] Patients may complain of dryness or tightness, and several washing-moisturizing cycles before observable signs of dryness appear.

Sensitive skin can occur in patients with atopic dermatitis (AD), allergic contact dermatitis (ACD), rosacea, acne, topical steroid damaged face (TSDF), aged and photoaged skin, and in sensitive skin syndrome. It is more frequently seen in those who undergo multiple dermatosurgical procedures involving peeling or abrasion of the skin. These patients often seek treatment for pigmentary changes and photoaging, and choosing the appropriate modality in them can be very challenging. Chemical peeling is a physician-controlled in-office procedure that can be carried out in such patients, albeit cautiously.

INDICATIONS

- Atopic dermatitis or ACD—postinflammatory hyperpigmentation
- Rosacea—postinflammatory hyperpigmentation
- Acne—excessive seborrhea, active acne, postacne hyperpigmentation
- Aged or photoaged skin—photoaging, melasma or dyschromias
- TSDF—hyperpigmentation, acneiform eruption.

DIFFICULTIES IN CHEMICAL PEELING IN SENSITIVE SKIN

Patients with sensitive skin may pose difficulties in chemical peeling not only due to a limited number of "safe" peels but also due to peculiarities in their skin:
- Choosing the right priming agent is tough as they may not tolerate most topical

Special Scenario: Chemical Peeling in Sensitive Skin

priming agents due to their irritation potential
- Sunscreens may also not find favor with them due to excessive occlusive feeling, greasiness or acneiform eruptions
- They may have exaggerated erythema after peeling
- Some may have thin skin, thus topical agents and peels can penetrate deeper than intended
- Some patients with TSDF have atrophic epidermis. This would make the skin more sensitive to photodamage especially in a hot sunny climate like ours, thus increasing risk of postinflammatory hyperpigmentation after peeling
- Unpredictable reactions of the skin are more likely to be encountered in such patients.

CONTRAINDICATIONS

- Patients with active infection or inflammation
- Patients who have undergone multiple aesthetic procedures and have unrealistic expectations from the procedure.

PATIENT PREPARATION

The following points need to be kept in mind in chemical peeling in all patients, but more so in patients with sensitive skin:
- Patient information sheets and counseling are of utmost importance and need to be individualized according to the characteristics and specific risks in such patients
- Some complications may occur only or more frequently in patients with sensitive skin—they should be clearly stated and highlighted
- List of precautions to be carried out by the patients should be explained carefully and reiterated repeatedly at every session
- Patients should be counseled about the slower response expected as milder peels would be used
- Physicians should be extremely cautious and should stop peels immediately if an unexpected response occurs and let it settle down before re-commencing peeling sessions
- Obvious peeling may not be visible in these patients as generally milder peels would be used; hence patients need to be counseled beforehand to avoid dissatisfaction
- The latest American Society for Dermatosurgery (ASDS) guidelines task force consensus recommendations concluded that there is insufficient evidence to justify delaying treatment with superficial chemical peels in patients on or exposed to isotretinoin within the past 6 months. Data on medium and deep chemical peels was insufficient to make recommendations. However, in patients with sensitive skin, it would be better to stick to the earlier guidelines and avoid even superficial peels while on or within 6 months after isotretinoin intake.

PRIMING

Priming is an indispensable part of the peeling process but is difficult in patients with sensitive skin due to low tolerance levels. Most priming agents are alpha-hydroxy acids, retinoid, or hydroquinone based and have high irritation potential. There are some agents that should be avoided and some that may be preferred as follows:

Priming agents to be avoided:
- Organic sunscreen agents
- Propylene glycol as base
- Combinations of two or more agents in the same formulation
- Tretinoin
- Glycolic acid

- Hydroquinone
- Mequinol.

Priming agents that are safer and preferable:
- Inorganic sunscreen agents
- Bland soap-free cleansers
- Noncomedogenic, free from fragrance (including masking fragrance) moisturizers
- Adapalene--for a couple of hours daily in microsphere gel (oily skin) or in cream base (if thin dry skin)
- Kojic acid, arbutin
- Newer agents.

CHOICE OF CHEMICAL PEEL

Mild peels are the peels of choice in patients with sensitive skin. The strength of a peel (depth of peeling) is determined by the chemical nature and size of the molecule, dissociation constant (pKa) and percentage of the peeling agent, duration of contact with skin, technique of application, and nature of action in the skin. Low percentage is a large molecule with high pKa, which penetrates the skin gradually, that would be the ideal peel in sensitive skin. Chemical peels that can be used in such patients are mandelic acid (10-40%), lactic acid (up to 40%) and low concentrations of salicylic acid (10-15%) and glycolic acid (up to 35%), arginine peel, citric acid peel, enzyme peels and kojic peels.

PRECAUTIONS

- Gel formulations would be preferable to alcoholic solutions due to slower penetration and less irritation potential
- Peeling agents should never be rubbed onto skin in such patients, especially if they have thin dry skin
- Vigorous degreasing should be avoided. Mild cetyl alcohol or stearyl alcohol based cleaning lotions can be used to clean the skin prior to peeling
- Contact time should be strictly monitored. Hotspots or unpredictable reactions may develop within the usual "safe" time for the peel and should be immediately terminated with cold water or neutralizer, if they do occur. Patients should be explained and reassured. Ice saline compresses can be useful in such cases.

COMPLICATIONS[3]

Patients with sensitive skin are more prone to developing complications. This is even more pertinent in type IV through type VI skins owing to the higher concentration of melanin in their epidermis. Treating physicians should be aware and be on the lookout for any possible complications. Complications can be immediate or delayed:

Immediate
- Burning sensation
- Irritation and tightness
- Intense and long-lasting redness
- Irritation and watering from eyes.

Delayed
- Hypertrophic or keloidal scarring
- Infections—bacterial and herpes simplex virus
- Milia
- Hyperpigmentation and hypopigmentation
- Acneiform eruptions
- Allergic contact dermatitis.

CONCLUSION

Patients with sensitive skin are best treated with very mild peels with large molecular weights so as to decrease the chances of deep penetration by the peeling agent. Mandelic acid and lactic acid are good peels in such patients. Others like low-strength salicylic and glycolic peels too can be used.

TAKE HOME POINTS

- Sensitive skin is a common and often self-diagnosed condition. It may also be secondary to cutaneous disorders. Chemical peeling needs to be done with extreme caution and by experienced clinicians only
- Patients with sensitive skin have varied symptoms like burning, stinging, itching, dryness and tightness usually without any clinical signs
- Chemical peeling in such patients is difficult as they may develop exaggerated or unpredictable responses post peeling
- The choice of priming agent and sunscreen has to be tailored to the individual patient
- Mild peels such as lactic and mandelic acid peels are preferred in patients with sensitive skin.

REFERENCES

1. Kligman AM, Sadiq I, Zhen Y, et al. Experimental studies on the nature of sensitive skin. Skin Res Technol. 2006;12(4):217-22.
2. Saint-Martory C, Roguedas-Contios AM, Sibaud V, et al. Sensitive skin is not limited to the face. Br J Dermatol. 2008;158:130-3.
3. Waldman A, Bolotin D, Arndt KA, et al. ASDS Guidelines Task Force Consensus recommendations regarding the safety of lasers, dermabrasion, chemical peels, energy devices, and skin surgery during and after isotretinoin use. Dermatol Surg. 2017;43(10):1249-62.

33
CHAPTER

Party Peels

Atula Gupta

INTRODUCTION

Party peels are very superficial chemical peels and are synonymous with "instant glow", "office peels", "lunch time", "freshening peels" and "red carpet" peels.

A party peel typically has the following features:
- No visible peeling or downtime
- Safe for all skin types
- Repeated often, as desired by the patient.

In the current scenario, the concept of party peels is more verbally discussed among dermatologists or patients but lacks any concrete published literature. In view of an almost nonexisting literature on this subject, the author shall discuss party peels based on personal experience, discussion with other peel professionals, in addition to a few internet sources and inputs from the manufacturers of these chemical peels.

A party peel may contain a single peeling agent or a combination of lower concentrations of multiple superficial peels.

LACTIC ACID

Lactic acid (LA) is an alpha-hydroxy acid (AHA), naturally occurring in tomato juice, sour milk and yogurt. Being one of the largest molecules among the AHAs, its cutaneous penetration is relatively slower thus causing lesser skin irritation. The hydration effect of LA adds to its role as an "instant" peel and makes it an ideal peel choice for sensitive, dry and dull skin.[1] LA has shown to inhibit tyrosinase enzyme activity directly in a dose-dependent manner.[2] As a peeling agent, LA reduces scaling and evens texture, rendering the skin smoother.[3] It is one of the most popular lunch-time peels.

Key Advantages as a Party Peel

- Superficial and gentle
- Instant turgor improvement and skin lifting effect stemming from a strong humectant property
- Very good tolerance profile in patients with sensitive skin and rosacea.

Utilizing Lactic Acid as a Party Peel

- *Mono peel:* Pure full strength LA (92% pH 3.5) works as an instant glow professional peel. It can be applied and left for 15–30 minutes followed by neutralization
- *Combination peel*: LA is also used in many combination peels along with arginine, kojic, glycolic and other hydroxy acids in

order to provide added advantages like better penetration, safety in periocular area and skin lightening.

PHYTIC ACID

Phytic acid has a larger molecular weight because of which it does not pass easily through the epidermis. It has efficacy at a low pH, does not require neutralization and has progressive and sequential therapeutic action in a nonaggressive manner. Phytic acid has antioxidant properties and provides a mild superficial peeling that is safe for all skin types.[4]

Key Advantages as a Party Peel

- Superficial and gentle when used at optimal concentration and pH
- Excellent molecule for a party peel as it reduces the postpeel inflammation caused by other hydroxy acids
- Marked tightening effect which has been subjectively appreciated by patients and objectively observed by the author.

Utilizing Phytic Acid as a Party Peel

- Easy phytic solution is a slow-release peel and a low pH formulation (between 0 and 1) which contains three AHAs (glycolic, lactic and mandelic) along with phytic acid. It is also referred to as the "Hollywood-style peel". Phytic acid is well known for its anti-tyrosinase and antioxidant action
- The peel is applied and left on the skin for 18-24 hours before being washed away. It can be repeated as frequently as every week.

CITRIC ACID

Citric acid is an AHA, the particularity of which is that it comprises three carboxylic functions.[5] Tolerance is considered better than that of smaller AHAs.

Key Advantages as a Party Peel

- Citric acid is more effective than glycolic acid at the same pH in reducing signs of photoaging.[5] Lower concentrations can be left on the skin without any risk of adverse reactions. Citric acid (20-70%) can be used as an effective lunchtime peel
- Astringent property, which helps to close dilated pores and gives a finer complexion (a property widely recognized and in general related to the traditional use of lemon). The best results are obtained with high concentrations like 20% and at a pH of less than 4.

Utilizing Citric Acid as a Party Peel

The peel is applied and left for about 2-5 minutes until the patient develops a minor pink appearance following which the peel can be neutralized with sodium bicarbonate or water. 30% citric acid peel (NeoStrata ProSystem) and is one of the author's commonly used instant brightening peel.

ASCORBIC ACID

L-ascorbic acid (LAA) is the chemically active form of vitamin C. Vitamin C interacts with copper ions at the tyrosinase-active site thereby inhibiting the enzyme tyrosinase and decreasing melanin formation. It also acts on the perifollicular pigment.[6-9] It is well known that LAA has anti-inflammatory action and increases collagen production in young as well as aged human skin (Fig. 1).[10]

Utilizing Ascorbic Acid as Party Peel

Vitamin C peel (Sesderma Laboratories) is wonderful as an instant glow treatment.

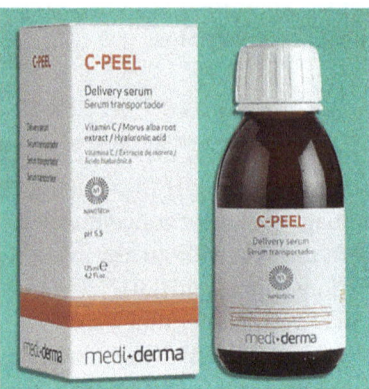

FIG. 1: L-ascorbic acid-based C-peel by Mediderma.

C-peel Delivery Serum

C-peel delivery serum contains ascorbyl glucoside, hyaluronic acid [very low molecular weight (VLMW) <50 kDA], mulberry extract, Syn-Coll and panthenol.
- *Ascorbyl glucoside (stable form of vitamin C)*: Antioxidant and tyrosinase inhibition
- *Hyaluronic acid (VLMW, encapsulated in liposomes)*: Anti-inflammatory and moisturizing
- *Mulberry extract*: Tyrosinase inhibition
- *Syn-Coll (Palmitoyl tripeptide-3)*: Stimulates collagen.

Peel Additives

- *Glowing powder*:
  - It contains 23% ascorbic acid and can be added to the C-peel delivery serum. It increases brightness and youthfulness for all skin types.

Peel Application

About 3 mL C-peel delivery serum is taken. Approximately 0.75 g or one fourth of ascorbic acid powder or glowing powder is added to the serum and mixed in a bowl (the serum and the powder have to be mixed in a ratio 4:1) till it forms a uniform mixture. The mixture is then applied as 2–3 coats over the face for 10–20 minutes following which it can be removed with water.

Peel additives are powdered heterogenous mixtures with different particle sizes that are mixed with gel-based AHAs to provide an instant glow before special occasions. They enhance the unique qualities of the various gel-based peels and diminish unwanted side effects.
- Luminous powder (23% ascorbic acid)
- Antioxidant powder (20.20% ascorbic acid, 3.40% thioctic acid and isoflavones)
- Depigmenting mix (12% kojic acid, 1.6% emblica)
- Depigmenting powder (15.2% kojic acid).

POLYHYDROXY ACIDS

Polyhydroxy acids (PHA) are a new generation of AHAs without irritant reactions. They are potent antioxidants, humectants and moisturizers. PHAs used in peels are gluconolactone and lactobionic acid.

Key Advantages as a Party Peel

- Antiaging benefits comparable to AHAs[11-16]
- Marked improvements in skin clarity and notable skin plumping
- Compatible with sensitive and dry skins[17,18]
- *Hygroscopic properties*:[16,19]
  - Lactobionic acid retains up to 10 times more water than glycolic acid whereas gluconolactone retains thrice as much as glycolic or LA.
- Better barrier conditioning[20]
- Antioxidant and free radical scavenging action[21]
- Absence of sun sensitivity.

Utilizing Polyhydroxy Acids as Party Peels

- Polyhydroxy acids have a larger molecular structure, resulting in slower epidermal

penetration, thereby reducing the potential of irritation
- Due to their multiple hydroxy groups, they bind water, have moisturizing properties and are potent antioxidants.

ARGININE

Arginine (2-amino-5-guanidinopentanoic acid) is a basic amino acid with anti-inflammatory and rehydrating properties.

Key Advantages as a Party Peel

- Gentle peeling agent. Perfect for sensitive skins and periorbital area
- Improves turgor, microcirculation and fine lines
- Ideal for providing a flash effect before parties.

Utilizing Arginine as a Party Peel

- Arginine in combination with LA is one of the safest party peel options. Arginine 20%, LA 20%, urea, aloe vera and allantoin (Argipeel from Sesderma Laboratories) offers a perfect "instant glow" for skins prone to irritation and sun sensitivity
- Arginine-based peels can be applied for 10–20 minutes over face and neutralized thereafter.

FERULIC ACID

Ferulic acid is a phenol derivative with antioxidant, anti-inflammatory and photoprotective properties. In combination with vitamin C, ferulic acid may provide 2–4 times as much photo protection. Ferulic acid also improves the stability of vitamin C and vitamin E.[22]

Key Advantages as a Party Peel

- All season party peel.

Utilizing Ferulic Acid as a Party Peel

Professional ferulic acid-based party peel system (Sesderma).

Ingredients

- Ferulic acid
- Phloretin
- AHAs (Malic, citric and lactic)
- Nicotinamide
- Retinol.

This is a superficial peel system based on ferulic acid, phloretin, fruit acids and retinoids. It optimizes the effectiveness of the ingredients with nanosome delivery and penetration. Ferulic acid has strong antioxidant properties which fight against reactive oxygen species (ROS). Its depigmenting effects derive from its function as a noncompetitive inhibitor of tyrosinase. Phloretin is a powerful antioxidant and also blocks melanin synthesis, inhibits the activity of elastase and potentiates the effect of other peel agents. The malic, citric and lactic acids add exfoliation, and enhance penetration of other ingredients. Nicotinamide maintains the cutaneous barrier and improves vascularization (Fig. 2).

- After the skin is cleaned and degreased, 2–3 coats of ferulic peel classic solution

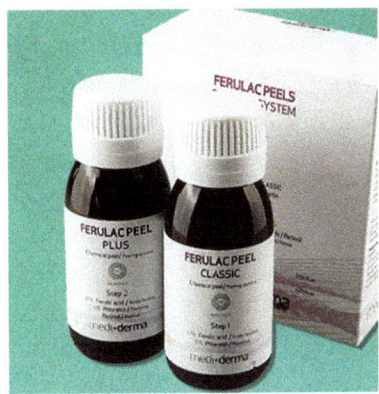

FIG. 2: Ferulac professional peel system by Mediderma.

(ferulic acid 12% and phloretin 5%) is applied to the skin. When the solution has dried, appearing as a light white mask, two coats of ferulic peel plus solution (ferulic acid 8%, phloretin 5%, mix of AHAs and retinol 0.25%) are applied and allowed to dry. After approximately 12 hours, the treated area can be washed.

KOJIC ACID

Kojic acid is produced from fungi like *Aspergillus* and *Penicillium* species. It is an important component of many combination peels by virtue of its skin lightening effect and functions more of an additive. Kojic acid inhibits tyrosinase.[23,24] Although there are no studies, kojic acid has been incorporated in many superficial combination peels. According to author's experience, a combination peel consisting of arginine 20%, LA 20%, kojic acid 5%, arbutin 2% and citric acid 2% works as an instant skin brightening peel.

COMBINATION PEELS

Combination peels combine two or more agents in a single formulation. There is a plethora of combination peel systems for instant glow from various manufacturers. Some of them are obviously suited for specific skin types. Further, choosing a party peel from the widespread available options is more often than not based on the dermatologist's personal experience and preference. Some of the popular combinations are listed below. Readers are advised to preferably stick to manufacturer's protocol when trying a new system (Table 1).

ILLUMINIZE PEEL (SKIN-MEDICA)

The Illuminize peel utilizes a novel approach to chemical peeling with a newer generation of AHAs (mandelic acid and malic acid) in combination with phytic acid and commonly used peeling agents (salicylic acid and resorcinol) to maximize skin rejuvenating

TABLE 1: Combination chemical peels being used as party peels

Peel name	Contents	Manufacturer
Mandelac C	30% citric acid and 20% mandelic acid	Sesderma
Mandelac L	35% mandelic acid and 20% lactic acid	Sesderma
Mandelac T	20% mandelic acid, 5% thioglycolic acid, 2.5% phytic acid	Sesderma
Azelac gel peel	20% azelaic acid, 4% lactic acid, 2% milk thistle extract	Sesderma
Argipeel	20% arginine, 20% lactic acid	Sesderma
Lactipeel	80% lactic acid, 11% dimethylamino ethanol	Sesderma
Sesglicopeel K	33% glycolic acid, 7% kojic acid, 9% lactic acid, 5% citric acid, 3% salicylic acid	Sesderma
Easy phytic peel	Phytic acid, glycolic acid, lactic acid and mandelic acid	
Pigment balancing peel	Vitamin C, 40% glycolic acid	Skinceuticals
Cosderma gel party peel	Lactic acid 20%, citric acid 10%, alpha arbutin 5%, ariginine 5% and bearberry extract 10%	Cosderma
ZO stimulator peel	10% salicylic acid, 10% lactic acid, 10% citric acid	Zein Obagi

effects with low irritation. Often described as the "red carpet peel," the Illuminize peel is a very light peel delivering immediate results.

ENZYME PEELS

Enzyme peels are gentler in many ways than acid-based chemical peels. The main plant enzymes are proteases found in papaya, pineapple, coconut, kiwi fruit, fig, mango, pumpkin, lemon and pomegranate.

- *Papain*: Proteolytic enzyme derived from the latex fluid of the papaya fruit
- *Sorbain*: Combined enzymes of lemon and papaya
- *Ficin*: Proteolytic enzyme from the stems and leaves of fig tree
- *Actinidin*: Derived from kiwi fruits
- *Arbutin*: Extracted from leaves of bearberry, red bilberry, etc.

Pumpkin Peel

Pumpkins contain proteolytic enzymes that break down keratin between epidermal cells leading to a superficial exfoliation of the stratum corneum. Pumpkin peel is applied to the skin, left for 5–10 minutes and subsequently neutralized. Stinging, warmth and redness are the desired endpoints of this peel.

Key Advantages of Enzyme Peels as Party Peels

- Offer an improvement in turgor, adding to the tightening effect
- Good alternative to skin intolerant to acid-based peels

HOME PARTY PEELS

Revitalize Personal Peel Program (Sesderma)

Revitalize personal peel program is also used as a flash treatment before special occasions. This formula includes 14 active ingredients, including stabilized vitamin C, ginkgo biloba, ferulic acid and phloretin that protect the skin from the action of free radicals. In addition, it contains AHAs such as glycolic and mandelic acid. Because of its active antioxidant cocktail, it functions as a perfect party peel solution and is ideal for those times when the skin needs an immediate brightening effect.

POSTPEEL CARE

Most party peels being very superficial have minimal postpeel care requirement. Standard precautions such as sun protection and avoidance of irritant topical applications are similar to other peels. Makeup can be applied immediately after the treatment in most peels.

CONCLUSION

Party peels are mild peels that use varying combinations of AHAs, botanicals and soothing emollients aimed at providing instant luminosity to the treated skin with lack of visible flaking, and minimal downtime. When used judiciously ensuring a close match between the peel system, skin type and patient's expectations, these superficial peels can be extremely gratifying for patients as well as dermatologists.

TAKE HOME POINTS

- Party peels are very superficial hydroxy acids, enzymes or other botanicals which cause minimal irritation, have no downtime and provide the key advantage of offering an instant "glow"
- A party peel entails a "micro-peeling process" meant to cause only a very superficial exfoliation of the area to be treated
- Party peels are not meant to provide long-term results and are typically done at short notice

- They can be single ingredient peels but are usually a combination of multiple chemical peel agents.

REFERENCES

1. Smith WP. Epidermal and dermal effects of topical lactic acid. J Am Acad Dermatol. 1996;35:388.
2. Usuki A, Ohashi A, Sato H, et al. The inhibitory effect of glycolic acid and lactic acid on melanin synthesis in melanoma cells. Exp Dermatol. 2003;12(Suppl. 2):43-50.
3. Sharquie KE, Al-Tikreety MM, Al-Mashhadani SA. Lactic acid chemical peels as a new therapeutic modality in melasma in comparison to Jessner's solution chemical peels. Dermatol Surg. 2006;32:1429-36.
4. Deprez P. Easy phytic solution: A new alpha hydroxy acid peel with slow release and without neutralization. Int J Cosmet Surg Aesthetic Dermatol. 2003;5(1):45-51.
5. Bernstein EF, Underhill CB, Lakkakorpi J, et al. Citric acid increases viable epidermal thickness and glycosaminoglycan content of sun damaged skin. J Dermatol Surg. 1997;23:689-94.
6. Telang PS. Vitamin C in dermatology. Indian Dermatol Online J. 2013;4:143-6.
7. Matsuda S, Shibayama H, Hisama M, et al. Inhibitory effects of novel ascorbic derivative VCP-IS-2Na on melanogenesis. Chem Pharm Bull. 2008;56:292-7.
8. Draelos ZD. Skin lightening preparations and the hydroquinone controversy. Dermatol Ther. 2007;20:308-13.
9. Inui S, Itami S. Perifollicular pigmentation is the first target for topical vitamin C derivative ascorbyl 2-phosphate 6-palmitate (APPS): randomized, single-blinded, placebo-controlled study. J Dermatol. 2007;34:221-3.
10. Burke KE. Interaction of Vit C and E as better Cosmeseuticals. Dermatol Ther. 2007;20:314-9.
11. Green BA, Edison BL, Sigler ML. Antiaging effects of topical lactobionic acid: results of a controlled usage study. Cosmet Dermatol. 2008;21(2):76-82.
12. Briden ME, Green BA. The next generation hydroxyacids. In: Draelos Z, Dover J, Alam M (Eds). Procedures in Cosmetic Dermatology: Cosmeceuticals. Philadelphia, PA: Elsevier Saunders; 2005. pp. 205-12.
13. Edison BL, Green BA, Wildnauer RH, et al. A polyhydroxy acid skin care regimen provides antiaging effects comparable to an alpha-hydroxyacid regimen. Cutis. 2004;73(suppl 2):14-7.
14. Grimes PE, Green BA, Wildnauer RH, et al. The use of polyhydroxy acids (PHAs) in photoaged skin. Cutis. 2004;73(suppl 2):3-13.
15. Green BA, Edison BL, Wildnauer RH, et al. Lactobionic acid and gluconolactone: PHAs for photoaged skin. Cosmet Dermatol. 2001;9:24-8.
16. Bernstein EF, Green BA, Edison B, et al. Poly hydroxy acids (PHAs): clinical uses for the next generation of hydroxy acids. Skin Aging. 2001;9(Suppl):4-11.
17. Rizer R, Turcott A, Edison B, et al. An Evaluation of the Tolerance Profile of a Complete Line of Gluconolactone-Containing Skin Care Fomulations in Atopic Individuals. Suppl Skin Aging. 2001;9:18-21.
18. Green B, Wildnauer R, Edison B. Lactobionic Acid- a Novel Polyhydroxy Bionic Acid for Skincare. San Francisco: Amer Acad of Derm Poster Exhibit; 2000.
19. Green B. Lactobionic Acid. Skin Inc. 2000;11:62-5.
20. Berardesca E, Distante F, Vignoli GP, et al. Alpha hydroxy acids modulate stratum corneum barrier function. British J Dermatol. 1997;137:934-8.
21. Bernstein EF, Brown DB, Schwartz MD, et al. The Polyhydroxy Acid Gluconolactone Protects Against Ultraviolet Radiation in an In Vitro Model of Cutaneous Photoaging. Dermatol Surg. 2004;30:1-8.
22. Lin, Fu-Hsiung et al. Ferulic Acid Stabilizes a Solution of Vitamins C and E and Doubles its Photoprotection of Skin. J Invest Dermatol. 2005;125(4):826-32.
23. Lim JT. Treatment of melasma using kojic acid in a gel containing hydroquinone and glycolic acid. Dermatol Surg. 1999;25(4):282-4.
24. Garcia A, Fulton JE Jr. The combination of glycolic acid and hydroquinone or kojic acid for the treatment of melasma and related conditions. Dermatol Surg. 1996;22(5):443-7.

34

CHAPTER

Extra-facial Peeling

Meenaz Khoja, Sourabh Jain

INTRODUCTION

Chemical peeling as a treatment modality is being explored in variety of dermatological and cosmetic concerns. Use of peeling agents on nonfacial skin (NFS) is increasing day-by-day; however, due to regional differences in skin, the safety and efficacy parameters of chemical peels on face cannot be simply extrapolated to that of NFS. There are often no specific guidelines or instructions to follow, when one wants to use a particular product over NFS. Conditions like striae, macular or lichen amyloidosis that are recalcitrant to medicines, peeling can be offered as an adjuvant cost-reasonable therapy for better treatment outcome. In this chapter, we attempt to discuss various skin conditions affecting the NFS where chemical peeling has been used as a treatment modality with its safety, efficacy and current opinion, in light of the peculiarities of NFS.

Before we proceed, it is important to understand how and why the NFS differs from facial skin.

DIFFERENCES BETWEEN FACIAL AND NONFACIAL SKIN[1]

- Chemical peeling is based on principle of controlled wounding where a limited number of epidermal or dermal layers are removed and regeneration of healthy epidermis takes places from the undamaged appendageal epidermis. The density of pilosebaceous units is thirty and forty times lower on the neck and trunk and the dorsa of arms and hands, respectively, as compared to face. Due to this regional variation of distribution of glands, healing post chemoexfoliation is delayed which increases the downtime and the risk of complications, e.g., scarring, postinflammatory hyperpigmentation (PIHr) and postinflammatory hypopigmentation as compared to facial skin. Figure 1 illustrates prolonged exfoliation after peel over extensors of forearms

FIG. 1: Desquamation or "peeling" beyond 3 weeks.
Courtesy: Dr. Meenaz Khoja, Consultant Dermatologist and Trichologist, Pune, India.

- Deep peels are not preferred over NFS for the reason mentioned above and superficial peels are not very effective due to poor penetration through thicker epidermis. Therefore, multiple superficial or sequential peels need to be carried out for good efficacy with minimal risk. Some medium-depth peels give balanced results too. Deep peels are usually avoided for fear of complications
- Upper chest, back and arms are sites prone for keloids and scarring; hence, deeper peels should be done cautiously and a history of such scarring tendencies must be elicited during counseling
- As NFS is much larger than the face, systemic toxicity of peeling agents from transcutaneous absorption should not be ignored in cases of peels with agents like salicylic acid (SA), phenol and resorcinol. In single session, peel should not be applied on more than 25% body surface area.[2] Wallace's "rule of nines" can be used to assess the body surface are
- Increased inflammation due to friction from clothes, sweating, difficult-to-access areas, and an overall lesser compliance with pre- and postpeeling care are other aspects that differ.

CHEMISTRY AND CHEMICAL FORMULATIONS USED

Just like we have a variety of peels for the face, various chemical agents are being tried on NFS. Selection of peeling agent depends upon the site, clinical indication and its severity, skin type and personal preference of the patient and the dermatologist. The authors have used some of the most commonly used peels viz. glycolic acid (GA), SA, phenol, trichloroacetic acid (TCA) and combinations thereof.

Glycolic Acid

Glycolic acid is the commonest α-hydroxy acid (AHA) used in peeling solutions. GA has keratolytic, anti-inflammatory and antioxidant properties. Depending on concentration and contact time, Fabbrocini classified GA peels as: very superficial (30–50% GA, 1–2 minutes); superficial (50–70% GA, 2–5 minutes); and medium depth (70% GA, 3–15 minutes).[4] NFS usually tolerates GA concentration of 50–70% for 5–10 minutes. However, it should be started at lower concentration and gradually increased in subsequent sessions. In authors' experience, time of onset of erythema after 35% GA on back or hands is longer than that when done over the face. In some patients, erythema or burning is not noticeable, but improvement is seen on subsequent visits. It is suggested that a 50% concentration for 1–3 minutes is effective on face, while a 70% concentration for 4–8 minutes is required to show results over NFS.[5]

Trichloroacetic Acid[1]

Trichloroacetic acid, an inorganic compound, is available as hygroscopic crystals. It brings about coagulative necrosis of cells through extensive protein denaturation that manifests clinically as frosting. It self-neutralizes and depth of penetration depends only on the concentration of the solution. A 10–15% solution is very superficial; 15–25% is superficial while 35–50% is a medium-depth peel. More than 50% TCA should be rather avoided on NFS due to high incidence of scarring and PIHr, especially in skin of color. Repeated superficial peels are efficacious and safe for dyschromias and mild rhytides.[6]

Salicylic Acid

Salicylic acid, a β-hydroxy acid, has keratolytic and lipophilic properties. It is very safe for all skin types and areas. It is an excellent peeling agent for truncal acne and has lightening effect on acne-induced PIHr,[7] which is otherwise recalcitrant to medical management. Higher concentration (50%) in ointment base is useful in thicker NFS.[8] SA is safer than GA as the vehicle evaporates giving an anesthetic effect and the peel does not penetrate deeper. SA is more predictable and causes more desquamation than GA making it more effective.[9]

Phenol Peel

Crude phenol (88%) or traditional Gordon-Baker formula[1] are not commonly used due to fear of its systemic toxicity and irreversible local side effects like chemical leukoderma. Use of phenol as a peeling agent for NFS has been rarely documented. Newer modifications like Stone Venner-Kellson formula[10] or Litton formula (Exoderm)[11] are medium-depth peels showing promising results in facial dermal melasma (even in darker skin types), thus may be tried in certain recalcitrant conditions like acanthosis nigricans (AN), macular amyloidosis (MA), striae distensae, etc. One of the authors has used 8% phenol-based peel (combined with TCA, SA, retinol and other AHAs) for MA of upper back and truncal acne with PIHr with good results.

INDICATIONS[12]

- *Acne*:
  - Truncal acne
  - Superficial acne scars
  - Postacne pigmentation (Fig. 2)
  - Comedonal acne (Fig. 3).
- *Hyperpigmentation disorders*:
  - Extra-facial melasma
  - Frictional melanosis (Fig. 4)
  - PIHr (Fig. 5)
  - Lentigines and freckles
  - Ashy dermatosis
  - Pigmented contact dermatitis (not active)
  - Macular amyloidosis (Fig. 6)
  - Acanthosis nigricans (Fig. 7)
  - Lichen planus pigmentosus (Fig. 8).
- *Epidermal growths*:
  - Seborrheic keratoses
  - Acrochordons
  - Dermatosis papulosa nigra
  - Warts
  - Sebaceous hyperplasia
  - Keratosis pilaris.
- *Aesthetic indications*:
  - Fine rhytides
  - Dilated pores
  - Skin rejuvenation
  - Photoaging.

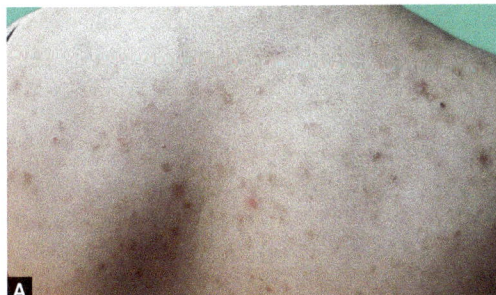 

FIG. 2: A, Truncal acne, superficial acne scars and pigmentation (Before peel); **B,** Lightening of pigmentation post acne and improvement in superficial scars after two sessions of 8% phenol peel done 3 weeks apart (After peel).
Courtesy: Dr. Meenaz Khoja, Consultant Dermatologist and Trichologist, Pune, India.

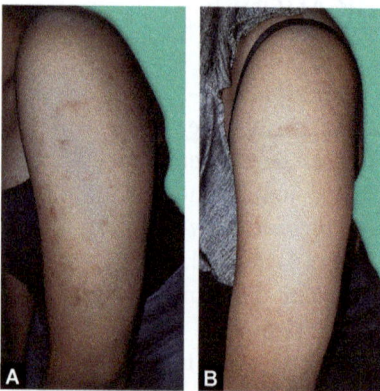

FIG. 3: A, Grade 2 acne with comedones before peel; **B,** Improvement in active acne as well as comedones after two sessions of 8% phenol peel done 3 weeks apart. The skin looks smoother than before.

Courtesy: Dr. Meenaz Khoja, Consultant Dermatologist and Trichologist, Pune, India.

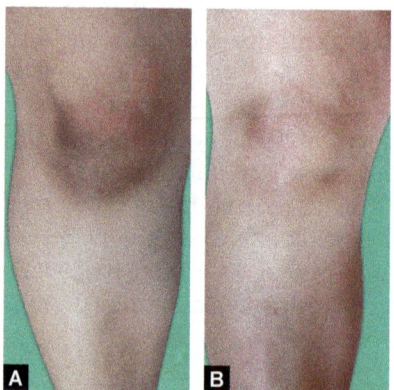

FIG. 4: Frictional melanosis of the knees. **A,** Before; and **B,** after five sittings of 30% TCA peel done at monthly intervals.

Courtesy: Dr. Meenaz Khoja, Consultant Dermatologist and Trichologist, Pune, India.

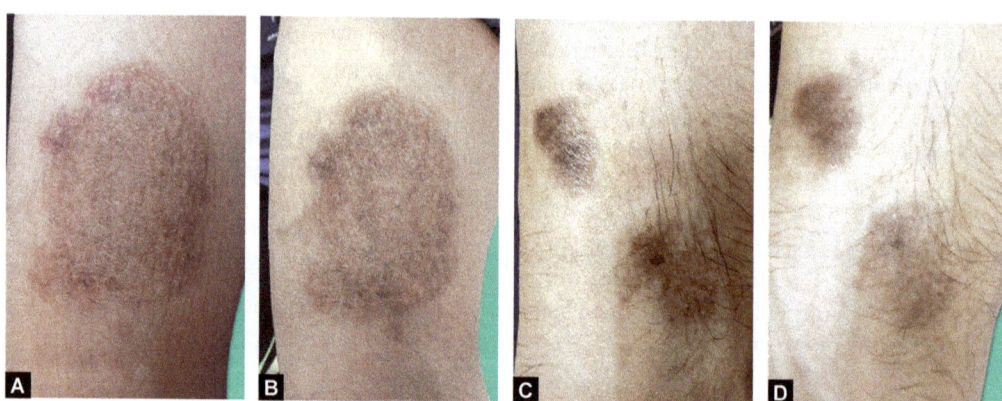

FIG. 5: Postinflammatory hyperpigmentation (following irritant contact dermatitis due to self-medication with dithranol for dermatophytosis) treated with GA 50% solution two sessions 15 days apart. **A** and **C,** Before peel; **B** and **D,** After peel.

Courtesy: Dr. Sourabh Jain, Senior Resident, All India Institutes of Medical Sciences, Bhopal, India.

- *Scars and striae*:
  - Superficial scars
  - Striae distensae
  - Topical steroid-induced striae.
- *Miscellaneous*:
  - *Nevoid conditions:* Generalized linear epidermal nevus, congenital melanocytic nevi and bathing trunk nevi.
  - Tumor prophylaxis in xeroderma pigmentosum
  - *Precancerous and cancerous conditions:* Actinic keratoses (AKs), Bowen's disease (BD), nevoid basal cell carcinoma (NBCC).

There are numerous indications for extra-facial peeling (EFP) and discussing

Extra-facial Peeling

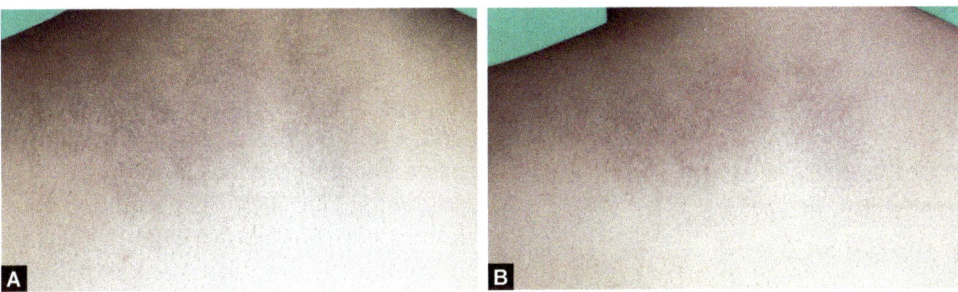

FIG. 6: **A,** Macular amyloidosis showing rippled pattern (Before peel); **B,** Significant improvement in macular amyloidosis using 8% phenol (with trichloroacetic acid, salicylic acid, various alpha-hydroxy acids and retinol) combination peel four sittings 1 month apart. Note that the treatment regimen consisted only of topical sunscreen and the peels. No other topical treatments were given (After peel).
Courtesy: Dr. Meenaz Khoja, Consultant Dermatologist and Trichologist, Pune, India.

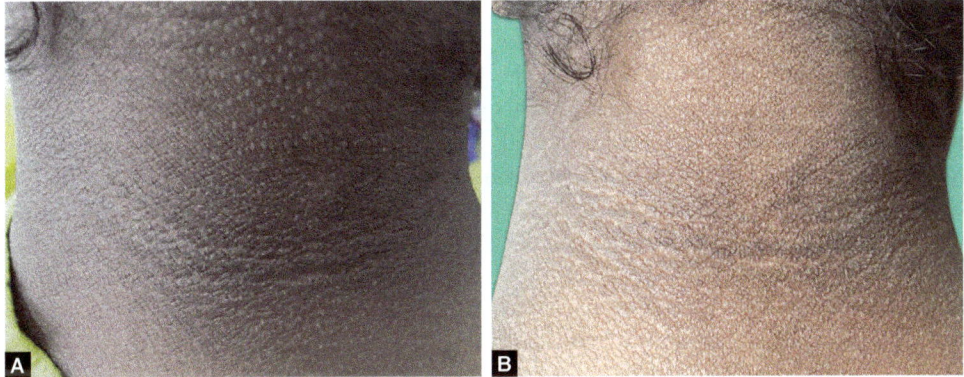

FIG. 7: **A,** Acanthosis nigricans over the neck before trichloroacetic acid peels; **B,** Significant improvement in acanthosis nigricans after two sittings of 15% trichloroacetic acid peel done 1 month apart.
Courtesy: Dr. Dharmendra Dave, Consultant Dermatologist, Patan, Gujarat, India.

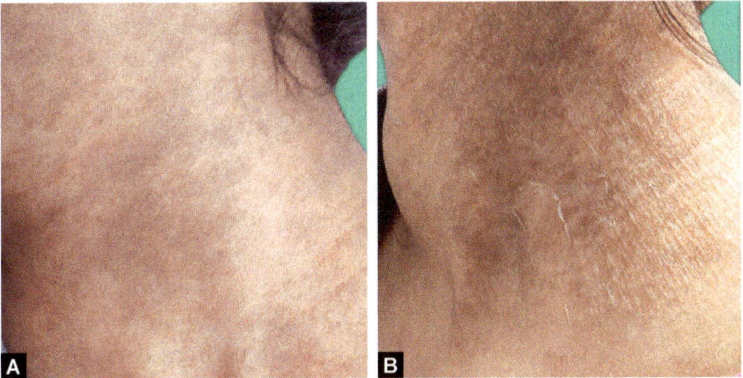

FIG. 8: Lichen planus pigmentosus over neck treated with sequential glycolic acid 35% solution and 15% trichloroacetic acid solution. Mild improvement and exfoliation noted within 5 days of first session. **A,** Before peel and **B,** after peel.
Courtesy: Dr. Sourabh Jain, Senior Resident, All India Institutes of Medical Sciences, Bhopal, India.

each of them in detail is beyond the scope of this chapter. Following is a brief highlight of studies reporting use of various peeling agents in different skin conditions.

Use of Chemical Peeling in Dermatoses Affecting Extra-facial Skin

Use of chemical peeling in various dermatoses affecting extrafacial skin—a literature search with current opinion is described as follows.

Truncal acne, pigmentary disorders and photoaging are the commonest indications for EFP.

There is level A evidence for use of SA and GA peels for facial acne[12] but there are no published comparative studies for the same in truncal acne. However, positive results of the reports on use of short contact foam-based preparations on trunk offers hope for studying peels for truncal acne.[13,14] In our experience, both SA 30% and GA 35–70% gives good results in 4–7 biweekly sittings. Improvement is seen in form of reduction of existing lesions, fewer new lesions and lightening of acne-induced PIHr.

Glycolic acid, TCA, SA and various combinations are being used for extra-facial pigmentary disorders. Sacchidanand et al. demonstrated equal efficacy of 15% TCA and 50% GA in frictional melanosis of forearms without any major side effects.[15] PIHr is a common indication for EFP. Figure 5 demonstrates improvement in PIHr with two sessions of 50% GA peel. Pigmentation in inguinal region is a common and often neglected complaint in patients of tinea cruris. SA or GA peels may not only treat pigmentation but may also reduce the risk of recurrence or reinfection because of its keratolytic activity.

Photodamaged skin has two pathological components, namely: thickened dermis due to breakdown of elastin fiber network and thinned, ironed out epidermis with cellular atypia.[16] To address both these components of photoaging, a combination of superficial and medium-depth peels or sequential peels should be used. Use of 70% GA gel augmented by 40% TCA solution (Cook's body peel) has shown significant results in nonfacial photodamaged skin (refer to "Peel Technique" for details).[6] Efficacy of peels for treatment of photodamaged facial skin has been repeatedly reported, but documentation of their effects on NFS are lagging behind.

There is a report of successful use of TCA 20% in 25 cases of MA, where more than 50% improvement was noted in half of the patients over 3–5 sessions.[17] Figure 6 demonstrates use of 8% phenol-based peel for MA.

A combination of treatments including peeling may offer solution for striae distensae and superficial scars. A recent study showed that combination of microdermabrasion, SA and retinol (yellow) peel resulted in improvement in 60% patients of striae rubra.[18]

Use of peeling agents in nevoid and neoplastic diseases holds promise in palliation of such difficult-to-treat conditions. Clinical and histological evaluation supports successful use of phenol and TCA-based peels in AKs, BD, NBCC, verrucous epidermal nevus and congenital pigmented nevi.[19-23] Hantash et al. conducted a randomized 5-year trial to conclude that peeling with 30% TCA offered prophylaxis and significantly reduced AKs and was associated with a longer time to develop new AKs compared with that of a control group.[24]

Interestingly, chemical peeling can be used in nail rejuvenation.[25] 70% GA and phenol peel has shown improvement in nail pitting and surface irregularities (Fig. 9). Although peels may not treat the nail pathology, they offer better cosmesis.

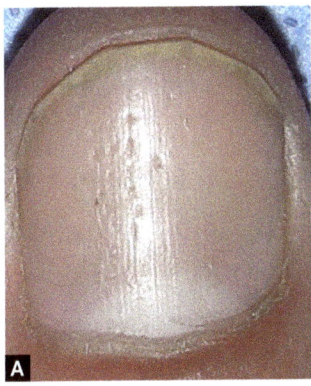 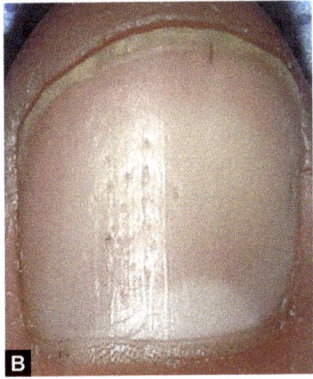 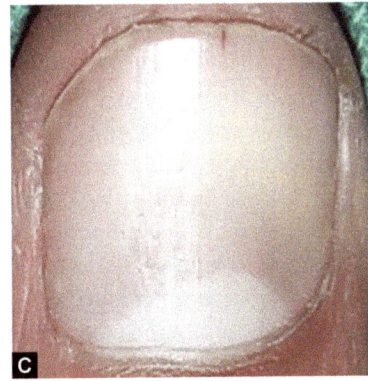

FIG. 9: Sequential improvement in nail pitting. 70% GA was used 3 weeks apart for three sessions.
Courtesy: Dr Soni Nanda, Consultant Dermatologist, New Delhi, and Dr Chander Grover, Professor, Department of Dermatology, University College of Medical Sciences and Guru Teg Bahadur Hospital, Delhi.

PATIENT PREPARATION

Patient assessment and counseling before the peel is of utmost importance. Following factors are to be considered:

- *Indication for the peel:* The type of peel to be done according to the indication should be discussed with the patients. The downtime and the pros and cons of each peel and its alternative options must be discussed so that the patient can make an informed choice
- *Patient history:*
    - Any past history of herpes simplex virus (HSV) infection should be elicited. Prophylactic antiviral therapy may be started 1 day before the peel and continued up to 1–2 weeks post peel
    - History of keloidal tendency should be elicited
    - Peels penetrate more deeply on areas that have an altered barrier function, viz. areas affected with inflammatory eczematous dermatoses. Hence, it is essential to bring the inflammation under control before the patient undergoes peels[9]
    - Diseases like psoriasis and lichen planus may koebnerize post peels
    - History of systemic diseases especially cardiac, renal and liver disease is important when planning peeling with resorcinol (cardiotoxic) and phenol (cardiotoxic and nephrotoxic)
    - History of radiation or recent surgery and drug history is important because it may interfere with collagen remodeling and healing post peel
    - Photosensitizers like perfumes, tricyclic antidepressants, minocycline, thiazide, amiodarone and oral contraceptive pills may make the patient prone to PIHr
    - Immunocompromised patients should be treated only after discussing the due risks of infections
    - History of addictions is important. Smoking delays healing to any injury[26]
    - Patients with unrealistic expectations should not be treated.
- *Patient examination*:
    - Examine the non-sun-exposed areas to know the patient's original skin type and degree of photodamage.[26]
    - Most patients say their sun exposure is minimal because they do not go out in the sun. Comparing the skin tan to

the non-sun-exposed areas helps in counseling the patient for a religious use of sunscreen.
- *Photographs*: Photographic documentation is absolutely necessary for evidence of improvement or lack thereof, and for the safety of the dermatologist. It helps the patient to appreciate the effect of the peel and saves unnecessary drama later on. Photographs of the face as well as the area to be treated should be taken before the peel. The authors suggest photographs in natural light (when available) or one each of with and without flash. Consent should be taken for photographs
- *Consent*: Every patient undergoing a peel should give a written informed consent before the procedure. This ensures that they have understood the procedure, the results to be expected and the complications that may occur. This also safeguards the dermatologist in case things go wrong due to unforeseen conditions
- *Counseling*: Patient should be informed "what to expect" from the procedure. It should be stressed upon that it may take months and multiple sessions for appreciable results, more so over NFS. Significance of postpeel care should be stressed upon to achieve best outcome.

Priming

Priming with moisturizer, broad-spectrum sunscreen and any one of retinoic acid, hydroquinone or AHA is advisable for EFP to activate the skin, control the peel depth and ensure uniform penetration, to shorten the healing duration by enhancing the epithelialization and to decrease the chances of PIHr. Priming should be done for at least 2-6 weeks before peel.[27] The priming agents are withheld for 2-3 days before the peel so that the skin is hydrated and the peel is well tolerated.

Prepeel

The area to be treated is "degreased" using alcohol or acetone. Kaminaka et al. used light curettage to remove the superficial crust or keratin over AKs and BD before applying phenol.[23]

Sedation or Anesthesia

Required for deeper peels like TCA and 88% phenol over larger areas. Topical anesthesia with eutectic mixture of local anesthetics under occlusion for 45-60 minutes usually suffices. Lorazepam 1 mg sublingually 30 minutes before the peel may be used for very anxious patients.[27]

Materials

Desired peel in a ceramic bowl, multiple sterile gauzes 3 × 3 inches, sodium bicarbonate solution, cool water and ice packs, and fan should be kept handy.

PEEL TECHNIQUE

Factors that affect the depth of the peel during application are: acid concentration, number of coats, skin color, degree of cotton gauze saturation and the duration of contact.[27] "Strip technique" is a recently published, standardized and reproducible method of TCA application which controls the depth of the peel and minimizes complications, especially in darker skin types.[27] The evaluation of the peel depth was based on the frost sign (whitening of the peeled skin). Although the strip technique was described for the face, it can be extrapolated to the NFS too. Similar number of coats are given on either side of the treated area and then evaluated for frosting. Extra coats may be given on areas with lesser frosting.

"Cook's total body peel" uses 70% GA gel followed by 40% TCA solution to NFS such

TABLE 1: Visual staging to determine the endpoint for chemical peel of the skin[6]

Stage	"Level of frost" (Rubin)	Description	Clinical implication
I	0	Pink or erythematous skin	Dark skin with minimal actinic damage; face and/or body
II	1	Small white speckles	Fair-to-medium skin with medium actinic damage; face and/or body
III	2	"Frosted" appearance with pink skin showing through	Fair skin with moderate-to-severe actinic damage; face and/or body
IV	3	"Blanched" appearance with an opaque white color	Fair skin; face only, or fair skin of upper neck blending into face
V	–	"Blanched" appearance with a yellowish-white color	Severe actinic damage; face only (rarely needed since laser peels may be preferred)
VI	–	"Blanched" appearance with a grayish-white color	Severe actinic damage; face only (rarely needed since laser peels may be preferred)

as the balding scalp, neck, chest, abdomen and extremities. This technique combines the benefits of gel-based GA (which acts as a partial barrier to deeper penetration of 40% TCA and decreases chances of PIHr) with advantages of TCA (which penetrates uniformly and deeply into photodamaged skin). Rubin's scale for "levels of frosting" is utilized to determine the endpoint (Table 1). Cook and Cook reported success of their technique in 3,100 patients with minimal side effects; however, they did not describe the patient characteristics and the number of sessions, and there was no randomization and comparison.

POSTPEEL CARE[5]

- The patient may use ice-packs or cold compresses for 1–2 days post peel to reduce the burning sensation, if any. Wet technique includes frequent washing of the peeled area with lukewarm water and application of bland emollients such as petrolatum jelly[27]
- No soap, makeup or scrubs to be used for 1–2 days post peel. No clean up, bleaching, waxing or steaming to be done over treated area at least for 1 week
- Disinfectants like Dettol or Savlon, and loofahs or bathing brushes to be avoided for at least a week
- The patient should be informed that the peel will have a downtime (desquamation) of 1–4 weeks
- Liberal use of moisturizers may be needed during the "peeling" phase. The patient should be asked not to pick or pull out the peeling skin
- Strict photoprotection using clothes or broad-spectrum sunscreen every 3–4 hours is essential to enhance results and decrease chances of PIHr
- Loose fitting cotton clothes should be worn during desquamation phase. Ornaments should be avoided for 2–3 weeks in neck peels to avoid friction and discomfort
- The patient should be advised to avoid contact with chlorinated water for 2–3 days post peel.

COMPLICATIONS

Common complications include erythema, persistent hyperpigmentation, HSV infection (in those with prior history) and hypopigmentation. Mild telengiectasia (if peel was deeper than ideal), *Staphylococcus* infection, keloids and hypertrophic scarring (seen in cases of deep TCA peel 40–45%) are rare side effects.[27]

Systemic absorption of phenol peels can lead to cardiac toxicity, respiratory depression, liver and kidney damage.[22] Cardiac toxicity of phenol peels may be reduced by intra-procedure monitoring, proper hydration, ventilation and prophylactic administration of oral propranolol.[28]

Development of keratoacanthomas has been reported after body peel with Jessner's + TCA peel and Cook's body peel.[29]

PRACTICAL TIPS

Extra-facial peeling may be done for specific areas to treat them or as a wholesome treatment along with a facial peel to ensure there is lesser unnatural contrast between treated and nontreated skin after peel.[6]

After priming, the change of skin color to a medium pink hue indicates the effectiveness of priming.[27]

The degree of desquamation postpeel is a good indicator of the efficacy of the peeling agent.[9]

Hypertrophic scarring after TCA peels is usually preceded by persistent induration and erythema. This can be taken as a warning sign and early intervention with intralesional corticosteroids may limit the progression.

Herpes simplex virus activation may or may not be accompanied by a prodrome but stinging or burning sensation within 7 days is used as an indicator. Prophylactic antivirals prevent reactivation.[27]

CONCLUSION

Extra-facial peels are becoming increasingly common for various indications. When done with appropriate care and caution, they give excellent results with minimal or no side effects.

TAKE HOME POINTS

- Extra-facial peels are becoming increasingly common; hence, it is essential to understand about them for best results and patient satisfaction
- Nonfacial skin is different from facial skin, and hence the reaction to the same peel is different in these areas
- Common indications include pigmentation, acne, striae, AN, amyloidosis and photoaging
- Comparing the tan on sun-exposed areas to the non-sun-exposed areas helps in counseling the patient for religious use of sunscreen after the peel, especially those who claim "no sun-exposure"
- Desquamation and healing is prolonged on nonfacial skin due to lower density of pilosebaceous units
- There is an increased risk of scarring and hypopigmentation in skin of color
- When done properly, EFP can give wonderful results even in recalcitrant diseases like MA and AN
- Extra-facial peeling is emerging as a minimally invasive therapy in conditions like BD, AKs and giant melanocytic nevi, especially when surgery is not an option
- When done over larger surface areas, it is essential to monitor the patient for untoward systemic consequences.

REFERENCES

1. Khunger N. Nonfacial peels. In: Khunger N (Ed.) Step by Step Chemical Peels, 2nd Edition. New Delhi: Jaypee Brothers Medical Publishers; 2010. pp. 169-77.
2. Small R, Dalano H, Linder J. In: Practical guide to chemical peeling, microdermabrasion and topical products. New Delhi: Wolters Kluwer; 2014. p. 64.
3. Tung RC, Bergfeld WF, Vidimos AT, et al. Alpha-hydroxy acid-based cosmetic procedures. Guidelines for patient management. Am J Clin Dermatol. 2000;1:81-8.
4. Fabbrocini G, De Padova MP, Tosti A. Chemical peels: what's new and what isn't new but still works well. Facial Plast Surg. 2009;25:329-36.

5. Khunger N, Taneja D, Khunger M. Glycolic acid peels. In: Mysore V (Ed.) ACS(I) textbook on cutaneous and aesthetic surgery. New Delhi: Jaypee Brothers Medical Publishers; 2013. pp. 580-6.
6. Cook KK, Cook WR Jr. Chemical peel of nonfacial skin using glycolic acid gel augmented with TCA and neutralized based on visual staging. Dermatol Surg. 2000;26:994-9.
7. Ahn HH, Kim IH. Whitening effect of salicylic acid peels in Asian patients. Dermatol Surg. 2006;32:372-5.
8. Swinehart JM. Salicylic acid ointment peeling of the hands and forearms. Effective nonsurgical removal of pigmented lesions and actinic damage. J Dermatol Surg Oncol. 1992;18:495-8.
9. Kligman D, Kligman AM. Salicylic Acid Peels for the Treatment of Photoaging. Dermatol Surg. 1998;24:325-8.
10. Stone PA. Use of modified phenol for chemical face peeling. Clin Plast Surg. 1998;25:21-44.
11. Park JH, Choi YD, Kim SW, et al. Effectiveness of modified phenol peel (Exoderm) on facial wrinkles, acne scars and other skin problems of Asian patients. J Dermatol. 2007;34:17-24.
12. Khunger N. Standard guidelines of care for chemical peels. Indian J Dermatol Venereol Leprol. 2008;74 (Suppl.):S5-12.
13. Del Rosso JQ. Management of truncal acne current perspective of management and treatment. Cutis. 2006;77:285-9.
14. Hoffman LK, Del Rosso JQ, Kircik LH. The Efficacy and Safety of Azelaic Acid 15% Foam in the Treatment of Truncal Acne Vulgaris. J Drugs Dermatol. 2017;16:534-8.
15. Sacchidanand S, Shetty AB, Leelavathy B. Efficacy of 15% trichloroacetic acid and 50% glycolic acid peel in the treatment of frictional melanosis: A comparative study. J Cutan Aesthet Surg. 2015;8:37-41.
16. Rendon MI, Berson SD, Cohen JL, et al. Evidence and Considerations in the Application of Chemical Peels in Skin Disorders and Aesthetic Resurfacing. J Clin Aesthet Dermatol. 2010;3:32-43.
17. Nandini AS, Sharath Kumar BC, TCA Peel in the Treatment of Macular Amyloidosis. J of Evolution of Med and Dent Sci. 2014; 3:11090-5.
18. Karia UK, Padhiar BB, Shah BJ. Evaluation of various therapeutic measures in striae rubra. J Cutan Aesthet Surg. 2016;9:101-5.
19. Bazex J, El Sayed F, Sans B, et al. Shave excision and phenol peeling of generalized verrucous epidermal nevus. Dermatol Surg. 1995;21:719-22.
20. Hopkins JD, Smith AW, Jackson IT. Adjunctive treatment of congenital pigmented nevi with phenol chemical peel. Plast Reconstr Surg. 2000;105:1-11.
21. Nelson BR, Fader DJ, Gillard M, et al. The role of dermabrasion and chemical peels in the treatment of patients with xeroderma pigmentosum. J Am Acad Dermatol. 1995;32:623-6.
22. Kaminaka C, Yamamoto Y, Furukawa F. Nevoid basal cell carcinoma syndrome successfully treated with trichloroacetic acid and phenol peeling. J Dermatol. 2007;34: 841-3.
23. Kaminaka C, Yamamoto Y, Yonei N, et al. Phenol peels as a novel therapeutic approach for actinic keratosis and Bowen disease: prospective pilot trial with assessment of clinical, histologic, and immunohistochemical correlations. J Am Acad Dermatol. 2009;60:615-25.
24. Hantash BM, Stewart DB, Cooper ZA, et al. Facial resurfacing for non-melanoma skin cancer prophylaxis. Arch Dermatol. 2006;142:976-82.
25. Grover C. Chemical peels in nail disorders. J Cutan Aesthet Surg. 2014;7:201-2.
26. Salam A, Dadzie OE, Galadari H. Chemical peeling in ethnic skin: an update. Br J Dermatol. 2013;169 Suppl 3:82-90.
27. Fanous N, Zari S. Universal TCA application technique. JAMA Facial Plast Surg. 2017;19:212-9.
28. Landau M. Cardiac complications in deep chemical peels. Dermatol Surg. 2007;33:190-3.
29. Cox S. Rapid development of keratoacanthomas after a body peel. Dermatol Surg. 2003;29:201-3.

35 CHAPTER

Home-based Peeling Systems

Ishad Aggarwal, Manmit K Hora

INTRODUCTION

Chemical peeling with various agents is an excellent in-office treatment modality for a variety of indications and has stood the test of time over last couple of decades. When done in a clinic, in controlled manner the results are spectacular. Even though, advances in recent times have made the procedure safer and more predictable, a lot of our patients are still reluctant to undergo a chemical peel. Lack of time, fast pace of life, recovery from downtime and fear of complications are commonly cited reasons. However, people are still very interested in having a beautiful, ever glowing, blemish free, clean and clear skin. This demand is reflected in how the market and online retail stores are flooded with skin care products and home-based peeling systems. Cosmetic and cosmeceutical brands have their own versions of home-based skin peeling systems. Elizabeth Arden,[1] lancome, cosmoderma, REJSOL, etc. are few such companies who have different home-based peels with different compositions.

CHEMISTRY

The concept of home-based peeling is not altogether new. Traditionally different forms of natural exfoliants have been used to enhance the beauty of skin. Lactic acid in milk and yogurt, fruit acids, lemon, sugar, honey, almonds, etc. have been used from centuries in form of mechanical scrubs. However, with refinement of beauty industry and technological innovations, sophisticated products are now available. There has been a shift from mechanical scrubbing to inclusion of alpha-hydroxy acids (AHAs), beta-hydroxy acids (BHAs) and even enzyme-based peeling agents in the home-based peeling systems.

Currently available home-based peeling solutions have ingredients like lactic acid, glycolic acid (GA), salicylic acid, mandelic acid, vitamin C and retinol. Although the ingredients in both the home-based and in-office peeling solutions are similar, the essential difference however lies in pH of the products. Commercially available in-office peels have a pH <2. Most of the home-based peeling systems have pH >3.5. This feature essentially makes them safer for people to use at the convenience of their homes without supervision of an expert dermatologist.

The various peels brands along with their products are listed below in table 1.

Home-based Peeling Systems

TABLE 1: Various peels brands along with their products

Brands	Products
Neutrogena	Advanced solutions facial peel, containing celluzyme
Elizabeth Arden	Visible difference peel and reveal revitalizing mask
Lancome	Visionnaire crescendo progressive night peel
Kaya	Insta Brightening Micro Mask
Peter Thomas Roth	• Firmx peeling gel • 20% glycolic solutions jumbo peel scrub • Professional strength 40% triple acid peel
Boscia	• Exfoliating peel gel • Charcoal deep pore exfoliating peel
Skin Inc.	Pure revival peel
Dr Dennis Gross skin care	• Alpha beta ultra-gentle daily peel for sensitive skin • Alpha beta universal daily peel • Alpha beta medispa peel • Ferulic + Retinol recovery peel
Dr Jart	Dermaclear micromilk peel
Kielh's	Kielh's dermatologist solutions nightly refining micropeel concentrate.
Kate somerville	Biometric peel pads
Care + Austin	Acne restructure pads
Murad	Rapid resurfacing peel (GA 10%)

GA, glycolic acid

INDICATIONS

Typically home-based peels are used in two scenarios—either as maintenance post or in-between a few sessions of in-office peels or other procedures to maintain results or for patients who seek better skin but do not wish to undergo skin peels at the clinic. A lot of information about home-based peels is available for patients on the internet and they are very easily procurable from the market, retail stores and online commerce portals such as Amazon, Flipkart, Nykaa, etc. More often than not, it leaves patients baffled and confused and they might ask the dermatologist or esthetic esthetic practitioner about the home based peeling systems. Hence, it becomes important for us to analyze our patient's skin condition, understand their expectations, assess their compliance and help them choose or prescribe the right products for them.

Home-based peels are sought for improving the texture of the skin, to reduce pigmentation, fine lines and other signs of aging, for acne control.

Choosing the right product for right skin type and for right concern is important. Salicylic acid and mandelic acid containing products may be beneficial for patients with acne. Similarly azelaic acid containing products may be used to improve postinflammatory hyperpigmentation, especially postacne marks. Retinol and GA may be used for aging skin and melasma. Lactic acid containing home-based peels can be prescribed for improving the texture of skin and to give it the coveted glow. One may even prescribe different formulations to same patient to address different needs. It is prudent to prepare a comprehensive skin plan for such patients.

Procedure of Application

The frequency of usage is determined depending upon skin type of an individual, the concerns as elicited by the dermatologist and sensitivity toward the product. In usual cases, these products may be used once to up to three times a week. One may even prescribe two different products to be applied as spot home peels only to be applied on area of concerns. Since most of the products cause exfoliation of skin, they are generally applied in night and sensitive areas like corners of eyes, corners of lips, lips, under eye area and upper eyelid are best avoided or applied with caution.

Postpeel Care

Needless to say that a prescription of a home-based peeling system should be done by a dermatologist after having evaluated all the factors that can affect the patient both in positive and negative manner.

Since home-based peels are used on a continuous basis contrary to the in-office peels, postpeel care is also usually an ongoing process. Therefore, patient education and counseling should be meticulous. Patients should be made aware of need for strict sun protection. They should also be advised about adequate moisturization and skin barrier repair. It is important for them to identify red flags such as erythema, extensive exfoliation, extreme sensitivity and development of postinflammatory hyperpigmentation.

It is imperative for the treating physician to also review other skin care products which the patient may be using while prescribing home-based peeling systems, because they may complicate the results. Due consideration should always be given to stoppage of products before any procedure like lasers, injectables, medical facials and other parlor activities such as depilation of hair.

CONTRAINDICATIONS

Products containing retinoids are contra-indicated in pregnancy.[2] Since the systemic absorption of GA after topical application is minimal, it is considered to be safe in pregnancy.[2] Although no study exists about effect of topical salicylic acid on pregnancy, it is better avoided. Azelaic acid can be safely used in pregnancy for acne and melasma.

Patients with sensitive and irritable skin, atopic dermatitis, herpes infection and bacterial infections should avoid homecare peels.

Patients who are on isotretinoin should take homecare peels with caution because they precipitate excessive dryness and exfoliation.

CONCLUSION

While health care strives to become less invasive while we speak, our patients constantly demand of simpler, less invasive procedures with lesser downtime. Home-based peeling systems definitely have augmented our bucket of choices that we can offer our patients, and as dermatologists it is important to be aware of such products, because they are easily available to our patients and there is increasing demand for them.

TAKE HOME POINTS

- Home-based peels are easily available and there is a huge demand for them in esthetic practice

- Different formulations have varying degrees of AHA, BHA and enzyme peels
- They have higher pH than the conventional peels, hence safer to use by people at home
- Choosing right product for right skin is most important
- They can be used frequently as maintenance postprocedures, bride therapy between different modalities, or for people who do not want to go for in-office peels
- Patient education, assessment of their lifestyle, skin care regimen, concomitant usage of other products, skin types, skin irritability is key to successful outcomes and safety.

REFERENCES

1. Cavegn B. Home peeling: a combined technique. In: Tosti A, Grimes P, Padova M (Eds). Colour Atlas of Skin Peels, 2nd Edition. Berlin: Springer; 2012.
2. Bozzo P, Chua-Gocheco A, Einarson A. Safety of skin care products during pregnancy. Can Fam Physician. 2011;57(6):665-7.

CHAPTER 36

Innovations with Chemical Peels in Dark Skin

Geraldine Jain

INTRODUCTION

Chemical peeling can be traced back to Cleopatra, "mother of chemical peeling" as she bathed in sour milk, thereby utilizing the properties of lactic acid. The Egyptian women also applied salt and alabaster to their skin, apart from using urine, pumice stone and other agents to effectively peel their skin.[1]

Clinicians are faced with specific challenges when using peels on dark skin. Although darker skin confers the advantage of added photoprotection, it is often an unpredictable response of melanocytes to injury that can cause disfiguring postinflammatory pigmentary changes (Fig. 1).

MORPHOLOGIC AND HISTOLOGIC FEATURES OF DARK SKIN

There is a wide variation in structure and function of the skin and hair of darkly pigmented individuals as compared to lightly pigmented skin. These differences have a very significant importance in aesthetic practice. Fitzpatrick skin phototype system classifies the skin according to the individual response to ultraviolet radiation with respect to burning or tanning ability.[2] In this classification, ("melanocompetent") individuals with brown constitutive skin or darkly pigmented color are classified as type IV to VI (Table 1 and 2).

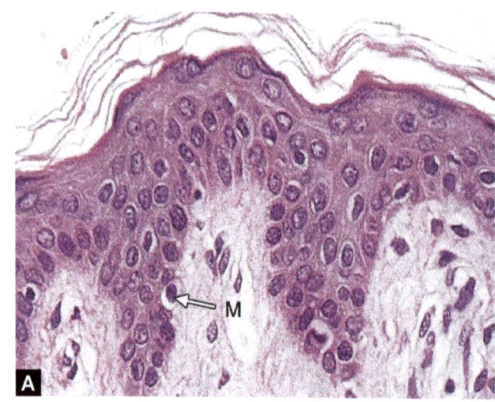
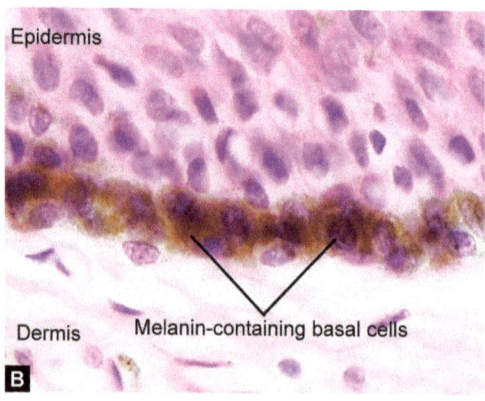

FIG. 1: Histology of fair skin and dark skin.

A thick stratum corneum, large melanosomes and a thick dermis with abundant fibroblasts constitute morphological features in a dark skin prototype.[3] Chemical peels facilitate improvement by thinning the stratum corneum and regenerating a compact epidermis which reflects light evenly across the skin surface and imparts a textural improvement and lightening effect as the elimination of epidermal melanin and prevention of transfer of melanin to keratinocytes occurs (Box 1). Skin color is influenced by the activity of protease-activated receptor 2 and this influences the ethnic skin color phenotypes.[4] Though dark individuals have minimal epidermal changes like wrinkles due to the protective nature of melanin, their aging is associated with soft tissue and gravitational changes. In dark skin, pigmentary changes are common features of photoaging.[5] The common clinical signs of photoaging in these patients include lentigines, keratosis, rhytides, telangiectasias and loss of elasticity (Table 3).

Unlike skin phototype (SPT) I and II, where peels are mostly used to treat skin changes associated with photoaging, SPT IV and V peels are mostly for mottled dyschromias, acne vulgaris, postinflammatory hyperpigmentation (PIH), melanoma and pseudofolliculitis barbae (PFB).[6]

BOX 1	Indications for chemical peels in dark skin

- Pigmentary abnormalities
- Photodamage
- Textural concerns

TABLE 1: Fitzpatrick's classification of skin types

Skin type	Color	Reaction to first summer exposure
I	White	Always burn, never tan
II	White	Usually burn, tan with difficulty
III	White	Sometimes mild burn, tan average
IV	Moderate brown	Rarely burn, tan with ease
V	Dark brown	Very rarely burn, tan very easily
VI	Black	No burn, tan very easily

ACNE AND DARK SKIN

Incidence of inflammatory acne is more common in Fitzpatrick type III-VI skin which resolves commonly with PIH, scars and keloid. Histopathological examination of acne lesions including noninflamed comedones in dark skin individuals revealed underlying

TABLE 2: Structural and functional differences and implications

Examples of contributing skin and structural or functional factor	Dermatologic implication
• Increased tyrosinase activity → increased melanin content • Larger individually dispersed melanosomes (stage IV) • Increased melanosomes • Dispersion of melanosomes throughout epidermis	• Greater photoprotection • Less prominent photoaging • Lower incidence of skin cancer
• Labile melanocytes • Slower melanin degradation	Dyschromias
• Larger, more numerous, binucleated and multinucleated fibroblasts • Fibroblast hyperreactivity • Larger mast cell granules • Increased tryptase	Greater prevalence of keloids and hypertrophic scarring

Chemical Peels: A Global Perspective

TABLE 3: Indications for chemical peeling

Fitzpatrick skin type	Actinic keratoses	Lentigines	Coarse rhytids	Fine rhytids	Acne vulgaris	PIH	Mottled dyschromias	Melasma	Scarring	PFB
I.	+	+	+	+	+	+	+	+	+	+
II.	+	+	+	+	+	+	+	+	+	+
III.	+	+	−	+	+	+	+	+	+	+
IV.	−	+	−	−	+	+	+	+	+	+
V.	−	−	−	−	+	+	+	+	+	+
VI.	−	−	−	−	+	+	+	+	+	+

PIH, postinflammatory hyperpigmentation; PFB, pseudofolliculitis barbae.

inflammatory infiltrate, though individuals with skin of color can also develop open and closed comedones or no inflammatory lesions.[7] The inflammation surrounding papules, pustules revealed foreign body granulomas with giant cells and epidermal melanin granules and melanophages extending to reticular dermis which was not consistent with the clinical findings. This exaggerated inflammatory lesions is responsible for the postinflammatory pigmentation in skin of color even in mild-to-moderate acne.[8] PIH can develop from irritant contact dermatitis from topical preparations for acne or cosmetics, sunlight and picking of lesions. Treatment of acne and scars in dark-skin patients should address the treatment for PIH simultaneously.

MELASMA AND DARK SKIN[9]

Even though dark skin confers better photoprotection due to the protective effect of melanin, it is by itself a risk factor for pigmentary disorders like melasma. Due to the faulty pathophysiological response to cutaneous injury by SPT IV–VI, these SPTs have an increased tendency for PIH after chemical peeling and laser resurfacing. So, when treating melasma with chemical peels in dark skin, care should be taken to prevent and manage PIH.

Deep peels are not addressed in Fitzpatrick skin types IV–VI.

The deeper the peelings, the more apparent the results; however, risks and discomfort in the period after the procedure will also increase.

ALPHA-HYDROXY ACIDS

The mechanism of action of alpha-hydroxy acids (AHAs) is desquamation of epidermis by epidermolysis within 3 minutes of application. Factors affecting the intensity of the AHA are listed in box 2.[10]

Glycolic Acid

Glycolic acid (GA) is a superficial peel with a concentration in between 30% and 70%. The

---

BOX 2: Factors affecting the intensity of the alpha-hydroxy acids[10]

- Concentration of the acid
- Vehicle of the acid (liquid solutions more than gel formulations)
- Amount of acid applied
- Technique used to deliver the acid

solution can be in the form of a water solution or a mixture of water, alcohol and propylene glycol or in gel form. GA acts on stratum corneum to cause enzymatic degradation, which results in thin, compact epidermis with dispersion of epidermal melanin. It also acts on dermis to improve the quality of elastin and collagen.[11] When used along with other depigmenting agents, GA enhances the efficacy of the topicals in melasma. GA is a less favorable peel for melasma and postinflammatory pigmentation in type V and VI as GA itself can cause PIH.[12] GA has recently been shown to be bactericidal against *Propionibacterium acnes*, having an anti-inflammatory effect on acne lesions. GA enhances the efficacy of topical regimens in melasma.

Mandelic Acid

Mandelic acid peels are low molecular weight AHA peels obtained from bitter almonds with strength of 20-50%. It is used for active acne lesions and postacne pigmentation due to the antibacterial and anti-inflammatory properties and due to their tolerability on dark skin. Because of the synergistic action, mandelic acid is used with salicylic acid and retinoic acid. The safety profile of this peel is high due to absence of postpeel irritation for dark skin types.[13]

Lactic Acid

An AHA with pH 3.5 in hydroalcoholic solution. It is used at 85%. Lactic acid inhibits tyrosinase enzyme activity directly in a dose-dependent manner. It can be used as a peeling agent in the treatment of melasma. It is a low cost and easy to use product. Lactic acid (92%) is a safe and effective peel in melasma and it improves the texture, pigmentation and general appearance of acne scar.[14,15]

Salicylic Acid

Salicylic acid is a naturally occurring beta-hydroxy acid derived from the bark of the willow tree. It is a noncaustic, keratolytic, anti-inflammatory, lipophilic and sebolytic peel causing epidermal exfoliation. At concentrations of 3-5%, it functions as a keratolytic agent. It produces desquamation of the upper, lipophilic layers of the stratum corneum, providing salicylic acid with its comedolytic effect in acne vulgaris. 20-30% salicylic acid function as a peel that is widely considered to be the safest in the ethnic skin population (Box 3).[16]

Salicylic and Mandelic Acid Peeling

This is a combination of a 20% salicylic acid with a 10% mandelic acid. Salicylic

---

BOX 3 | **Chemical peeling agents for ethnic skin[6]**

Very superficial peeling agents
- 30% glycolic acid, for 1–2 minutes
- Jessner's solution, 1–3 coats
- 30% salicylic acid
- 20–30% resorcinol, for 5–10 minutes
- 10% trichloroacetic acid, one layer
- Lactic acid
- Phytic acid

Superficial peeling agents
- Trichloroacetic acid 10–35%
- Glycolic acid solution 50–70%
- Jessner's solution (Combes' formula), 4–7 coats

Medium-depth peeling agents
- Trichloroacetic acid 50%
- Glycolic acid solution 70%
- Trichloroacetic acid 25% + glycolic gel 70%
- Jessner's solution and trichloroacetic acid

Trichloroacetic acid 25% + glycolic gel 70%, Jessner's solution and trichloroacetic acid

acid penetrates rapidly and mandelic acid penetrates the epidermis slowly and evenly. It is ideal for sensitive skin. It has the added benefit of preventing postinflammatory pigmentation, making it especially useful for ethnic skins. Indications for salicylic and mandelic acid are acne, postacne scars and dyschromias, including melasma. As compared to GA, salicylic–mandelic acid combination is more effective for active acne and PIH with fewer side effects.[17]

Jessner's Peel

Jessner's peel or Combes' peel is a combination of resorcinol 14 g, salicylic acid 14 g and lactic acid 14 g in a sufficient quantity of ethanol (95%) to make 100 cc of solution. Salicylic acid is a sebolytic, keratolytic agent; lactic acid acts by desquamating the corneocytes and resorcinol, which is structurally and chemically similar to phenol, disrupts the weak hydrogen bonds of keratin. Dr Max Jessner originally formulated this peel to reduce the concentration and toxicity of each of the individual ingredients while increasing efficacy.

To avoid the toxicity of resorcinol, modified Jessner's solution is formulated which contains lactic acid 17%, salicylic acid 17%, citric acid 8% in ethanol (95%) without resorcinol solution.

The combination of Jessner's solution with 35% trichloroacetic acid (TCA) known as Monheit's peel, achieves a more uniform penetration and is an excellent peel with a safe low concentration of TCA.[18]

The lighter variant of a medium combination peel, weekend peel by L Wiest is Jessner's peel with 15–25% TCA can be used for pigmentation and early signs of skin aging.

Modified Jessner's solution can be used as an adjuvant treatment with TCA in the treatment of melasma, improving the results and minimizing PIH.

The solution can be used in conjunction with other agents like GA and 5-fluorouracil (for actinic keratosis) as it enhances the effects of each.

Jessner's solution can also be combined with TCA. Jessner's solution can be combined with 7–15% TCA and 0.04% retinoic acid.

Retinol Peels

Tretinoin also known as all-transretinoic acid is a synthetic form of vitamin A. Topical tretinoin is known to induce increased collagen deposition, and inhibit the metalloproteinases responsible for degrading collagen. It promotes wound healing and collagen synthesis and corrects pigmentary abnormalities. The orange peeling solution is preserved in brown containers. The patient is advised to wash off the solution after 4-6 hours. One percent tretinoin peel is as effective as 70% GA for melasma with less erythema and desquamation in dark skin.[19] Tretinoin peel significantly reduces the need for longer duration of topical retinoids.

Trichloroacetic Acid Peel

Trichloroacetic acid is a crystalline organic compound, acts by denaturing the protein which causes coagulative necrosis of cell and precipitation of proteins, and appears externally as white frosting. As there is a risk of dyschromias and scarring, TCA is less preferred in type IV-VI SPT. The depth of necrosis correlates with the concentration of TCA, which at medium level concentrations of 35–50% will penetrate between the superficial papillary and midreticular dermis. When used, only a low concentration of TCA (10–35%) is preferred which reaches up to the upper papillary dermis, and hence TCA peels are not appropriate for treating dermal and mixed forms of melasma. When TCA is used in Indian skin for melasma, TCA shows similar effect to GA, but with increased incidence of postpeel cracking and burning sensation.[20] Focal application of higher TCA concentrations (10-65%) on the pigmented lesions is a safe and effective modality for the treatment of benign pigmented lesions with no significant complications.[21]

Obagi Blue Peel[22]

Obagi blue peel or TCA blue peel offers depth-controlled TCA peels. It contains fixed percentage of TCA (15% or 20%) mixed with blue peel base (saponins, glycerine and nonionic blue color). As the blue peel base decreases the surface tension, the peel will penetrate slowly. The blue peel allows to identify the area that has been treated. Frosting occurs more slowly which allows physician to control the depth of the peel.

Beta-lipohydroxy Acid

Lipohydroxy acid (LHA) is a salicylic acid derivative. It is a more lipophilic than salicylic acid and has a higher molecular weight. The highly lipophilic property of LHA slows its penetration and results in an exfoliation of individual corneosomes which mimics physiological desquamation. LHA has a high affinity for the pilosebaceous unit making it an excellent option as a comedolytic agent for acne vulgaris.[23]

Pyruvic Acid

Pyruvic acid is a potent medium-depth peel, which converts into lactic acid. The vapors of pyruvic acid have a pungent smell. There is no systemic toxicity, there are no studies reported till date on the use of pyruvic acid in skin of color. As it is a potent medium-depth peel and is associated with intense pain, caution should be taken if it is using in skin of color.[9]

NEWER PEELS

Phytic Peels[24]

Phytic acid (myoinositol hexaphosphate) is a natural plant antioxidant found in almost all grains, fibers and plants. It inhibits melanin production by acting as a chelating agent that inhibits entrance of iron and copper into the cell. It can act at low pH without causing stinging or irritation. Three percent phytic acid solution with pH 1.0 shows superior efficacy and increased mildness when compared with 10% AHA with pH 3. Phytic acid does not require neutralization. Easy phytic peel (EPP) (Skin rebirth SL, Spain) is a combination of GA, lactic acid, mandelic acid and phytic acid. The three AHAs in the EPP solution have different velocities of penetration through the skin, from GA, which penetrates first, to lactic and mandelic acids. Phytic acid scavenges the free radical oxygen, formed during the inflammatory process after chemical peeling.

Vi Peel

The Vi peel (a variation of the Apothe Peel) is a premixed formula containing TCA (10-12% in alcohol), phenol (10-12%), salicylic acid (10-12%) and tretinoin (0.4%). The home regimen consists of two nightly applications of a pad containing tretinoin oil and vitamin C.[11]

Amino Fruit Acids

Amino fruit acids are slightly alkaline chemicals, with a close to physiological pH. They are well tolerated, especially in those with dry and sensitive skin.[25] Amino fruit acids have been shown to be effective in the treatment of melasma and acne but further study in dark skin is required.

Miami AR Peel

The Miami AR peel is a superficial peel which contains acids derived from fruits and organic substances along with retinol ester which is three times more powerful than retinol. It contains retinol ester, retinyl linoleate, ethyl macadamiate, hydroxy phenoxy propionic acid, ascorbyl linoleate, tocopheryl linoleate and caprylyl glycol. Indications are photoaging, hyperpigmentation, melasma, PIH and skin rejuvenation.

The peel is applied all over the face after cleaning. It can be applied in 1-3 layers at an interval of 2 minutes. The peel is kept on the face for 4-5 hours and washed with cold water. Any excessive erythema can be washed after 5 minutes. The consecutive peels were done at an interval of 2 weeks (Fig. 2).

PATIENT PREPARATION

A detailed medical, drug and occupational history should be taken along the lines for other skin prototypes. History of PIH, keloids and scarring should be elicited. Detailed physical examination should be done to assess the type of skin, degree of photoaging, presence of infection, degree of PIH and keloidal scarring. Prepeel photographs should be taken. Discuss about the expected results, risk and complications. Counsel regarding treatment plan, expected outcome, complications, downtime, importance of adherence to the prepeel regimen and maintenance therapy.

PREPEEL REGIMEN

A religious regimen of priming should be started 3-4 weeks prior to the peel and discontinued 3 days before the peel. It helps to reduce healing time, complications, ensures uniform penetration of peeling agents, detects intolerance to any agent and enforces patient compliance. The agents used for priming depend upon the indication for chemical peeling and the type of individual's skin. Morning application of a gentle cleansing agent and a 10% AHA moisturizing agent. Photoprotection is the most important measure in the prepeel regimen. A broad-spectrum sunscreen with SPF more than 30 is given. Formulations can be adjusted according to the skin type.

Topical retinoids are given 2-4 weeks prior to the peel, which thins the stratum corneum and increases collagen deposition. Topical depigmenting agents are given to those patients with Fitzpatrick type III skin or more and those with facial pigmentary dyschromias. Four percent hydroquinone cream or kojic acid is given as depigmenting agents. Patients should be instructed not to bleach, wax, scrub, massage, use depilators, or schedule an important event 1 week before the peel. Peel technique is described in table 4.

CHEMICAL PEELS FOR ACNE (BOX 4)[6]

Both GA and salicylic acid can be used to treat acne and when used as superficial peels

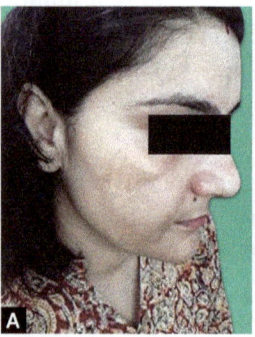 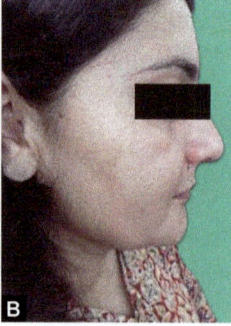

FIG. 2: A, Melasma in an Indian patient before treatment; and **B,** After two Miami AR peels.

TABLE 4: Peel technique

Step	Procedure
Prepeeling	
I.	• Prime face • Discontinue 2 days before treatment
Peeling	
II.	Choose peel according to patient characteristics and desired depth. Acne prone/oily skin: consider salicylic acid. Dry skin: glycolic acid
III.	Degrease to remove excess oils
IV.	• Remove hair from face, apply occlusive ointment to lips and protect ear canal. Test peel postauricular region. • Adapt technique to the desired depth of peel. Monitor volume of agent used, amount of pressure applied, contact time with skin and neutralization of peel. Apply to treatment area starting with low concentration and titrate to tolerability, spacing peels 4–6 weeks apart both the strength of peel and time to neutralization can be increased with each subsequent peel
Postpeeling	
V.	Commence with photoprotection and bland emollients immediately postpeel
VI.	2 days to 1 week postpeel restart hydroquinone and topical retinoid therapy

BOX 4 Benefits of chemical peels in acne

- Targets the factors contributing to the development of acne
- Enhances the absorption of other topical agents
- Improves postinflammatory hyperpigmentation, textural improvements and photodamage correction
- Speeds up the time taken to restore skin to normal
- Synergistic to lasers in treating atrophic scars

they have got an excellent safety profile in SPT IV-VI (Fig. 3).

In salicylic acid peel, the agent (20–30%) is applied, crystalizes forming a pseudofrost which is the endpoint. Salicylic acid is kept on the face for about 4–5 minutes. When discrete papules and pustules are present, salicylic acid can be directly applied over the lesions with a cotton-tip applicator. Peel is neutralized with cold water.

For glycolic peel, in skin of color, buffered or partially buffered 30–50% is used. The peel is left on the face for 2–4 minutes and neutralized with neutralizing solution. If there is any erythema, blisters, or grayish white appearance of epidermis, peel is neutralized immediately.

CHEMICAL PEELS FOR POSTINFLAMMATORY PIGMENTATION

Pigment deposition in the skin resultant from trauma caused by mechanical effects or from inflammatory skin disorders poses a therapeutic challenge.

Serial GA peels give good results in recalcitrant cases of pigmentation in skin of color, but caution must be exercised as overly aggressive peeling may result in PIH. Superficial salicylic acid peels (20–30%) are safe and efficacious for PIH in skin type IV-VI (Fig. 4).

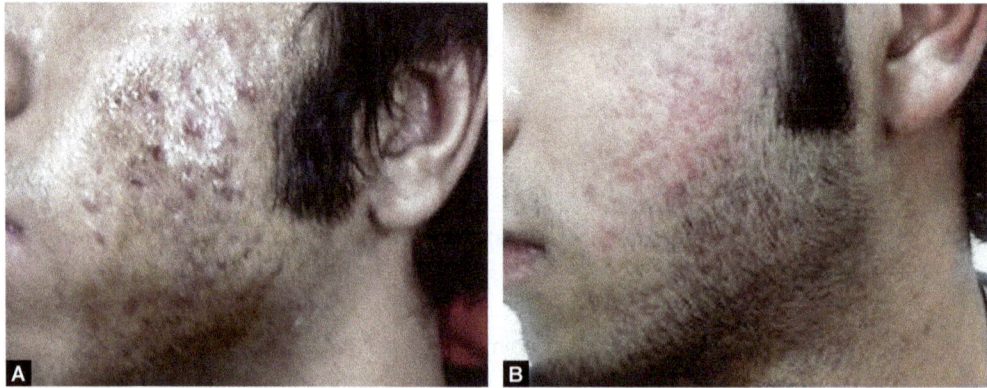

FIG. 3: A, Acne vulgaris in an Indian patient; and **B,** Clearance of acne vulgaris 5 weeks after two salicylic–mandelic peels.

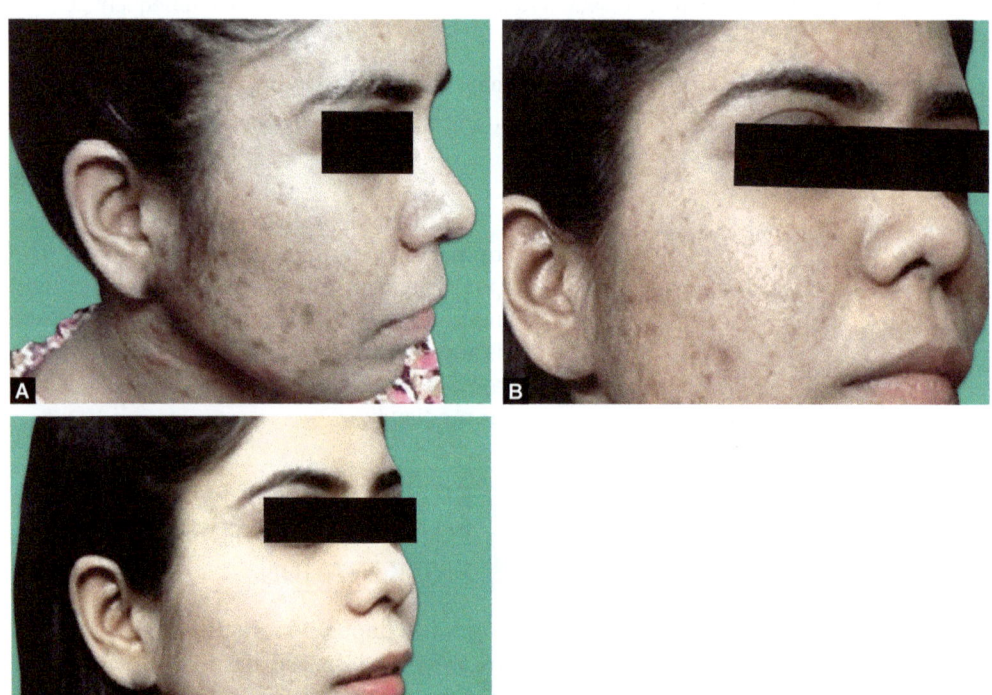

FIG. 4: A, Acne and postinflammatory pigmentation (PIH); **B,** Improvement of acne and PIH with a 30% salicylic acid; and **C,** At week 16 after to serial 50% glycolic acid full-face peel.

Jessner's Peel

For hyperpigmentation, in skin of color, another technique which can be used for peeling is "spot peel". Using this technique, the peeling agent is directly focused on the dark skin. When peel is applied on the entire face, overall lightening of face occurs. There

Innovations with Chemical Peels in Dark Skin

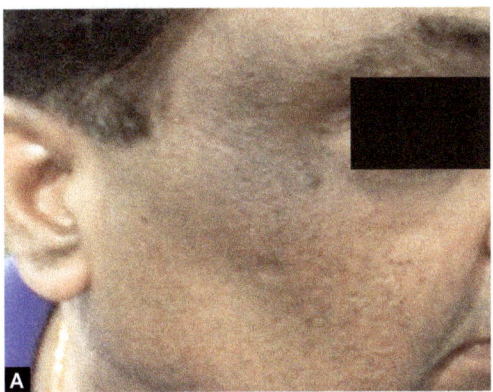 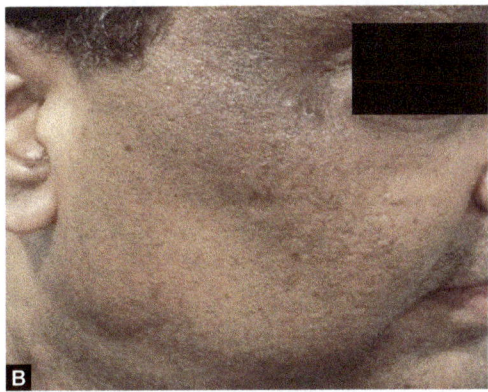

FIG. 5: **A,** Patient with skin type V before a Jessner's face peel and 25% trichloroacetic acid spot peel; and **B,** Patient after two treatments of the combined agents at week 10.

would still be color difference between affected and normal skin. When we use spot peeling, the hyperpigmented skin will match with normal skin.

Trichloroacetic acid, Jessner's solution and salicylic acid can be used for this "spot peel" technique (Fig. 5).

CHEMICAL PEELING FOR SCARRING

When preparing a dark-skinned individual for chemical peeling for acne scarring, certain precautions should be taken. Both the atrophic and the ice-pick form have a dermal component. Therefore, a medium-depth peel, which acts up to the upper reticular dermis is indicated when treating this type of acne scarring. The risk of transient hyperpigmentation is high, and as such, the patient must be accepting of this phase in the healing process.

In acne scarring, in skin of color, a combination peel of 70% GA gel with 25% TCA is used. After preparing the patient, 70% GA gel is applied on the affected part. When the patient feels a tingling sensation, 25% TCA is applied. It is allowed to remain for 2-4 minutes, and then the face is neutralized with sodium bicarbonate solution. The advantage of this combination peel is that gel vehicle limits the harshness of the TCA and the peel moves along a little slower with excellent control. An intramuscular injection of 40 mg triamcinolone acetonide is administered and the patient is sent home with postpeel instructions. The same procedure is typically repeated in 4-6 weeks. If tolerated well, the peeling agent may be left on 1-2 minutes longer the next time. After the last peel is completed, the patient is put back on their pretreatment regimen. This may continue for 12 weeks or until all dyschromia is resolved. These patients are maintained with monthly microdermabrasion.

CHEMICAL PEELING FOR PSEUDOFOLLICULITIS BARBAE

Alpha-hydroxy acid and salicylic acid are found to be effective in the treatment of PFB. Due to the high affinity for folliculosebaceous structures and due to its keratolytic and comedolytic action, salicylic acid is used in the treatment of PFB. The procedure is performed using 30% salicylic acid and the same technique as described for acne above. In between peels, the patient is maintained on a twice-daily application of a 15% glycolic cream or gel.

Serial GA peels is effective in PFB.[26] The GA acts as a potent exfoliating agent, preventing hyperkeratosis.

POSTPEEL CARE

After the peel, the patient is instructed not to wash the face for 24 hours. A regular cleansing routine may resume 24 hours after the peel. Emphasize on bland cleansers and moisturizers. Broad-spectrum sunscreen should be used judiciously.

Excessive peeling, erythema, or irritation post peel can be treated with low or mid- to high-potency steroids for 5–7 days, in the author's experience, if required. Use of such agents should be based on the extent of irritation and inflammation (Box 5).

The risk of complications can be significantly reduced with meticulous patient selection, peel selection (volume, combination, concentration and technique of application), patient education, adequate priming, and good intrapeel and postpeel care.

PRACTICAL TIPS

- Choose chemical peels according to the skin type
- Select peel according to the depth of the peel and the mechanism of action required
- Priming is the most important step in chemical peeling in the skin of color
- Postoperative maintenance regimen ensures long-term satisfaction
- Anticipate the complications
- Ensure the peeling effects of the previous peel is complete before the next session
- Newer peels or combination peels with less complication potential are to be considered in ethnic skin
- Spot peel technique is a good alternative method for applying medium-depth peel in dark skin
- Except EPP, all AHAs should be neutralized with sodium bicarbonate solution or water.

BOX 5	Complications of chemical peel is more common with dark skin

Immediate complications:
- Irritation or burning sensation
- Erythema and edema
- Spillage into the eyes

Late complications:
- Allergic reactions
- Acneiform eruptions
- Reactivation of the herpes infection
- Milia
- Scarring

Textural changes.
- Postinflammatory hyperpigmentation or hypopigmentation (more common in skin type IV–VI). Long standing postinflammatory pigmentation is commonly seen in skin of color

TAKE HOME POINTS

- Chemical peels to correct acne, acne scar, dyschromias and other conditions are recommended in patients with dark skin
- The choice of peeling agent, the concentration of the peel as well as the duration and frequency of peels all contribute to optimal results
- Dark skin needs special emphasis on primary photoprotection and need for maintenance peels along with adjuvant topical or interventional therapies
- Chemical peels in dark skin if used judiciously and with extreme caution,

- offer immense satisfaction to the patient and the treating physician
- Newer agents and combinations show promise and need more studies.

REFERENCES

1. Bryan CP. Ancient Egyptian medicine; the papyrus ebers. Chicago, IL: Ares Publishers; 1974.
2. Fitzpatrick TB: the validity and practicality of sun-reactive skin types I through VI. Arch Dermatol. 1998;124(6):869-71.
3. Taylor SC. Skin of color: physiology, structure, function, and implications for dermatologic disease. J Am Acad Dermatol. 2002;46(2 Suppl):S41-62.
4. Babiarz-Magee L, Chen N, Seiberg M, Lin CB. The expression and activation of protease-activated receptor-2 correlate with skin color. Pigment Cell Res. 2004;17(3):241-51.
5. Yosipovitch G, Theng CTS. Asian skin: its architecture, function and differences from Caucasian skin. Cosmet Toiletries. 2002;117(9):104-10.
6. Roberts WE. Chemical peeling in ethnic/dark skin. Dermatol Ther. 2004;17:196-205.
7. Callender VD. Acne in ethnic skin: special considerations for therapy. Dermatol Ther 2004;17:184-95.
8. Halder RM, Holmes YC, Bridgeman-Shah S, et al. A clinicohistopathologic study of acne vulgaris in black females (abstract). J Invest Dermatol. 1996;106:888.
9. Sarkar R, Bansal S, Garg VK. Chemical Peels for Melasma in Dark-Skinned Patients. J Cutan Aesthet Surg. 2012;5(4):247-53.
10. Brody H. Chemical peeling. St Louis, MO: Mosby-Yearbook; 1992.
11. Rullan P, Karam AM. Chemical Peels for Darker Skin Types. Facial Plast Surg Clin N Am. 2010;18:111-31.
12. Godse K, Sakhia J. Triple combination and glycolic peels in postacne hyperpigmentation. J Cutan Aesthet Surg. 2012;5:60-1.
13. Grimes PE, Rendon MI, Pellerano J. Superficial chemical peels: Aesthetics and Cosmetic Surgery for Darker Skin Types, 1st Edition. Philadelphia, USA: Lippincott Williams & Wilkins; 2008.
14. Sachdeva S. Lactic acid peeling in superficial acne scarring in Indian skin. J Cosmet Dermatol. 2010;9:246-8.
15. Sharquie KE, Al-Tikreety MM, Al-Mashhadani SA. Lactic acid as a new therapeutic peeling agent in melasma. Dermatol Surg. 2005;31:149-54.
16. Kodali S, Guevara IL, Carrigan CR, et al. A prospective, randomized, split-face, controlled trial of salicylic acid peels in the treatment of melasma in Latin American women. J Am Acad Dermatol. 2010;63:1030-5.
17. Garg VK, Sinha S, Sarkar R. Glycolic acid peels versus salicylic mandelic acid peels in active acne vulgaris and post-acne scarring and hyperpigmentation: a comparative study. Dermatol Surg. 2009;35:59-65.
18. Monheit GD. The Jessner's-trichloroacetic acid peel: An enhanced medium-depth chemical peel. Dermatol Clin. 1995;13:277-83.
19. Khunger N, Sarkar R, Jain RK. Tretinoin peels versus glycolic acid peels in the treatment of Melasma in dark-skinned patients. Dermatol Surg. 2004;30:756-60.
20. Kumari R, Thappa DM. Comparative study of trichloroacetic acid versus glycolic acid chemical peels in the treatment of melasma. Indian J Dermatol Venereol Leprol. 2010;76:447.
21. Chun EY, Lee JB, Lee KH. Focal trichloroacetic acid peel method for benign pigmented lesions in dark-skinned patients Dermatol Surg. 2004;30:512-6.
22. Obagi ZE, Obagi S, Alaiti S, et al. TCA-based blue peel: A standardized procedure with depth control. Dermatol Surg. 1999;25(10):773-80.
23. Zeichner JA. The Use of Lipohydroxy Acid in Skin Care and Acne Treatment. J Clin Aesthet Dermatol. 2016;9(11):40-3.
24. Deprez P. Easy Phytic Solution: A New Alpha Hydroxy Acid Peel with Slow Release and without Neutralization. Int J Cosmet Surg Aesthet Dermatol. 2003;5(1).
25. Sarkar R, Chugh S, Garg VK. Newer and upcoming therapies for melasma. Indian J Dermatol Venereol Leprol. 2012;78:417 28.
26. Perry PK, Cook-Bolden FE. Defining pseudofolliculitis barbae in 2001. J Am Acad Dermatol. 2002;46(Suppl.):113-9.

Chemical Peels in Dark Skinned Patients: Asian and African Skin

Nicole A Negbenebor, Kaveri Korgavkar, Kachiu C Lee

INTRODUCTION

Chemical peels are a popular cosmetic procedure performed by dermatologists today. Many patients seek fast, simple and minimally invasive cosmetic procedures with a short recovery time. Demand for these cosmetic procedures continues to increase in the general population especially in those with darker skin types (Fitzpatrick skin types IV–VI). There is a growing population of ethnic and racial minorities in the United States (US); the US census estimated that almost a third of the population identify as people of color.[1] Globally, patients with skin of color exemplify the majority of world outside of the US. Therefore, it is imperative that dermatology providers be well-versed in treating patients with skin of color and understands the unique challenges associated with current cosmetic procedures. Chemical peeling has been used for postinflammatory hyperpigmentation (PIH), melasma, pseudofolliculitis barbae, oily skin, acne vulgaris and scarring in skin of color. Most commonly, peels are used for patients who have PIH or melasma after failing treatment with topical hydroquinone bleaching. Peels involve applying chemical agents to the skin to target the epidermis or dermis. There are three levels of penetration for chemical peeling agents—(1) superficial [i.e., glycolic acid (GA), salicylic acid (SA), Jessner's solution and trichloroacetic acid (TCA) 10–30%], (2) medium-depth (i.e., TCA 35–50%, dry ice with TCA 35%, Jessner's with TCA 35%, GA 70% with TCA 35% and phenol 88%), or (3) deep (i.e., phenol-croton oil formulas). Other superficial peeling agents, such as lactic acid, mandelic acid (MA), kojic acid and phytic acid, are also used. Several of these peeling agents may also be used in combination such as the salicylic-MA variation.[2]

There are also relative contraindications to chemical peels including but not limited to: Active atopic dermatitis, inflammatory rosacea, or pregnancy. Absolute contraindications include—presence of ulceration or erosions, active infection (herpes, erysipelas), and a severe allergy to the chemical peel agent. The dermatologist should use his or her clinical judgment in conjunction with full patient evaluation before considering a chemical peel in patients with skin of color.

PREPEEL PREPARATION

Patients considering a chemical peel should have a complete skin type evaluation, interview and physical exam. The presence of any underlying medical issues should also be assessed prior to application.[3] The patient should begin preparation for a chemical peel by abstaining from depilatory creams or laser hair removal 1 week before and topical retinoids 3-7 days before the chemical peel. Retinoids increase penetration of peeling agents, so they potentially put skin of color patients at higher risk of PIH.[4]

For patients with sensitive skin or previous reaction to skin care products containing alpha-hydroxy acids (AHA) or beta hydroxy acid (BHA), an initial skin patch test may be warranted. If an initial skin patch test on the chin or neck does not reveal any adverse reactions, the patient can then be pretreated with hydroquinone 4-6% beginning 4-14 days before applying the peeling solution. An additional agent to help penetration, such as tretinoin, may also be used in combination with the bleaching agent but since this increases the risk of PIH, it should be first applied with an initial test patch on an area of the skin. Nonhydroquinone bleaching agents may also be used, typically alternating with or in combination with hydroquinone. Previous studies have concluded that adequate priming is the key to reducing complications and promoting healing and that this technique is cheap, safe and effective in reducing ice pick acne scars in darker skin.[5-7]

In general, the best technique is to use low concentrations of the chemical peeling agent initially and increase concentration at subsequent encounters based on tolerability. Stronger solutions should be introduced gradually to prevent scarring or other complications.

Trichloroacetic Acid

Trichloroacetic acid is a crystalline powder that has been heavily studied as a chemical peeling agent that can be used alone or in combination with other agents such as dry ice, Jessner's solution, GA, or SA.[8-11] TCA causes collagen necrosis in the upper reticular dermis and thickening of the epidermal and dermal proteins.[7] It has been used to improve facial pigmentation and acne scarring in patients with skin of color. TCA is a safer, more tolerated peel than phenol-croton oil peels since it is less painful, has a lower risk of systemic toxicity, and is less caustic. In darker skin tones, higher concentrations of TCA have been reported to increase the risk of scarring and PIH in areas of application.[12]

Jessner's Solution

Jessner's solution is a superficial peeling solution composed of ethanol 95%, SA 14%, resorcinol 14% and lactic acid 14%. Jessner's self-neutralizes into SA and can be applied along with other chemical peel agents. The resorcinol provides a brightening effect while the SA component is effective for acne. While Jessner's solution is listed as safe to use in all skin types, resorcinol has been reported to cause dermatitis and PIH in patients with Fitzpatrick skin type IV-VI.[13,14] In darker skin types, applying Jessner's solution before TCA 35% to create a medium-depth peel is effective for treating acne scars.[15-17] The use of Jessner's solution prior to the application of TCA 35% provides more even penetration of TCA without having to increase the percentage of TCA and risking hyperpigmentation in skin of color.[8,18]

Salicylic Acid

Salicylic acid is a BHA with a phenol ring. Derived from the willow tree bark, the crystalline organic acid is able to reduce corneocyte adhesion and is keratolytic.[19] The lipophilicity of the agent makes it able to penetrate the skin better than other chemical peel agents. This property allows it to decrease the intercellular connections of horny cells, improving the ease with which the outer skin layer is removed. SA also has anti-inflammatory properties that make it effective in treating acne and erythema with low systemic toxicity and minimal side effects. It comes in many different vehicles, with the ethanol solution of SA being the best vehicle for acne, melasma and hyperpigmentation in skin of color. Side effects such as dryness and burning after application have been reported in patients with skin of color.[19-23]

Glycolic Acid

Glycolic acid is the most widely used chemical peeling agent and has been used to treat melasma, hyperpigmentation and acne. It is AHA with exfoliative properties. Although it does not have the same anti-inflammatory effectiveness as SA, GA can still be used for improving acne and has been shown to decrease the bactericidal effect of *Propionibacterium acnes*.[19,24] It has been suggested that GA skin peels in skin of color, particularly Asian skin, are beneficial in treating melasma, lentigines and PIH.[12,25-31]

Phenol-croton Oil

Phenol or carbolic acid is an agent used in deep chemical peels. Used alone, it can be safe in Asian skin types or Fitzpatrick III. Croton oil is the most important ingredient in phenol-croton oil deep peels. It is reported that the effects of the phenol-croton oil deep chemical peel are able to last up to 20 years after application.[32] In the hands of an experienced physician, deep peels can be used on light Asian or Hispanic patients, but have a high risk of inducing hyperpigmentation in patients with darker skin tones.

Croton oil is a potent agent, derived from the seeds of the *Croton tiglium* tree. Even in small concentrations, it can cause skin vesiculation and injury into the dermal layers. It is dissolved into phenol, which serves as a solvent, for use in deep peels.

ETHNIC SKIN

East and South Asian

Although, it varies with country of origin, the most common skin conditions in Asian patients are acne and pigmentary disorders such as melasma.[33] There are limited data on the effects of chemical peels in Asian skin. Peels in this population can be chosen based on the underlying medical condition, as well as the overall texture of Asian skin. In general, Asian skin often tends to be more glabrous with enlarged pores compared to Caucasian skin. This feature is especially prominent on the cheeks and nose.

Common peels for active acne treatment include SA or GA. Acne scarring can be treated with TCA (35-100%) by itself or in combination with another peeling agent. Lower concentrations are utilized for atrophic boxcar scars, whereas higher concentrations are useful for hard-to-remove ice pick scars.[16] Higher concentrations should only be used for spot treatments of ice pick scars, as TCA in high concentrations can be volatile with uneven depth of penetration.

Chemical reconstruction of skin scars (CROSS) with TCA can be used to treat atrophic acne scars. The CROSS technique consists of focally applying a high concentration of TCA with a wooden applicator onto a depressed ice pick scar. Overtime, a frost will appear and healing is expected to be faster. It has been associated with lower complications since there is only localized application of the chemical agent.[6] One randomized clinical trial (RCT) recruited 65 patients with Fitzpatrick skin types IV-V with atrophic acne scars to evaluate the safety of focal CROSS with TCA 100% treatment on Asian patients with darker skin types.[7] About half of the patients were treated with TCA 65% CROSS and the other half of the cohort were treated with TCA 100% CROSS. There was decreased visibility of scars for all patients, but one patient reported that the peel was not as effective at decreasing scar appearance after 3 months with no further improvement until the 6th month follow up. 82% of the patients in the TCA 65% group and 94% of the TCA 100% group demonstrated a significant improvement of acne scars. Patients in the TCA 100% group who had 5-6 series of treatments reported a 65% satisfaction rate. The procedure was safe and tolerable even though there were cases of patients experiencing both temporary hypopigmentation and hyperpigmentation.

To study the effectiveness of a combination agent for a medium depth peel, one pilot study used TCA and Jessner's solution for treatment of crateriform and ice pick acne scars in 15 patients with a dark skin complexion. They gave 42 applications of Jessner's solution with TCA 35% over a course of 2 years. There was significant improvement for most patients. One patient had 75% clearance of acne scars but the majority of patients (53.5%) had moderate improvement. The only patient who did not have as robust of an effect was someone who had several deeply pitted and atrophic scars. Many of the darker skinned patients (73.4%) developed side effects of temporary erythema and hyperpigmentation more often than the lighter skinned patients.[17]

Another agent that has been explored for treatment of superficial ice pick and boxcar acne scars is the lactic acid 92% peel.[16] In a pilot study, seven patients with Fitzpatrick skin type IV-V with acne and superficial scarring received lactic acid chemical peeling biweekly with a maximum of four peels for 3 months. An improvement in the overall pigmentation and texture of the treated skin was seen, with the added feature of scar lightening. One patient reported 75% clearance of lesions, 3 patients had 51-75% clearance, two patients had 26-50% clearance and one patient had 25% clearance. No side effects were recorded and it was well tolerated, making this agent a promising chemical peel for darker skin.[34]

Next, a pilot study looked at 24 patients with acne who underwent full-face peels with 30% SA in ethanol twice a week for 3 months. Reflectance spectrophotometry was used to record the colorimetric changes of each patient's face. SA peels were found to significantly lighten the face of patients with acne even after the first peel in the 6 peel series.[22] In an investigator-blinded non-RCT, 35 Korean patients with facial acne vulgaris and skin type III-IV were treated with SA 30% peels biweekly for 12 weeks. They experienced significantly decreased inflammatory and noninflammatory acne. This showed that SA peels proved to be successful and safe for treating acne vulgaris in Asian patients. 77% of the cohort of patients reported either moderate or good improvement of their acne. The most common side effects were dryness, severe exfoliation, crusting and burning for more than 24 hours.[22]

Glycolic acid is safe to use for the treatment of acne in darker skin types as well as an adjunctive therapy for the treatment of acne scars.[16,35-40] Often, it can be combined with TCA to create a medium depth peel. One non-RCT used GA by itself in patients with moderate-to-severe acne while another study evaluated it in comparison to the combination peel of SA with MA and Jessner's solution. With the application of an increasing concentration of GA (15-50%) peels for acne treatment, there are significant decreases in acne comedones, papules and pustules in Asian skin. Patients experience better skin texture because of the lessening of acne scars and cystic lesions. In addition, there was increased lightening of the skin as a result of the GA chemical peel series. Out of 40 patients with skin type IV, 32% reported good improvement of comedones, 37.5% reported good improvement of papules, 17.7% had good improvement of pustules and only 45.5% had fair improvement of cysts. Transient PIH and herpes simplex activation were the side effects.[40] In a split-face randomized controlled clinical trial, 70% GA was compared to Jessner's solution in Korean patients with skin type III–IV. Although, both peeling agents significantly reduced the appearance of acne, the exfoliation on the side treated with Jessner's solution required a longer healing process and was rated as more bothersome by patients. Because of this downside, more patients preferred GA over Jessner's solution.[41]

Lastly, when GA was evaluated against the SA and MA combination peel, both were effective at reducing acne but the MA peel produced a more statistically significant decrease in acne than the GA peel. Both peels produced minimal side effects.[42]

Using the split face technique, Goyal et al. showed that more adverse events were seen with TCA 15% than GA 35% peels. GA only produced mild erythema and burning sensation in two patients as compared to TCA causing erythema, PIH, burning sensation and epidermolysis (Table 1). Another trial with series of six peeling sessions using increasing concentrations of GA (20–50%) also examined side effects of this peel when used for treatment of melasma. Comparing the two melasma patterns seen in their

TABLE 1: Side effects of chemical agents in patients with skin of color

Author	Skin type	Primary condition	Major finding	Peeling agent	Side effects
Asian					
Vavouli et al.	II, III, or IV	Periorbital hyperpigmentation	Physicians felt that 93.3% of the patients had fair, good, or excellent improvement while patients rated 96.7% had fair, good or excellent response to treatment	TCA 3.75% and lactic acid 15%	Telangiectasia, dryness and edema
Lee et al.	IV–V	Acne scars	Decreased visibility of scars for all patients	CROSS with 100% TCA	Hypopigmentation and hyperpigmentation
Al-Waiz et al.		Acne scars	One patient had 75% clearance of acne scars but the majority of patients (53.5%) had moderate improvement	Jessner's solution with 35% TCA	Hyperpigmentation
Handog et al.	IV–V	Acne scars	Improvement in pigmentation and texture, with the added feature of scar lightening	Lactic acid 92%	None reported
Lee et al.	III–IV	Acne vulgaris	77% of patients reported either moderate or good improvement of their acne	Salicylic acid 30%	Dryness, severe exfoliation, crusting and burning

Continued

Continued

Author	Skin type	Primary condition	Major finding	Peeling agent	Side effects
Goyal et al.	IV–V	Melasma	Melasma improved and glycolic acid has less side effects than 15% TCA	TCA 15% and glycolic acid	Erythema, PIH, burning sensation and epidermolysis
Landau et al.		Wrinkles, acne scars and precancerous skin lesions	deep chemical peels with full-face application caused cardiac arrhythmias	Phenol-croton	Cardiac arrhythmia, hyperpigmentation and hypopigmentation
African American					
Smita et al.	IV–VI	PIH	Significant improvement with no side effects	Salicylic acid 20–30%	Burning, dryness, hypopigmentation and hyperpigmentation
Burns et al.	IV, V, or VI	Melasma	Significant and fast improvement of hyperpigmentation	Glycolic acid 68%	Lightening of the normal skin
Sharquie et al.	IV	Melasma	Significant improvement and no side effects	Lactic acid 92%	None reported
Sobhi et al.	IV–V	Melasma	Improvement with a glycolic acid 70% peel but side effects like burning, dryness, blistering and PIH	Glycolic acid 70%	Electric shock and burning sensation
Sobhi et al.	IV–V	Melasma	Improvement with side effects such as stinging and burning sensation	Nanosome vitamin C	Burning sensation, PIH, dryness and blistering

TCA, trichloroacetic acid; CROSS, chemical reconstruction of skin scar; PIH, postinflammatory hyperpigmentation.

patients, malar distribution responded better as compared to the centrofacial pattern for the peels. However, a large range of complications included erythema (90%), peeling (70%), crusting (55%) and PIH (20%).[30] Typically, crusting and superficial erosions should not occur, if the appropriate strength GA peel is chosen and neutralized in a timely manner. GA is a good chemical peel agent to pair with resurfacing procedures because of its additive effect.[16]

A pilot study in Korea investigated the use of phenol-croton peels for small pox scars, which may be similar in presentation to acne scars. Unfortunately, the study revealed many side effects related to the use of phenol-croton chemical peels, including cardiac arrhythmias in 5 out of 30 patients (17% of subjects).[43] One study of 181 patients found that the deep chemical peel with full-face application caused cardiac arrhythmia in 6.6% of the patients during the procedure with a higher risk in patients who had pre-existing depression, hypertension and diabetes. Eight of the patients needed IV lidocaine to help control their arrhythmia.[44] Another 74% of patients experienced hyperpigmentation while one patient had persistent hypopigmentation in the treated areas of the skin. Phenol-croton as a deep peel was also not as effective at treating acne as compared to laser skin resurfacing.[16]

In addition to acne and acne scars, hyperpigmentation in the periorbital area is a common complaint in the Asian population.

TCA can also be used safely and effectively, for treatment of periorbital discoloration. In a nonrandomized controlled clinic trial, 30 patients with periorbital dark circles and skin types II, III, or IV had treatments of TCA 3.75% and lactic acid 15%. The TCA 3.75% and lactic acid 15% chemical peels improved periorbital hyperpigmentation. Chemical peels were applied once a week for a total of four treatments. After taking photos to document the changes, data were collected on the patient's and physician's global assessment of the effects of the chemical peeling. Physicians felt that 93.3% of the patients had fair, good, or excellent improvement while patients rated 96.7% had fair, good or excellent response to treatment. Side effects such as telangiectasia, dryness and edema were recorded.[45]

African American

One of the most genetically diverse populations, the black population in America encompasses people of color from Africa, the Caribbean and Europe. The most common skin diseases in black populations are acne and hyperpigmentation disorders.[46] Combination treatments are highly effective in treating hyperpigmentation in dark skin tones.[47] The concurrent usage of topical retinoids and topical or oral antibiotics with hydroquinone to manage the severity of hyperpigmentation has proved to be successful for most patients. If the patient has sensitive skin, providers should use lower concentrations of topical agents to reduce potential complications.[48] Tretinoin chemical peeling might be a very useful procedure for treating a large number of black patients with hyperpigmentation in addition to intense pulsed light (IPL) or fractional photothermolysis.[49]

In the evaluation of treatment for melasma, one study applied full strength lactic acid 92% as a chemical peeling agent to patients with skin type IV who had melasma. The sessions were conducted every 3 weeks for up to six sessions. The authors reported that all of the patients showed significant improvement and no side effects occurred.[50]

Patients with skin types IV-V with melasma have showed improvement with a GA 70% peel. They also showed improvement when treated with nanosome vitamin C. In one study comparing GA versus nanosome vitamin C, the GA group experienced side effects including burning, PIH, dryness and blistering while the vitamin C group experienced a stinging and burning sensation.[51]

In another trial examining treatment of melasma, 19 patients with Fitzpatrick skin type IV, V, or VI were randomized to a control group (hydroquinone 2%/GA 10% gel twice daily and tretinoin 0.05% cream at night) or peel group (same regimen plus six GA 68% peels). They found that both treatment groups had improvement of hyperpigmentation, but the patients who had GA peels showed faster and more significant improvement. The most common side effect was increased lightening of the normal skin as well in peel group patients. This adverse reaction was less significant in the group for the topical regimen.[52] Combining a series of GA peels, azelaic acid cream and adapalene gel are both effective and safe treatment for recalcitrant melasma in dark skin, and offers other treatment options for this patient population.[53]

Topical tretinoin is very effective at lightening PIH but may also lighten patches of normal skin in black patients. This causes uneven tone of skin that can lead to more follow-up treatments for correction.[54-60]

Patients with skin types IV-VI received two SA 20% peels followed by three SA 30% peels. The authors demonstrated that SA peels had transient side effects such as burning, dryness, hypopigmentation and hyperpigmentation. They concluded that these peels were safe in this population, with no permanent long-term side effects.[61]

In a split face comparison of chemical agents, 25 patients with Fitzpatrick skin types III–V with facial acne had TCA 25% applied to one side of the face and SA 30% to the other side at biweekly for 2 months. TCA was better at treating comedonal lesions, whereas SA was more effective at treating inflammatory lesions in dark skin.[62] The safety and efficacy of SA chemical peels has been studied in patients with types V and VI who had PIH, melasma, enlarged pores with oily skin and acne vulgaris. About 88% of patients showed moderate to significant improvement and side effects occurred in 16% of the cohort.[23]

Also, it has been reported that chemical peels containing phenol and TCA may cause keloids, hypertrophic scars, hyperpigmentation and sudden flares ups of latent herpes virus. Also, persistent erythema and rhytids in the treated areas have been reported with both ingredients.[63-65]

POSTPEEL CONSIDERATIONS

Patients should use gentle cleansers to wash the skin after the chemical peel and apply sunscreen sun protection factor (SPF) 30 or greater daily. Topical retinoids such as tretinoin should be used as maintenance therapy and can be used instead of hydroquinone. After completing the peel series, the patient should do a daily application of hydroquinone for 6–8 weeks to maintain initial results. However, consistent long-term use of hydroquinone has been found to cause lasting leukoderma, hyperpigmentation and exogenous ochronosis of nearby normal skin.[3] Although hydroquinone has been traditionally used, studies have discussed potential topical treatments including soy, licorice, rucinol, mulberry, niacinamide and resveratrol as alternatives.[49] Even when chemical peels are used in combination with consistent sun protection, sometimes melanosis can reappear. Therefore, frequent superficial- and medium-depth chemical peel applications be used as the safest way to treat dark-skinned patients with melanosis if tolerated (optimal management of recalcitrant disorders of hyperpigmentation in dark-skinned patients). This approach minimizes the risk of PIH. We also suggest the utility of topical steroids such as hydrocortisone 2.5% postpeel to decrease inflammation and try to limit the amount of PIH (Fig. 1).

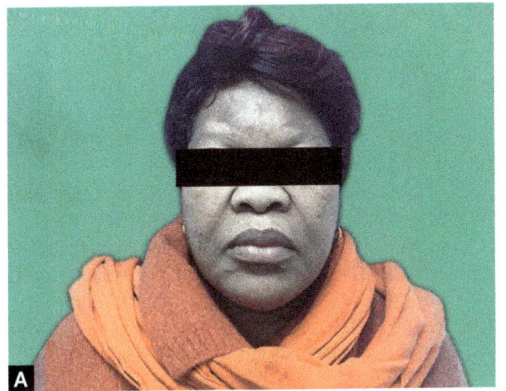 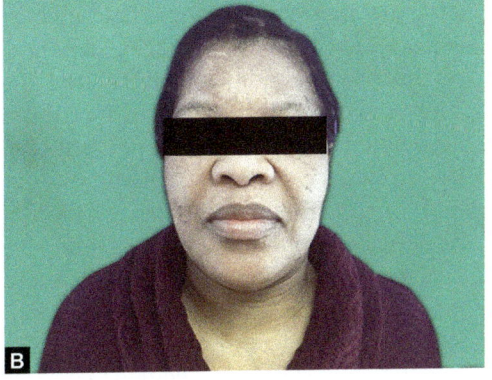

FIG. 1: **A,** Melasma, prepeel. Note the patchy hyperpigmentation at the forehead; **B,** melasma, postpeel with Jessner's solution + trichloroacetic acid 20%. Note lightening of hyperpigmentation of the forehead.

CONCLUSION

In conclusion, chemical peels are great for treating many conditions such as acne and pigmentary issues in patients with skin of color. As the population continues to diversify, it will be important for providers to know which chemical peels are best for various types of Fitzpatrick skin types. Patients should be counseled about treatment goals as well as potential complications of pigmentary changes and scarring before the application of the peel. Deeper peels have a higher risk of hyperpigmentation and should be avoided in darker skin types. Overall it is safe to use several types of chemical peels in Asian and African-American patients but a patch test should be performed before application.

TAKE HOME POINTS

- Chemical peels are a common cosmetic procedure sought by patients with skin of color for treatment of acne, melasma, PIH and other pigmentary concerns
- The population of people with skin of color is rapidly increasing and dermatologists will need to be able to understand which procedures are best on skin of color, along with their associated side effects
- It is safe to use chemical peels on Asian and African-American patients. The effectiveness of the chemical peel agent depends on the specific condition being treated
- The most common complications associated with chemical peeling are hyperpigmentation, hypopigmentation and scarring. Therefore, a patch test should be done before complete application
- Deeper peels such as the phenol-croton peel carry increased risk of cutaneous and systemic complications in skin of color, and therefore should be avoided in darker skin types. These peels have a high risk of causing PIH

REFERENCES

1. Vespa J, Armstrong DM, Medina L. Demographic turning points for the United States: Population projections for 2020 to 2060. U.S. Census Bureau Current Population Reports. 2018;25-1144.
2. Bureau USC. United States Quick Facts. United State: Bureau USC; 2015.
3. Shah SK, Alexis AF. Acne in skin of color: practical approaches to treatment. J Dermatolog Treat. 2010;21(3):206-11.
4. Shokeen D. Postinflammatory hyperpigmentation in patients with skin of color. Cutis. 2016;97(1):E9-E11.
5. Nikalji N, Godse K, Sakhiya J, et al. Complications of medium depth and deep chemical peels. J Cutan Aesthet Surg. 2012;5(4):254-60.
6. Ramadan SA, El-Komy MH, Bassiouny DA, et al. Subcision versus 100% trichloroacetic acid in the treatment of rolling acne scars. Dermatol Surg. 2011;37(5):626-33.
7. Khunger N, Bhardwaj D, Khunger M. Evaluation of CROSS technique with 100% TCA in the management of ice pick acne scars in darker skin types. J Cosmet Dermatol. 2011;10(1):51-7.
8. Lee JB, Chung WG, Kwahck H, et al. Focal treatment of acne scars with trichloroacetic acid: chemical reconstruction of skin scars method. Dermatol Surg. 2002;28(11):1017-21.
9. Monheit GD. The Jessner's-trichloroacetic acid peel. An enhanced medium-depth chemical peel. Dermatol Clin. 1995;13(2):277-83.
10. Coleman WP 3rd, Futrell JM. The glycolic acid trichloroacetic acid peel. J Dermatol Surg Oncol. 1994;20(1):76-80.
11. Brody HJ. Medium-depth chemical peeling of the skin: a variation of superficial chemosurgery. Adv Dermatol. 1988;3:205-19.
12. Brody HJ, Hailey CW. Medium-depth chemical peeling of the skin: a variation of superficial chemosurgery. J Dermatol Surg Oncol. 1986;12(12):1268-75.
13. Roberts WE. Chemical peeling in ethnic/dark skin. Dermatol Ther. 2004;17(2):196-205.
14. Fisher AA. Resorcinol—a rare sensitizer. Cutis. 1982;29(4):331-2.
15. Keil H. Group reactions in contact dermatitis due to resorcinol. Arch Dermatol. 1962;86:212-6.
16. Puri N. Efficacy of Modified Jessner's Peel and 20% TCA Versus 20% TCA Peel Alone for the Treatment of Acne Scars. J Cutan Aesthet Surg. 2015;8(1):42-5.
17. Handog EB, Datuin MS, Singzon IA. Chemical peels for acne and acne scars in asians: evidence based review. J Cutan Aesthet Surg. 2012;5(4):239-46.
18. Al-Waiz MM, Al-Sharqi AI. Medium-depth chemical peels in the treatment of acne scars in dark-skinned individuals. Dermatol Surg. 2002;28(5):383-7.

19. Monheit GD. The Jessner's + TCA peel: a medium-depth chemical peel. J Dermatol Surg Oncol. 1989;15(9):945-50.
20. Lee HS, Kim IH. Salicylic acid peels for the treatment of acne vulgaris in Asian patients. Dermatol Surg. 2003;29(12):1196-9.
21. Bae BG, Park CO, Shin H, et al. Salicylic acid peels versus Jessner's solution for acne vulgaris: a comparative study. Dermatol Surg. 2013;39(2):248-53.
22. Levesque A, Hamzavi I, Seite S, et al. Randomized trial comparing a chemical peel containing a lipophilic hydroxy acid derivative of salicylic acid with a salicylic acid peel in subjects with comedonal acne. J Cosmet Dermatol. 2011;10(3):174-8.
23. Ahn HH, Kim IH. Whitening effect of salicylic acid peels in Asian patients. Dermatol Surg. 2006;32(3):372-5; discussion 5.
24. Grimes PE. The safety and efficacy of salicylic acid chemical peels in darker racial-ethnic groups. Dermatol Surg. 1999;25(1):18-22.
25. Takenaka Y, Hayashi N, Takeda M, et al. Glycolic acid chemical peeling improves inflammatory acne eruptions through its inhibitory and bactericidal effects on Propionibacterium acnes. J Dermatol. 2012;39(4):350-4.
26. Dayal S, Sahu P, Jain VK, et al. Clinical efficacy and safety of 20% glycolic peel, 15% lactic peel, and topical 20% vitamin C in constitutional type of periorbital melanosis: a comparative study. J Cosmet Dermatol. 2016;15(4):367-73.
27. Sacchidanand S, Shetty AB, Leelavathy B. Efficacy of 15% trichloroacetic Acid and 50% glycolic Acid peel in the treatment of frictional melanosis: a comparative study. J Cutan Aesthet Surg. 2015;8(1):37-41.
28. Puri N. A study on fractional erbium glass laser therapy versus chemical peeling for the treatment of melasma in female patients. J Cutan Aesthet Surg. 2013;6(3):148-51.
29. Chaudhary S, Dayal S. Efficacy of combination of glycolic acid peeling with topical regimen in treatment of melasma. J Drugs Dermatol. 2013;12(10):1149-53.
30. Kumari R, Thappa DM. Comparative study of trichloroacetic acid versus glycolic acid chemical peels in the treatment of melasma. Indian J Dermatol Venereol Leprol. 2010;76(4):447.
31. Gupta RR, Mahajan BB, Garg G. Chemical peeling--evaluation of glycolic acid in varying concentrations and time intervals. Indian J Dermatol Venereol Leprol. 2001;67(1):28-9.
32. Moy LS, Murad H, Moy RL. Glycolic acid peels for the treatment of wrinkles and photoaging. J Dermatol Surg Oncol. 1993;19(3):243-6.
33. Park JH, Choi YD, Kim SW, et al. Effectiveness of modified phenol peel (Exoderm) on facial wrinkles, acne scars and other skin problems of Asian patients. J Dermatol. 2007;34(1):17-24.
34. Lee CS, Lim HW. Cutaneous diseases in Asians. Dermatol Clin. 2003;21(4):669-77.
35. Sachdeva S. Lactic acid peeling in superficial acne scarring in Indian skin. J Cosmet Dermatol. 2010;9(3):246-8.
36. Al-Talib H, Al-Khateeb A, Hameed A, et al. Efficacy and safety of superficial chemical peeling in treatment of active acne vulgaris. An Bras Dermatol. 2017;92(2):212-6.
37. Chandrashekar BS, Ashwini KR, Vasanth V, et al. Retinoic acid and glycolic acid combination in the treatment of acne scars. Indian Dermatol Online J. 2015;6(2):84-8.
38. Khunger N, IADVL Task Force.. Standard guidelines of care for acne surgery. Indian J Dermatol Venereol Leprol. 2008;74 (Suppl):S28-36.
39. Dreno B, Katsambas A, Pelfini C, et al. Combined 0.1% retinaldehyde/ 6% glycolic acid cream in prophylaxis and treatment of acne scarring. Dermatology. 2007;214(3):260-7.
40. Erbagci Z, Akcali C. Biweekly serial glycolic acid peels vs. long-term daily use of topical low-strength glycolic acid in the treatment of atrophic acne scars. Int J Dermatol. 2000;39(10):789-94.
41. Wang CM, Huang CL, Hu CT, et al. The effect of glycolic acid on the treatment of acne in Asian skin. Dermatol Surg. 1997;23(1):23-9.
42. Kim SW, Moon SE, Kim JA, et al. Glycolic acid versus Jessner's solution: which is better for facial acne patients? A randomized prospective clinical trial of split-face model therapy. Dermatol Surg. 1999;25(4):270-3.
43. Garg VK, Sinha S, Sarkar R. Glycolic acid peels versus salicylic-mandelic acid peels in active acne vulgaris and post-acne scarring and hyperpigmentation: a comparative study. Dermatol Surg. 2009;35(1):59-65.
44. Yoon ES, Ahn DS. Report of phenol peel for Asians. Plast Reconstr Surg. 1999;103(1):207-14; discussion 215-7.
45. Landau M. Cardiac complications in deep chemical peels. Dermatol Surg. 2007;33(2):190-3; discussion 3.
46. Vavouli C, Katsambas A, Gregoriou S, et al. Chemical peeling with trichloroacetic acid and lactic acid for intraorbital dark circles. J Cosmet Dermatol. 2013;12(3):204-9.
47. Halder RM, Grimes PE, McLaurin Cl, et al. Incidence of common dermatoses in a predominantly black dermatologic practice. Cutis. 1983;32(4):388, 90.
48. Molinar VE, Taylor SC, Pandya AG. What's new in objective assessment and treatment of facial hyperpigmentation? Dermatol Clin. 2014;32(2):123-35.
49. Callender VD. Acne in ethnic skin: special considerations for therapy. Dermatol Ther. 2004;17:184-95.
50. Konda S, Geria AN, Halder RM. New horizons in treating disorders of hyperpigmentation in skin of color. Semin Cutan Med Surg. 2012;31(2):133-9.

51. Sharquie KE, Al-Tikreety MM, Al-Mashhadani SA. Lactic acid as a new therapeutic peeling agent in melasma. Dermatol Surg. 2005;31:149-54; discussion 54.
52. Sobhi RM, Sobhi AM. A single-blinded comparative study between the use of glycolic acid 70% peel and the use of topical nanosome vitamin C iontophoresis in the treatment of melasma. J Cosmet Dermatol. 2012;11(1):65-71.
53. Burns RL, Prevost-Blank PL, Lawry MA, et al. Glycolic acid peels for postinflammatory hyperpigmentation in black patients. A comparative study. Dermatol Surg. 1997;23(3):171-4; discussion 5.
54. Erbil H, Sezer E, Tastan B, et al. Efficacy and safety of serial glycolic acid peels and a topical regimen in the treatment of recalcitrant melasma. J Dermatol. 2007;34(1):25-30.
55. Kligman DE. Tretinoin peels versus glycolic acid peels. Dermatol Surg. 2004;30:1609.
56. Kligman DE, Draelos ZD. High-strength tretinoin for rapid retinization of photoaged facial skin. Dermatol Surg. 2004;30(6):864-6.
57. Kligman AM. Side-effects of topical vitamin A: what's new? J Eur Acad Dermatol Venereol. 2004;18(3):260.
58. Kligman DE, Sadiq I, Pagnoni A, et al. High-strength tretinoin: a method for rapid retinization of facial skin. J Am Acad Dermatol. 1998;39(2 Pt 3):S93-7.
59. LaVoo EJ. Tretinoin for hyperpigmentation in black patients. N Engl J Med. 1993;329(20):1503.
60. Bulengo-Ransby SM, Griffiths CE, Kimbrough-Green CK, et al. Topical tretinoin (retinoic acid) therapy for hyperpigmented lesions caused by inflammation of the skin in black patients. N Engl J Med. 1993;328(20):1438-43.
61. Kligman AM, Grove GL, Hirose R, et al. Topical tretinoin for photoaged skin. J Am Acad Dermatol. 1986;15(4 Pt 2):836-59.
62. Joshi SS, Boone SL, Alam M, et al. Effectiveness, safety, and effect on quality of life of topical salicylic acid peels for treatment of postinflammatory hyperpigmentation in dark skin. Dermatol Surg. 2009;35(4):638-44.
63. Abdel Meguid AM, Elaziz Ahmed Attallah DA, Omar H. Trichloroacetic Acid Versus Salicylic Acid in the Treatment of Acne Vulgaris in Dark-Skinned Patients. Dermatol Surg. 2015;41(12):1398-404.
64. Polano MK. Chemexfoliation: indications and cautions. J Am Acad Dermatol. 1988;18(5):1149.
65. Lober CW. Chemexfoliation—indications and cautions. J Am Acad Dermatol. 1987;17(1):109-12.

CHAPTER 38

Chemical Peels in Ethnic Skin: Latin American Skin

Carlos G Wambier

INTRODUCTION

Chemical peels, when indicated for skin beautification of a Latin American patient usually presents higher risks of pigmentary skin changes because of high miscegenation of ethnicity. In the last decades, it is rare to find a person with a single ethnicity, or that could be classified uniquely as Caucasian, Asian, African, or Native tribal skin in Latin America. Nevertheless, chemical peels are among the most performed esthetic procedures among dermatologists and estheticians in Latin America. When performed with adequate technique and chemicals, these procedures have a very low potential for adverse effects.

ETHNIC SKIN: LATIN AMERICAN PATIENTS

Latin America is probably the most ethnically diverse places in the world, not only by the intense migration that occurred from Europe, Africa and Asia, but also by the previous diversity of Native tribes. The skin melting pot is further enhanced by the real miscegenation of ethnicities in Latin America, thus, a Brazilian patient may have more than four ethnicities, for example, Native American, German, Italian, African and Portuguese. Habits, costumes and cultural appraisal to sun tanning may also change phenotypes, creating hardening and difficulty to set the Fitzpatrick's phototype based on color and burning from the sun. So, someone originally phototype II may have a skin that behaves like phototype III or IV. Another perspective is the increased risk for unexpected postinflammatory hyperpigmentation (PIH) by patients with African, Asian and Native American ascendency. The assessment of the real phototype of a Latin American should be undertaking by evaluating non-sun-damaged skin, for example, by examining axillary or inframammary skin.

Chemical peels may be used either for improving conditions such as melasma, PIH, freckles and lentigines; epidermal growths such as seborrheic keratoses, actinic keratoses and sebaceous hyperplasia among others; acne and acne scars; superficial scars; photoaging changes; wrinkles and textural alterations can be treated with this procedure.

PEELING IN DARK SKIN

Prepeel Preparation

Priming the skin with bleaching agents such as hydroquinone 2–4%, or alternative agents, such as azelaic acid 15–20%, associated with broad-spectrum sunscreen may increase safety by decreasing the individual tendency to PIH. Also, during this period the physician may experience the tolerability of the individual skin and adhesion to the treatment plan. In patients with melasma, if the patient has no background of thrombophilia, the physician may consider prescribing tranexamic acid 250 mg BID.

Postpeel Considerations

Immediate postpeel regimen should include a hypoallergenic moisturizer and sunscreen. Patients are instructed to wash their faces only with baby shampoo or use only micellar water rich in essential fatty acids to remove make-up and sunscreen.

CHEMICAL PEELS

For phototypes IV–VI, the safest peels are superficial peels. The author recommends peels based on the pathology to be treated. For acne, salicylic acid 30% in ethanol (for patients who like to peel off)[1] or salicylic acid 30% in polyethylene glycol (PEG, Fig. 1).[2] For melasma, the author recommends modified Jessner's solution (MJS) (Rohrich and Herbig 2009), containing 17% lactic acid, 17% salicylic acid, 8% citric acid in ethanol (Fig. 2).

When the patient has PIH, the author recommends associating Q-switched 1,064 nm with low intensity, for example, using Revlite at PTP 8 mm or 6 mm with very light MJS combined with trichloroacetic acid (TCA) 10–20% (Puri 2015). Sometimes, only laser can result in substantial improvement, so, the author only associates chemical peels in refractory cases (after at least two laser sessions, Fig. 3).

For body peels, the author's preferred chemical peel for lentigines and photoaging is the Cook's peel,[5] which consists on fast application of 70% glycolic acid followed by 40% TCA, neutralizing at the endpoint of erythema or minimal light frosting for dark skin types. For lighter skin, the endpoint may be reticular to uniform frosting (Fig. 4). For improvement of diffuse facial melanosis due to tanning, the author prefers 40% pyruvic acid combined with 25–35% TCA (Fig. 5).

For deep wrinkles, the author considers the only effective treatment available is deep peeling, using one of Hetter's formulas,[6,7] however the risks of PIH and permanent discoloration should be well discussed with the patient (Fig. 6).

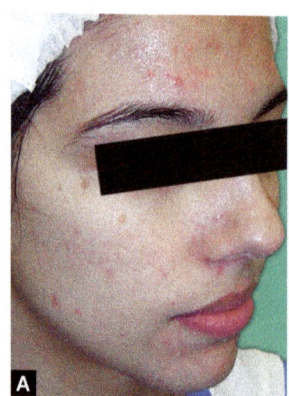 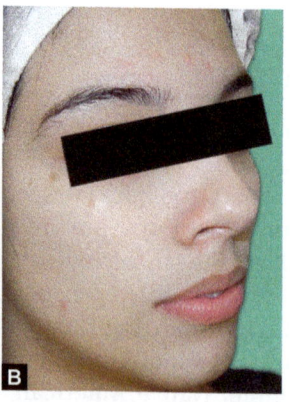

FIG 1. Before **A,** and after 7 days of superficial peel with salicylic acid in polyethylene glycol; **B,** Improvement of acne after a single session.

Chemical Peels in Ethnic Skin: Latin American Skin

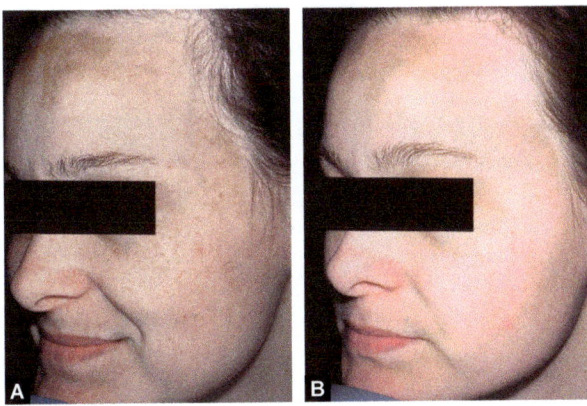

FIG. 2: Superficial peel with modified Jessner's solution for melasma. **A,** Before; **B,** After three sessions.

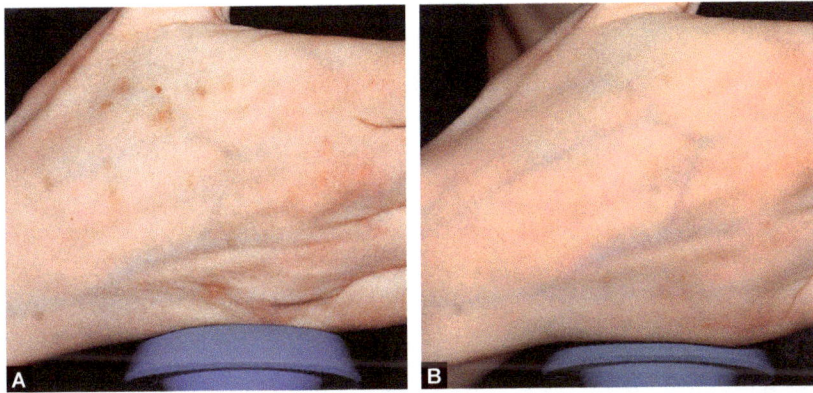

FIG 3. Treatment of postinflammatory hyperpigmentation due to treatment of solar melanosis with Q-switched 532 nm. **A,** Before; **B,** After two monthly sessions of Q-switched Nd-YAG 1064 nm at PTP 6 mm.

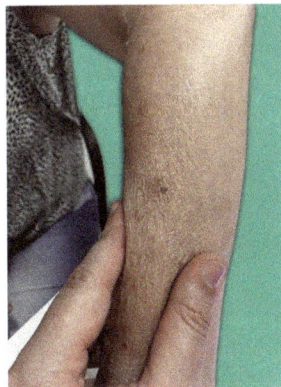

FIG. 4: . Medium depth body peel using Cook's peel at 10th postoperative day. Thick scales start to peel at the second week for arms, forearms and hands.

Adverse Effects

Chemical peels are usually classified by the depth of penetration into the skin. The possible adverse effects correlate to the depth of penetration of the chemicals, as shown in table 1. In general, the deeper the peel the higher the possibility of permanent pigmentary changes and scars. Whereas the superficial peels may cause more transient pigmentary changes. PIH may be prevented to a certain level by adequate sun protection on the months after peels, use of hydroquinone priming before the procedure.

Chemical Peels: A Global Perspective

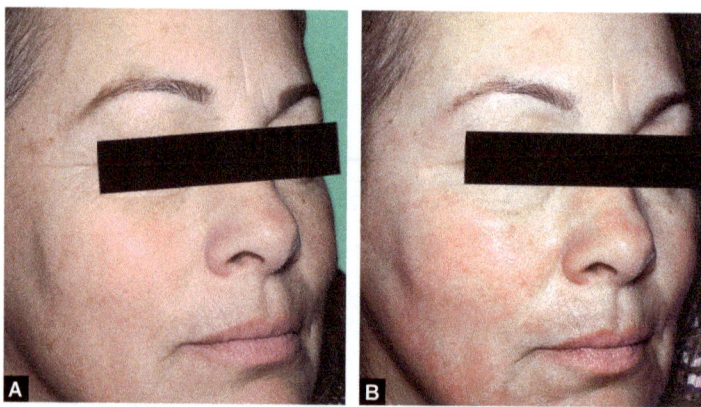

FIG 5. **A,** Before; **B,** After two weeks of 40% pyruvic acid followed by 25% trichloroacetic acid for diffuse melanosis. Note improvement of fine perioral and periocular wrinkles. This peel is also safe for higher phototypes and requires no previous skin priming.

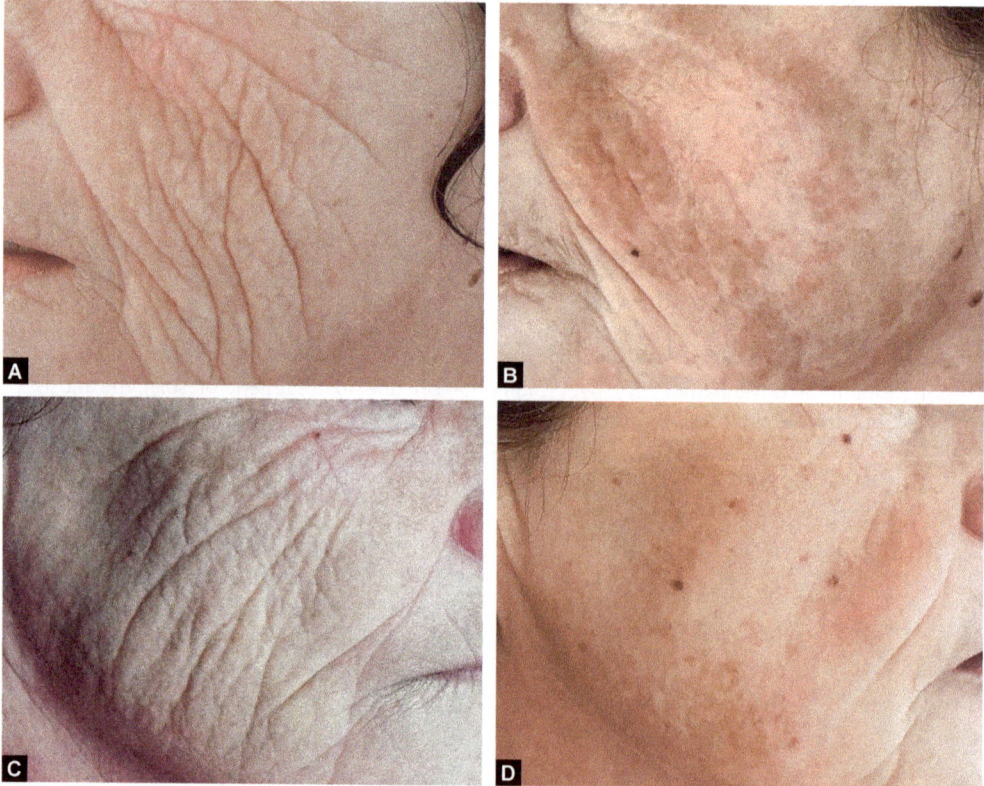

FIG 6. Deep peeling to the cheeks using Hetter's 1.6 croton oil in 35% phenol, with perfect meticulous feathering to the malar and perioral region. **A** and **C,** Before; **B** and **D,** After 6 months. Note residual postinflammatory hyperpigmentation in the feathering zone, which will still last 1-2 months.
Courtesy: Dr. Jaqueline Peres, MD.

TABLE 1: Chemical peels and possible adverse effects in higher phototypes

Depth of the peel	Possible adverse effects in higher Latin American phototypes
Very superficial	None
Superficial	Postinflammatory hyperpigmentation, prolonged erythema
Medium	Hypopigmentation, postinflammatory hyperpigmentation, prolonged erythema
Deep	Keloids, hypopigmentation, postinflammatory hyperpigmentation, prolonged erythema

CONCLUSION

Chemical peelings are indicated based on patient's indication by diagnosis, each condition has the right depth of peeling. Patient selection should be prioritized during the indication of a peel. If the physician and the patient are willing to endure the perioperative period, and accept possible adverse effects, chemical peels may be used. When treating Latin American skin, the physician must take proactive prophylactic measures for prevention of pigmentary changes.

TAKE HOME POINTS

- Most superficial chemical peels are safe for ethnic skin
- Medium depth peels may be safe
- Adequate patient selection is key to successful outcomes.

REFERENCES

1. Kligman D. Technologies for cutaneous exfoliation using salicylic acid. Dermatol Ther. 2001;14(3):225-7.
2. Dainichi T, Ueda S, Imayama S, et al. Excellent clinical results with a new preparation for chemical peeling in acne: 30% salicylic acid in polyethylene glycol vehicle. Dermatologic Surg. 2008;34(7):891-9.
3. Rohrich RJ, Herbig KS. The role of modified Jessner's solution with 35% trichloroacetic acid peel. Plast Reconstr Surg. 2009;124(3):965-6.
4. Puri N. Efficacy of modified Jessner's peel and 20% TCA versus 20% TCA peel alone for the treatment of acne scars. J Cutan Aesthet Surg. 2015;8(1):42.
5. Cook KK, Cook WR. Chemical peel of nonfacial skin using glycolic acid gel augmented with TCA and neutralized based on visual staging. Dermatol Surg. 2000;26(11):994-9.
6. Hetter GP. An examination of the phenol-croton oil peel: part IV. Face peel results with different concentrations of phenol and croton oil. Plast Reconstr Surg. 2000;105(3):1061-83.
7. Wambier CG, de Freitas FP. Combining phenol-croton oil peel. In: Issa MC, Tamura B (Eds). Lasers, Lights and Other Technologies. Chem Phys Proced. Cham: Springer International Publishing; 2017. pp. 1-13.

CHAPTER 39

Complications of Chemical Peels and How to Deal with Them

Shehnaz Z Arsiwala

INTRODUCTION

Chemical peels are more than two decades old and are the most commonly conducted procedure globally. Over a decade, a variety of peeling agents are available in various formulations and combinations and these are used for multiple indications from therapeutic to esthetic, conducted on face or extra-facial sites and used for acne, marks, scars to pigmentation and textural improvement. Although peels are seemingly safe and easy to do procedure there is high potential for adverse effects with peels. Complications from peels can range from mild and transient to severe and long lasting. It is critical to recognize, characterize and report complications in order to acknowledge the limits of therapeutic efficacy. The chapter deals with the adverse effects of peels and how to deal with them.

COMPLICATIONS OF PEELS

Chemical peels are associated with certain unwanted side effects. Inappropriate peeling agent, and high pH and high concentration peels are associated with more frequent side effects, etc.[1] Treating skin of color demands additional consideration as one has to focus on preventing pigmentary altercations, so adequate priming and achieving right depth of peel is essential. This is simply achieved by getting the right choice of peel agent, right priming, adequate sunprotection, inter-peel vigilance and optimum postpeel care.

Factors influencing peel complications can be divided into patient factors, technical factors and peeling agent factors (Table 1).

The multiple factors listed in table 1 are very pertinent and can easily predict an untoward outcome of a chemical peel.

TABLE 1: Factors influencing peel complications

Patient factors	Technical factors	Peeling agent related factors
• Skin type • Degree of tan • Priming • Skin barrier compromise • Sensitive skin • Concomitant applications • Concomitant procedures • Postpeel care	• Degreasing • Method of application	• Choice of peeling • Mechanism of action of peel • inflammatory profile of peeling agent • pH of peel • Peel base—aqueous or alcohol or gel based • Combination of formulation

PATIENT FACTORS

Skin type of patient is very crucial predictor for peel outcome and side effect while potential for erythema with an inflammatory peel is high in skin type 1-4, potential for pigmentary altercation is high in skin type 4-6. Darker skin types have higher risk of postinflammatory hyperpigmentation (PIH) after a single session of chemical peel and this has to be considered while choosing a patient.[2,3]

The degree of tan influences the risk of pigmentary sequelae even after a superficial to medium depth peel.[4] The tanned skin has high amount of melanin content and a recent tan signifies a high stimulation of precursor melanin which can result in PIH after peel. In dark skin types it is a mandatory protocol to prime a patient with broad spectrum sunscreen cream at least 2-3 weeks before peel. This ensures adequate control of neomelanogenesis and ensures less risk of PIH after peel.[5-7]

Priming is a mandatory requirement before any kind of peels on any skin type for any indication. Priming not only determines patient tolerance but also establishes patient compliance. Priming introduces sunprotection, prelightening of normal or tanned skin to a particular degree, adequate hydration and repair of barrier if compromised. Poor priming is associated with high risk of pigmentary side effects.[7,8] Sun protection and lightening agents prevent pigmentation after peel and hydration during priming phase prevents severe dryness in postpeel phase. Priming also unmasks sensitive skin to certain sun creams and lightening agents, can unmask retinoid dermatitis and enables the physician to be judicious about undertaking peels in these patients.[8,9] Peels should be conducted on well informed, sun protected, primed, compliant, patients with realistic expectations! Choose a newer photostable sunscreen with an inorganic sunscreen. Start sun protection earliest.[8,9]

Skin barrier compromise—when barrier is compromised a transgradient for water loss is created which leads to dryness and also inadvertent absorption of peeling agent.[10] Situations where barrier is compromised such as dry skin, retinoid dermatitis, atopic eczema, psoriasis, etc. warrant judicious use of peeling. Increased or rapid absorption of an inflammatory peel leads to stinging, excess burning, flaking, oozing and even bacterial colonization.[11,12]

Sensitive Skin

Peels on a sensitive skin may amplify the subjective and objective symptoms of burning, stinging, irritation and intolerance especially if the peel base is acidic and nonaqueous. Peels should be conducted with utmost caution and deferred if necessary for sensitive skin patients with alternative therapeutic options.

Concomitant Applications and Procedures

Concomitant steroids used topically or retinoids or photosensitizing agents which alter the skin barrier and behavior should be withheld at least a week before the peels. Shaving, waxing and depilatory creams should be avoided at least 3-5 days before peel depending on skin type. Concomitant procedures including microdermabrasion, derma roller and lasers should be carefully considered while conducting a peel on the same day sequentially. Any product or procedure which can alter the skin barrier should be withheld before conducting aggressive peels.[13]

Postpeel Care

This is the most crucial patient factor which influences not only outcome but also the peel side effects. Avoidance of sun, picking, shaving, scratching will alter the ability of epidermal repair and increase risk of pigmentation and infections, use of mandatory sun protection is of utmost importance. Reintroduction of barrier altering creams in-between the peel sessions have to be explained to patients and retinoids, and lightening agents can be reintroduced a few days after the peels.[9]

TECHNICAL FACTORS WHICH INCREASE RISK OF PEEL SIDE EFFECTS

Degreasing and Technique

Aggressive degreasing can lead to irritation of skin and result in increased uptake of a peel, subsequent hot spots and epidermolysis. Adequate degreasing and cleansing should be undertaken before peels.

Technique

Peel technique is important. Peel technique is often specific to the type of peeling agent chosen and its mechanism of action, e.g., in trichloroacetic acid (TCA) peels number of coats increase the depth of penetration of peel and the frost achieved is an indicator, one has to be zealous in applying quick and multiple coats for TCA peels.[14] In glycolic peels where contact time and endpoint of peel is important, in cross TCA focal peel where high strength TCA has to be carefully applied with the toothpick point and accidental application to outside the scar crater may accentuate scarring and invite risk for discoloration.[15] Protection of eye and mouth corners are important to prevent peel pooling and accidental spillage into eye can be prevented by semi-reclined patient position. Usage of cotton balls over brush is preferred during peel application as the bristles of brush harden and cause abrasion of the skin while application.

If applied by an assistant staff or nurse vigilance and supervision is important.

PEELING AGENT DEPENDENT FACTORS

The choice of peeling agent has to be right, the pH, the base and inflammatory profile of the peeling agent as well as mechanism of action are important characters of an agent and interplay of these on the target tissue defines the outcome. If the peel is acidic and skin is dry potential for irritation exists, if the peel is toxic it may absorb systemically and lead to side effects like in phenol or salicylic peels.

The peeling process can result in certain mild transient effects and sometimes moderate or permanent complications especially while dealing with dark skin patients (Table 2).

The mild complications include erythema and edema which lasts for 2-3 days to a week depending on inflammatory profile of the peeling agent, its strength and depth of peels. A strong keratolytic peel like salicylic acid (SA) can cause significant dryness which manifests at 2-3 days and may persist up to a week. Adding emollients and avoiding drying agents topically for a week can easily solve this.

TABLE 2: Chemical peel complications

Complications	
Mild and transient	• Irritation • Dryness • Edema • Erythema
Moderate	• Pigmentary complications • Contact dermatitis • Bacterial infections • photosensitivity • Reactivation of herpes • Flare of acne vulgaris • Acneiform eruptions
Severe	• Hypopigmentation • Scarring and atrophy • Hypertrophy/Keloids

Erythema and edema are the standard endpoints of some peels like glycolic acid and TCA, and this should not be mistaken for a complication of a peel. The patient should be counseled for the same. An endpoint, erythema and edema usually clear within a week. Intense or persistent erythema and edema beyond 3-5 days and up to 2 weeks or more can be considered as a peel side effect, this may be seen with medium depth peels and inflammatory peeling agents such as SA, phenol, high strength GA and TCA. A deep peel can produce more long-lasting edema and erythema than a superficial peel. This can be managed by adding mild topical steroid cream or pimecrolimus for a couple of days along with emollients in the postpeel phase. Any erythema or edema persisting for more than 2 weeks should generate alarm as this may herald a pigmentary sequelae. In such a situation, the next peel should be postponed till this resolves and the strength or peel type should be changed if necessary to prevent escalation of side effects.[9,13]

Dryness and irritation may be seen in postpeel phase with all peeling agents, more so in winter and patients with dry or sensitive skin. Gel peels are less drying than low pH based aqueous peels; in predictive situations stinging on immediate application of peel is an indicator for potential for dryness, irritation erythema and edema in immediate postpeel phase. Leave in peels can sometimes cause dryness and itching for a few days. Often when patient is on topical retinoids, peeling can cause excessive dryness and irritation, this can be avoided by deferring the peel procedure till dryness is corrected. A topical retinoid regimen should be withheld a week before peels to avoid dryness, any glycolic or salicylic based face washes should be taken off the prescription a few days before the peels and reintroduced 3-4 days later.[9,13] Contact dermatitis can occur with GA, resorcinol and even LA peels should be avoided in patients with dry and sensitive skin types.

Infections like herpes reactivation can occur if adequate prophylaxis is not obtained while treating predisposed patients with moderate to deep peels. Secondary bacterial colonization can occur from an infected focus in patients who are treated with peels with an active infection. This can result in erosions, slow re-epithelization, delayed healing and subsequent scarring. Any potential risk of herpes reactivation should be identified and acyclovir/valacyclovir prophylaxis should be initiated. Any active bacterial infection should be well controlled or covered with prophylactic oral or topical antibacterial. Any manifest signals of infection should be handled immediately to reduce risk of scarring.[16,17]

Acne flare may happen in some cases with any type of peels. These can happen if comedones exposed to peels evoke an inflammatory effect due to influx of inflammatory mediators. These are seen as papular and pustular lesions mainly on chin, jawline and cheeks. In the postpeel phase, picking of lesions or scratching may act as a trigger.

Acneiform eruptions seen as erythematous follicular papules may be evident in few cases. These may be exacerbated by any oil-based creams or moisturizers and should be withheld. Only emollients which are noncomedogenic should be recommended after peels. The acne and acneiform eruptions respond to oral antibacterials. Milia usually appear 2-4 months after peels in up to 20% of patients undergoing medium and deep peels and may be treated with extraction or electrosurgery.[14,18]

Pigmentary side effects are the most distressing complications of chemical peels, especially in dark skin types IV to VI. TCA, high strength GA, phenol peels and other medium depth to deep peels are often associated with pigmentary complications. Postpeel hyper- or hypopigmentation can be temporary or persistent.[2,9,13]

After TCA, peels, a transient PIH, may be seen and needs to be alleviated before next session. In such situations rotational intermittent alternative lightening peels with lightening agents should be conducted to overcome PIH after a TCA peel. Hyperpigmentation may be focal or seen as demarcatory lines or blotchy and pan facial. Lines of demarcation are technique related, seen mostly in TCA peels and can be avoided by gentle feathering of the peel. Erythema which lasts for more than 2-3 weeks in postpeel phase is likely to result in hyperpigmentation. In some cases hyperpigmentation may persist for longer periods and can be improved by introducing high strength hydroquinone, topical retinoid, vitamin C or azelaic acid in between the peels.[19] Adequate priming is often the key to prevent PIH after peels and importance of adequate sunscreen usage should be emphasized time and again to the patient. Also picking, scratching and application of peels on a broken skin increases risk of hyperpigmentation.[20] QS lasers are sometimes used to achieve faster clearance of hyperpigmentation after peels and are also replacing peels for pigmentary conditions.

Hypopigmentation after a peel is a more concerning side effect as it depicts damage to melanocytes, often seen after TCA and phenol peels in high strength and dark skin types. It can be temporary but known to last for 12-24 weeks in some patients and rarely permanent. Treatment of hypopigmentation is often difficult and includes use of calcineurin inhibitors, and sometimes 308 excimer lamp treatments till complete repigmentation is established.[21]

Scarring and keloidal tendency after a peel can happen in predisposed individuals with deep peels and are reported in patients with high dose isotretinoin. In patients with pre-existing keloids or hypertrophic scars, deep peels are best avoided.[21]

Exacerbation of pre-existing dermatoses can occur in sensitive, atopic, psoriatic or photosensitive individuals. This should be handled by discontinuation of further peels and treatment of underlying skin disorder.[14,22]

SYSTEMIC EFFECTS OF CHEMICAL PEELS

Certain peels have toxic actions when absorbed systemically.[14,18,22] Salicylic peels in large volume can be absorbed systemically and lead to systemic symptoms such as dizziness, renal compromise, etc.[18] large amount of water consumption to improve body hydration while doing a large area salicylic peel is precautionary. Cardiac arrhythmias are reported with toxic peels like phenol and can be fatal.[23-25] Phenol absorption into systemic circulation results in cardiac toxicity. Tachycardia, premature ventricular beats, bigeminy and atrial as well as ventricular tachychardia are reported.[18,23-25] Hypersensitivity to any ingredient in peel formulation can lead to focal rash or even rarely systemic hypersensitivity.[14,22]

Superficial peels can result in itching, irritation, dryness and transient hyperpigmentation very rarely scarring, with medium depth peels risk for hyperpigmentation amplify and persistent erythema can be experienced, scarring is another risk with medium depth or deep peels and should be done with utmost caution in dark skin individuals.[16,22]

CONTRAINDICATIONS FOR PEELS

The contraindications for peels are actually indicators for poor outcomes or risk of

Complications of Chemical Peels and How to Deal with Them

enhanced side effects. These include any active bacterial/viral/fungal infections, tendency for keloids, presence of pre-existing inflammatory or photosensitive dermatoses, patients on oral steroids and immunosuppressant, and within 6 months of oral isotretinoin therapy in case of deep peels, patients with unrealistic expectations and unprimed or poorly primed patients. Identifying patients at potential risk and choosing an appropriate peel agent with understanding of the depth and efficacy versus adverse effects helps one to avert major complications.

Prepeel preparation is actually meant to prevent complications and in addition to mandatory broad spectrum sunscreen creams and lightening agents, the following help to pave a better peel outcome. These include:

- *Test peel*: A patch test behind the ear/inner arm to gauge tolerability to peeling agent
- Stop electrolysis, waxing, depilatories, masks, hair dyes, bleaching, straightening, etc.
- Glycolic and SA based face washes
- No makeup/cologne/shaving/remove contact lenses on the day of the peel.

TIPS TO HANDLE PEEL COMPLICATIONS (TABLE 3)

- Excellent priming
- Sheer vigilance
- Readiness to handle complications
- Rough predictability of peel outcome
- Understanding the peel formulation, pH and mechanism of action
- Rational realistic discussion with patient
- Prophylaxis for herpes and bacterial infections if indicated.

TABLE 3: Management of complications from peel

Complications	Management
Edema	Mild topical steroids/tacrolimus
Erythema	
Pain	Analgesics
Acne flare	• Topical antibiotics/retinoids
Acneiform eruptions	• Oral antibiotics
Hyperpigmentation	• Topical lightening agents (dual or triple combinations)
	• Sun protection
	• Light superficial peels/QS lasers
	• Oral and topical antioxidants
Hypopigmentation	Tacrolimus/pimecrolimus, excimer laser, beta fibroblast growth factor
Irritation	• Bland emollients/sunscreen agents
Dryness	• Noncomedogenic moisturizers, topical hyaluronic acid
Infection	• Bacterial: Topical and oral antibiotics, guided by culture reports if severe
	• Viral: Oral acyclovir or valacyclovir
	• *Candida*: Topical/oral antifungal
Scarring—atrophic	Fractional ablative/nonablative laser resurfacing, microneedling, radiofrequency
Allergic reactions/hypersensitivity	Oral or topical steroids and immunosuppressive agents
Keloid/hypertrophic scar	Topical or intralesional steroids/silicone gel sheet/cryotherapy. Pulse dye laser, fractional laser, nonablative and ablative, intense pulsed light, 5-fluorouracil

CONCLUSION

No skin intervention is sans adverse effects and complications. Sheer vigilance is of utmost value during peel procedure as most of the adverse effects result from poor priming, noncompliance, wrong peeling agent, etc. Treating skin of color demands additional consideration as one has to focus on preventing pigmentary altercations, so adequate priming and achieving right depth of peel is essential. This is simply achieved by getting the right endpoint of the peel.

TAKE HOME POINTS

- Complications from peels are challenging in dark skin types
- Complications from peels may be transient or long-standing
- Recognition of potential peel complications and management is crucial for successful outcomes
- Superficial peels are relatively safer than medium depth and deep peels in dark skin types.

REFERENCES

1. Brody HJ. Complications of chemical resurfacing. Dermatol Clin. 2001;19(3):427-37.
2. Khunger N, Arsiwala S. Step by Step Chemical Peels. In: Khunger N (Ed). Combination and Sequential peels. New Delhi: Jaypee Brothers Medical Publishers (P) Ltd.; 2008. pp. 201-18.
3. IAA Consensus Document. Acne scars. Indian J Dermatol Venereol Leprol. 2009;75 (suppl 1):52-3.
4. Bari AU, Iqbal Z, Rahman SB. Tolerance and safety of superficial chemical peeling with salicylic acid in various facial dermatoses. Indian J Dermatol Venereol Leprol. 2005;71:87-90.
5. Hexsel D, Arellano I, Rendon M. Ethnic considerations in the treatment of Hispanic and Latin-American patients with hyperpigmentation. Br J Dermatol. 2006;156 (Suppl 1):7-12.
6. Sarkar R, Arsiwala S, Dubey N, et al. Chemical peels in melasma: A review with consensus recommendations by Indian pigmentary expert group. Indian J Dermatol. 2017;62:470-6.
7. Roberts WE. Chemical peeling in ethnic/dark skin. Dermatol Ther. 2004;17:196-205.
8. Shehnaz AZ. Chemical peels for post acne hyperpigmentation in skin of color. Pigmentary Disorders. 2015;2:162.
9. Khunger N. Standard guidelines of care for chemical peels: IADVL task force. Indian J Dermatol Venereol Leprol. 2008;74:S5-12.
10. Song JY, Kang HA, Kim MY, et al. Damage and recovery of skin barrier function after glycolic acid chemical peeling and crystal microdermabrasion. Dermatol Surg. 2004;30:390-4.
11. Dewandre L, Tenenbaum A. The chemistry of peels: A hypothesis of action mechanisms and a proposal of a new classification of chemical peels. In: Tung RC, Rubin MG (Eds). Chemical Peels, 2nd edn. London: Elsevier Saunders; 2011. pp. 1-16.
12. Jackson A. Chemical peels. Facial Plast Surg. 2014;30(1):26-34.
13. Arsiwala S. Acne Scars: complications of Treatment and their management: Step by step treatment of acne scars, 1st edition. New Delhi: Jaypee Brothers Medical publishers (P) Ltd; 2014. p. 13.
14. Monheit GD, Chastain MA. Chemical peels. Facial Plast Surg Clin North Am. 2001;9:239-55.
15. Lee JB, Chung WG, Kwahck H, et al. Focal treatment of acne scars with trichloroacetic acid: chemical reconstruction of skin scars method. Dermatol Surg. 2002;28:1017-21.
16. Clark E, Scerri L. Superficial and medium-depth chemical peels. Clin Dermatol. 2008;26:209-18.
17. Cernik C, Gallina K, Brodell RT. The treatment of herpes simplex infections: an evidence-based review. Arch Intern Med. 2008;168:1137-44.
18. Rubin MG. A peeler's thoughts on skin improvement with chemical peels and laser resurfacing. Clin Plast Surg. 1997;24:407-9.
19. Grimes P. Chemical peeling in dark skin: Color Atlas of chemical peels, 2nd edition. India: Springer; 2013.
20. Burns RL, Prevost-Blank PL, Lawry MA, et al. Glycolic acid peels for postinflammatory hyperpigmentation in black patients. A comparative study. Dermatol Surg. 1997;23:171-4.
21. Landau M. Chemical peels. Clin Dermatol. 2008;26:200-8.
22. Zakopoulou N, Kontochristopoulos G. Superficial chemical peels. J Cosmet Dermatol. 2006;5:246-53.
23. Landau M. Cardiac complications in deep chemical peels. Dermatol Surg. 2007;33(2):190-3.
24. Truppman F, Ellenbery J. The major electrocardiographic changes during chemical face peeling. Plast Reconstr Surg. 1979;63(1):44.
25. Finsti Y LM. Exoderm: phenol-based peeling in olive and dark-skinned patients. Int J Cosm Surg Aesthet Dermatol. 2001;3:173-8.

Recent Advances in Treatment with Chemical Peels

Sakshi Srivastava, Sidharth Sonthalia

INTRODUCTION

Chemical Peeling is among the oldest and most widespread used aesthetic procedures worldwide.[1] Chemoexfoliation is probably the most often done procedure in present day practice, even though it is often necessary to combine chemical peeling with other skin rejuvenating and resurfacing techniques for better results. In this chapter, we shall dwell upon the latest trends in chemical peeling based on evidence and our own innovation and experience.

NOVEL MOLECULES

Lipohydroxy Acids

Hitherto, the two major chemical groups of peeling agents comprise of alpha-hydroxy acids (AHA) like glycolic acid and beta-hydroxy acids like salicylic acid (SA). The latest development is the use of lipohydroxy acids (LHA). Lipohydroxy acid molecule detaches individual corneosomes from adjacent corneocytes without fragmentation by acting at the corneosome/corneocyte interface. Lipohydroxy acid does not affect keratin fibers or the corneocyte membrane. Similar to the effect of retinoic acid, LHA also stimulates renewal of epidermal cells and the extracellular matrix. In contrast to many other peeling chemicals, LHA has a pH that is similar to that of normal skin (5.5) and does not require neutralization.

Chemical Properties of Lipohydroxy Acid

- A derivative of SA (beta-hydroxy acid), with an added fatty chain
- Also known as C8-LHA
- *Chemical formula*: 2-hydroxy-5-octanoyl benzoic acid
- *Molecular weight*: Higher than SA
- *Solubility*: More in oil, lipophilic (more lipophilic than SA)
- *pH*: 5.5 (similar to skin).

Exfoliating Properties

The chemical structure of LHA results in less skin penetration than its parent SA; in fact with respect to skin penetration, it exhibits a profile similar to glycolic acid. Hence there is a larger reservoir effect in the stratum corneum with use of LHA compared to SA. It is an excellent chemoexfoliant. Process of exfoliation does not affect keratin; however, involves breakage of intercellular desmosomes. Probably it acts on transmembrane glycoproteins and corneocytes are shed. Both SA and LHA have been shown to increase corneocyte desquamation, reducing the overall thickness of stratum corneum. Salicylic acid penetrates more rapidly into the skin than LHA, desmosomes are also more rapidly broken resulting in exfoliation of sheets of cells. The penetration of LHA is slow and results in exfoliation of individual corneosomes. This cell by cell exfoliation is thought to more closely mimic the physiologic desquamation than the more global exfoliation that results from use of other hydroxy acids and SA. In contrast to other chemical peeling agents, LHA has a pH similar to that of normal skin (5.5) and it does not require neutralization. Whether exfoliating ability of LHA more closely mimicking physiologic desquamation results in better tolerance, needs further evaluation.

While LHA use results in stratum corneum thinning, it is associated with dermal thickening. In study by Piérard et al. dermal stimulatory effect was found to be equivalent to that of tretinoin.[2] The antiaging effects are thought to be largely due to LHA's stimulation of structural skin proteins and lipids.

Comedolytic Properties

Due to extremely lipophilic nature of the LHA, it has a high affinity for pilosebaceous unit, making it an excellent option as a comedolytic agent for acne vulgaris. In a study, Uhoda E, et al. reported a significant decrease in size and number of comedones after use of LHA.[3] Draelos et al. in their study demonstrated comparable efficacy and greater tolerability compared to benzoyl peroxide.[4]

Indications

- *Photoaging*: Roughness, fine lines, keratosis, solar lentigines
- *Pigmentary disorders*: Melasma, post-inflammatory hyperpigmentation
- *Retention acne*: Comedones.

Contraindications

- *Absolute*: Pregnant, nursing patients, active herpes simplex, six months of isotretinoin treatment.

Relative
- *Cold sores*: 6-8 weeks after healing
- *Botulinum toxin*: 1-2 weeks
- *Collagen injections*: 2 weeks prepeel and postpeel
- *Facial surgery*: 6 weeks after edema settles down
- *Lasers*: 4-6 weeks before and after
- *Electrolysis and dying*: 7 days before and after
- *Waxing and depilators*: 2-3 weeks after.

Side Effects and Complications

Redness, transient hyperpigmentation and pimples (sometimes).

Peeling Treatment Steps

Priming
- *Timing*: 1-2 weeks prior to first session.
- *Purpose*: To prepare the skin by starting the exfoliative process. To optimize and homogenize the penetration of peel solution
- *Solution to be used*: LHA cleansing gel or LHA solution (0.25% of LHA) and LHA serum (0.45%)
- *Procedure*: Daily cleaning gel or solution and LHA serum application.

Pretreatment Preparation Essentials
- Cleaning or degreasing of skin prior to treatment to achieve homogenous peeling results
- No sedation or analgesia/topical anesthesia needed
- *Solutions used*: LHA solution and degreasing wipes
- Eye protection (patient and physician)
- Cleaning and degreasing and protection of sensitive areas with vaseline-occlusion.

During Treatment
- *Purpose*: Exfoliation of epidermal layer
- *Solutions*: Cotton tip applicator is used, LHA solution 5% or 10%.
- *Procedure*: Application all over face, 1-3 coats, depending upon skin type
- *Neutralization*: Not required
- *Frequency*: Once in fifteen days.

Post-treatment
- *Time for meticulous care*: 7-15 days
- *Purpose*: To stabilize and enhance the exfoliating process. To prepare skin for next peeling procedure
- *Home-based maintenance regime components recommended*: LHA cleansing gels, LHA solution (0.25%), LHA serum (0.45%)
- Daily meticulous application of broad-spectrum sunscreen.

CHEMICAL PEELS WITH CONCOMITANT ORAL ISOTRETINOIN: A NEW APPROACH

The notion that if systemic isotretinoin taken within 3-6 months of cutaneous peels contributes to abnormal scarring or delayed wound healing is taken into consideration and practiced a lot. A systemic review with evidence based consensus recommendation by Leah K. et al reviewed that physicians and patients may have an evidence based discussion regarding the risk of cutaneous procedure in the setting of systemic isotretinoin therapy. For some patients and some conditions, an informed decision may lead to earlier and potentially more effective interventions.[5] Waldman et al in their study also concluded that there is insufficient evidence to justify delaying treatment with superficial peels.[6] Kar et al. in their study also concluded that oral isotretinoin along with salicylic acid peel has a significantly better outcome in moderate to severe acne than oral isotretinoin therapy.[7] In conclusion, patients on oral isotretinoin therapy may be offered the privilege of superior results by not delaying the initiation of chemical peels treatment for them, but definitely with signed and informed consent by adding on concomitant chemical peels, in terms of better acne control, early prevention and treatment of acne-associated and postacne pigmentation and scarring. However, careful patient selection, preferential use of only superficial chemical peels, ruling out a definite history of keloidal tendency, generous postpeel moisturization and specially designed consent form are important parameters to ensure safety of this combination.

In our personal experience, we have found that stopping oral isotretinoin for around 7 days around the peel session (3-4 days before as well as after the peel), increases the safety factor, probably by temporarily reducing isotretinoin induced facial dryness and desquamation. Additionally, we suggest that the timed superficial peels should be left on for a lesser duration of time, i.e., neutralized earlier in patients on oral isotretinoin, compared to those who are not on oral isotretinoin.

RECENT TREND IN CHEMICAL PEEL

Combining Superficial Peels and Microdermabrasion in Single Session

Hexsel et al. in their study concluded that combining retinoic acid 5% and microdermabrasion (MDA) gave better results than retinoic acid peels alone.[8] The study was further supported by Briden et al. who concluded that MDA combined with superficial glycolic acid peels are commonly performed aesthetic procedures.[9] Microdermabrasion *per se* provides the benefits of exfoliation but its overall aesthetic benefit can be substantially enhanced by combining it with superficial peels. Combining superficial peels with MDA is more effective as the removal of superficial stratum corneum leads to an increase in penetration of topical product applied after it. It is important to note that MDA is contraindicated for those suffering with active pustular acne, impaired barrier function and rosacea.[10] It can be well inferred that combining MDA with superficial peels yield better results, but informed consent of patient should be taken prior to the session and rigorous postpeel care should be followed. Conclusively, in carefully selected patients, conducting a sequential session of MDA followed by a superficial peel is likely to yield better results provided, postprocedure care, especially meticulous sun-protection and moisturization are followed. Informed consent of the patient undergoing combination therapy is essential.

MOLECULES FOR SENSITIVE SKIN

Polyhydroxy Acids: Home Care Products

Poly Hydroxy Acids (PHA): Function are same as alpha-hydroxy acid (AHA), but cause less irritation and burning due to their bigger molecular size. They are especially advantageous in treating sensitive skin types that may not tolerate AHA. They provide anti-inflammatory and antioxidant benefits and also contribute to exfoliation. They are excellent postpeel home care agents. Some common polyhydroxy acids are:

- *Lactobionic acid*: Derived from lactose found in cow's milk acts as a humectant, antioxidant and calming agent
- *Galactose*: A sugar utilized in glycosaminoglycan and collagen synthesis and cell movement, may also enhance wound healing
- *Gluconic acid*: A naturally occurring ingredient in cells, also known as gluconolactone in skin care products, is an antioxidant and anti-inflammatory agent, while holding AHA properties.

For those with dry, sensitive skin, antiaging procedures can be a challenge. That's where the role of PHAs comes into play. Polyhydroxy acids reinforce skin's barrier function and help fight the signs of aging without irritation. Polyhydroxy acids offer a distinct advantage over conservative AHAs when used on sensitive skin, such as rosacea, atopic dermatitis and eczema. In addition to their gentleness, PHAs are natural hygroscopic agents and can attract and bind atmospheric water, helping to keep dry skin well hydrated. Polyhydroxy acids such as gluconolactone lightly exfoliate to reinstate feel without irritation, while improving clarity and diminishing the look of lines and wrinkles.[11,12] These agents have also been shown to reduce redness, making them an ideal choice for postprocedure use.

NEXT LEVEL OF POST PEEL COOLING WITH LIQUID NITROGEN (UNDER EVALUATION)

This practice innovated by one of the authors (Srivastava S), has yielded good results. The technique involves replacement of ice-packs for cryoslush with liquid nitrogen to cool the skin after the superficial chemical peel has been neutralized.

Technique, Effect and Proposed Advantages

After neutralizing the superficial peel, a sterile gauze dipped in liquid nitrogen is gently swiped on the face with an ultra-short contact time (15–20 s). In comparison to ice-packs, the cooling effect of liquid nitrogen is better and provides immediate uniform cooling on the entire face. Except for a transient stinging sensation, the procedure is very comfortable for the patient. Although, the author has observed that the overall postpeel glow is better with this technique, compared to the use of ice-packs, the same is currently under objective evaluation under a project.

IMMEDIATE REPAIR WITH RECOMBINANT EPIDERMAL GROWTH FACTOR

The most dreaded adverse effect of a chemical peel is a burn, which is signaled by appearance of a hot-spot (level 3 frosting or postpeel severe persistent erythema with burning sensation). This unfortunate event, although rare, may happen with the most expert dermatologists and in peel-experienced patients. However, if a localized burn, heralded by the postpeel appearance of a "hot-spot" is suspected, the repair of the epidermal damage may be expedited by the use of commercially available gels containing recombinant epidermal growth factor (rEGF).[13] Since rEGF is very temperature-sensitive, the tube containing the gel has to be maintained at 2–8°C (not to be frozen). A discovery and propagation by the second author (Sidharth Sonthalia), the use of this gel on any suspected hot-spot, almost always prevents a burn and postpeel PIH and scarring. After initial application in the clinic, immediately postpeel, the gel may also be suggested for home use over the hot-spot. It should however, not be routinely applied on otherwise optimally peeled skin as its epidermal healing effect would interfere with the desirable epidermal desquamation effect of the peel. It is to be noted that the primary indication of these gels is for healing of diabetic foot ulcers and burns.

GLUTATHIONE PEEL

- Glutathione is a simple molecule, a strong antioxidant which protects the cells in our body from harmful toxins and oxidative injuries and is beneficial to us. It is produced naturally in our body. A tripeptide, it is composed of glycine, glutamic acid and cystine[14]
- Glutathione has been used as an alternative to hydroquinone due to its skin lightning properties.[15] This is also one of the accepted peel in the world cosmetic dermatology. The pH range is 1.3–1.5
- Glutathione peel is available as a combination peel. It contains glutathione, kojic acid, trichloroacetic acid, retinoic acid, phenol, salicylic acid and vitamin C.

Properties

- It is a medium depth peel
- Glutathione is a strong antioxidant, it takes care of the free radicals
- Kojic acid is a lightning agent, also makes the skin more radiant and firm
- Trichloroacetic acid reduces fine lines and pigmentation
- Phenol improves skin texture, appearance, reduces fine lines and works on pigmentation as well
- Retinoic acid reduces fine wrinkles, exfoliates skin and eliminates acne
- Salicylic acid exfoliates skin and reduces pigmentation.

Prepeel Priming

No prepeel conditioning is required.

Peel Application

- Can be used on all skin types
- Peel to be applied on skin after degreasing the face with acetone or alcohol

- A slight tingling or stinging sensation may be felt by the patient
- After the first pass itself, slight numbing takes place which makes it pain free
- Peel once applied can be left on face for 4–6 hours and then can be washed off (it is a self-limiting peel).

Repeat Sessions of Peel Treatment

- For normal skin, glutathione peel can be done 2–3 times a year
- For acne scars, melasma and fine lines, peel may be done once a month
- Series of 2–3 peel treatments can be done once in 4 weeks may help to get desired results, in conditions like melasma and acne.

Postpeel Care

A good sunscreen should be used regularly as with any other peel. Moisturization for scaling and dryness may be required.

Indications

- Enhances texture and tone of skin
- Lightens and brighten the skin
- Works on pigmentation
- Decreases the appearance of pore size
- Reduces fine line and wrinkles
- Stimulates collagen production
- Reduces freckles and sun damage
- Lightens post-acne scars.

Contraindications

- Pregnancy and lactation
- Those who are allergic to aspirin
- Active herpes or infected lesions
- Need to stop oral isotretinoin, as discussed earlier.

Side Effects

- Slight stinging or tingling may be felt when the peel is applied
- Some redness may be seen which is normal
- Skin may be slightly itchy and mildly swollen for few days postpeel
- Skin may feel dry and peeling can be visible for 6–7 days
- Makeup can be applied after 2 days
- Skin may be sensitive for about a week.

5-FLUROURACIL PEEL FOR ARMS AND ACTINIC KERATOSIS AND SEBORRHEIC KERATOSIS

- Fluorouracil solutions topical preparation contains the fluorinated pyrimidine
- It is an antineoplastic antimetabolite. Available as 5% or 2% solution
- Chemical formula: 5-fluoro-2,4 (1-H,3H)-pyrimidinedione.

Appearance

White crystalline powder, sparingly soluble in water and slightly soluble in alcohol. One gram of fluorouracil is soluble in 100 mL of propylene glycol. The molecular weight is 130.08 g/mol.

Mechanism of Action

It blocks the methylation reaction of deoxyuridylic acid to thymidylic acid. Fluorouracil blocks the synthesis of deoxyribonucleic acid (DNA) and also to an extent blocks ribonucleic acid (RNA). The DNA and RNA are essential for cell division and growth, the effect of fluorouracil creates a thymine deficiency which causes unbalanced growth and death of the cell. The effects of DNA and RNA deprivation is more on the cells which grow faster and take up fluorouracil at higher rate. The catabolic metabolism of fluorouracil results in degradation products, which are inactive. Systemic absorption with topical application is negligible.

Contraindications

- Application to mucous membrane should be avoided, it may result in local inflammation and ulceration
- Pregnancy and lactation
- Hypersensitivity to product
- Active herpetic infection.

Postapplication Effects on Lesions

When fluorouracil is applied to a lesion, a response that follows are—Erythema, vesiculation, desquamation, erosion and re-epithelialization. Fluorouracil should be applied preferably with a nonmetal applicator.

Bagatin et al. in their trail also found that fluorouracil topical peels proved to be helpful in clearance of actinic keratosis lesions and also it had excellent effect on overall improvement of photodamaged skin.[16] They concluded that 5-fluorouracil superficial pulse peel is safe, well tolerated, very effective and highly inexpensive therapeutic option for treatment of multiple, diffuse actinic keratosis lesions.

Guimarães et al. in their studies also observed that 5-fluorouracil peels are safe and effective in the treatment of photodamaged skin.[17]

Dini et al. in their comparative study on treatment of large actinic keratoses with glycolic acid peeling and 5-fluorouracil versus cryopeeling also concluded that both techniques studied can be used in the treatment of extensive actinic keratosis; however, with cryopeeling there is intense and persistent erythema.[18] One of the authors (Sonthalia S) has found the approach of 5-FU peeling for actinic keratosis equally useful for seborrheic keratosis, which are much more common in darker skin types.

Technique Used for Peeling by Dini et al.[18]

After cleansing and degreasing the skin with acetone, a coat of 70% glycolic acid gel was applied until the appearance of erythema or frosting of actinic keratosis lesion, then neutralization was done with sodium bicarbonate solution.[18] Later 5% 5-fluorouracil solution was applied for 12 hours. Patients were instructed to wash the solution after 12 hours.

FUTURE TRENDS

Tranexamic acid, an agent well-established as an effective adjuvant therapy for melasma in oral and topical formulations as well as when given through mesotherapy[19], is now commercially available as a combination peel. As per the limited experience of the authors, the initial results have been encouraging. Nail peeling, a concept introduced by Banga and Patel,[20] has been improvised upon and is expected to evolve into a safe and effective therapy for not only surface abnormalities of the nail plate, but also as an adjuvant treatment for onychomycosis.[21,22]

CONCLUSION

Despite rapid advancements in light, laser and thermal-based approaches for skin rejuvenation, acne and pigmentary disorders like melasma, chemical peeling continues to be the most commonly performed procedure in a busy dermatologist's clinic, owing to its simplicity, need for minimal infrastructure and investment, decades of established efficacy and safety. With the empowerment of the aesthetic patient by the internet and social media, it has become imperative that cosmetic dermatologists keep themselves updated about the latest advances in chemical peeling pertaining to new agents and/or new approaches.

TAKE HOME POINTS

- Latest advances in chemical peeling may involve introduction of a new molecule/agent as a peel ingredient and/or a novel approach to enhance the efficacy or safety of existing peel protocols
- Lipohydroxy acid (LHA) is an addition after the alpha- and beta-hydroxy acids. The LHA form of salicylic acid serves as an excellent chemoexfoliant, results in epidermal thinning and dermal thickening. In contrast to the global exfoliation effected by standard chemical peels, LHA results in exfoliation of individual corneosomes that closely mimics the physiologic desquamation. Further, LHA has a pH similar to that of normal skin (5.5) and does not require neutralization
- Patients on oral isotretinoin therapy for whom any physical procedure including peels were contraindicated, can now be offered the privilege of superior results by concomitant chemical peeling for better acne control, early prevention and treatment of acne-associated and post-acne pigmentation and scarring. Careful patient selection, taking informed consent, using superficial peels only, and avoidance of oral isotretinoin therapy for a few days before and after the peel constitute the key to ensuring safe and better patient outcome
- Combining superficial peels with MDA is more effective as the removal of superficial stratum corneum leads to an increase in penetration of topical product applied after it. But the combination therapy should be undertaken in selected patients ensuring meticulous post-procedure skin care
- Poly hydroxy acids (PHA) such as lactobionic acid, gluconic acid, etc. are large molecular-sized agents that function similar to alpha-hydroxy acids but cause less irritation and burning and provide excellent skin hydration, making them specially useful for chemical treatment of sensitive skin types. They are also useful as postpeel home care agents
- Postpeel cryoslush with liquid nitrogen is an innovative approach of not only rendering the peeling procedure more comfortable for the patients, it has also been observed to enhance the peel-associated facial glow
- Recombinant epidermal growth factor (rEGF)-based gels, otherwise indicated for ulcers and burns, can be used to prevent/expedite healing due to chemical peel-induced epidermal burn. It can dramatically reduce the possibility of PIH and scarring resulting from an inadvertent peel-induced burn
- Glutathione-based combination peels are medium-depth peel combinations that may be used for all skin types. The anti-oxidant, depigmenting and anti-inflammatory properties of glutathione make such peels especially useful for pigmentary disorders
- 5-FU based peel protocols are being used for treatment of actinic keratoses. The same may be used for seborrheic keratoses as well
- Tranexamic acid, hitherto used orally/topically/as mesotherapy for melasma is now available in combination peels. Initial results are encouraging
- Nail peeling is a revolutionary advancement in chemical peeling. It may be used for superficial textural abnormalities of the nail (rough nails) or as adjuvant treatment for onychomycosis.

REFERENCES

1. Fischer TC, Perosino E, Poli F, et al. Chemical peels in aesthetic dermatology: An update 2009. J Eur Acad Dermatol Venereol. 2010;24(3):281-92.
2. Piérard G, Leveque JL, Rougier A, et al. Dermoepidermal stimulation elicited by a salicylic acid derivative: A comparison with salicyclic acid and all trans-retinoic acid. Eur J Dermatol. 2002;4:XLIV-VI.
3. Uhoda E, Piérard-Franchimont C, Piérard GE. Comedolysis by a lipohydroxy acid formulation in acne-prone subjects. Eur J Dermatol. 2003;13:65-8.
4. Draelos ZD, Shalita AR, Thiboutot D, et al. A multicenter, double-blind study to evaluate the efficacy and safety of 2 treatments in participants with mild to moderate acne vulgaris. Cutis. 2012;89:287-93.
5. Spring LK, Krakowski AC, Alam M, et al. Isotretinoin and timing of procedural interventions. A systematic review with consensus recommendations. JAMA Dermatol. 2017;153(8):802-9.
6. Waldman A, Bolotin D, Arndt K, et al. ASDS Guidelines Task Force: Consensus recommendations regarding the safety of lasers, dermabrasion, chemical peels, energy devices, and skin surgery during and after isotretinoin use. Dermatol Surg. 2017;43(10):1249-62.
7. Kar BR, Tripathy S, Panda M. Comparative study of oral isotretinoin versus oral isotretinoin + 20% salicylic acid peel in the treatment of active acne. J Cutan Aesthet Surg. 2013;6(4):204-8.
8. Hexsel D, Mazzuco R, Dal'Forno T, et al. Microdermabrasion followed by a 5% retinoid acid chemical peel vs. a 5% retinoid acid chemical peel for the treatment of photoaging - a pilot study. J Cosmet Dermatol. 2005;4(2):111-6.
9. Briden E, Jacobsen E, Johnson C. Combining superficial glycolic acid (alpha-hydroxy acid) peels with microdermabrasion to maximize treatment results and patient satisfaction. Cutis. 2007;79:13-6.
10. Dudelzak J, Hussain M, Phelps R, et al. Evaluation of histologic and electron microscopic changes after novel treatment using combined microdermabrasion and ultrasound-induced phonophoresis of human skin. J Cosmet Laser Ther. 2008;10(4):187-92.
11. Edison BL, Green BA, Wildnauer RH, et al. A polyhydroxy acid skin care regimen provides antiaging effects comparable to an alpha-hydroxyacid regimen. Cutis. 2004;73(2 Suppl):14-7.
12. Grimes PE, Green BA, Wildnauer RH, et al. The use of polyhydroxy acids (PHAs) in photoaged skin. Cutis.2004;73(2 Suppl):3-13.
13. Wong WKR, Ng KL, Lam CC, et al. Review article: Reasons for underrating the potential of human epidermal growth factor in medical applications. J Anal Pharm Res. 2017;4(2):00101.
14. Sonthalia S, Daulatabad D, Sarkar R. Glutathione as a skin whitening agent: Facts, myths, evidence and controversies. Indian J Dermatol Veneeol Leprol. 2016;82:262-72.
15. Watanabe F, Hashizume E, Chan GP, et al. Skin-lightening and skin-condition-improving effects of topical oxidized glutathione: A double-blind and placebo-controlled clinical trial in healthy women. Clin Cosmet Investig Dermatol. 2014;7:267-74.
16. Bagatin E, Teixeira SP, Hassun KM, et al. 5-Fluorouracil superficial peel for multiple actinic keratoses. Int J Dermatol. 2009;48(8):902-7.
17. Guimarães CO, Miot HA, Bagatin E. Five percent 5-fluorouracil in a cream or for superficial peels in the treatment of advanced photoaging of the forearms: A randomized comparative study. Dermatol Surg. 2014;40(6):610-7.
18. Dini LY, Stangarlin CT, Pessanha ACA, et al. Comparative study of the treatment of large actinic keratoses with glycolic acid peeling and 5-fluorouracil vs. cryopeeling. Surg Cosmet Dermatol 2013;5(1):52-4.
19. Zhang L, Tan WQ, Fang QQ, et al. Tranexamic Acid for Adults with Melasma: A Systematic Review and Meta-Analysis. Biomed Res Int. 2018;2018:1683414.
20. Banga G, Patel K. Glycolic acid peels for nail rejuvenation. J Cutan Aesthet Surg. 2014;7:198-201.
21. Sonthalia S, Tosti A. Innovative physical approaches for onychomycosis – Peeling, Lasers and beyond. Skin Appendage Disord. [In Press].
22. Sonthalia S, Jakhar D, Yadav P, Kaur I. Chemical Peeling as an Innovative Treatment Alternative to Oral Antifungals for Onychomycosis in Special Circumstances. Skin Appendage Disord. [In Press].

41 CHAPTER

Chemical Peel Pearls

Wendy E Roberts

INTRODUCTION

Pearls for chemical peeling can be divided into seven categories:
1. Patient selection
2. Patient education
3. Prepeel care
4. Peel plan
5. Peel preparation technique
6. Peeling technique
7. Postpeel care.

PATIENT SELECTION

- *Know your indications*: Photo aging, superficial acne scarring and hyperpigmentation
- Avoid patients, who have failed with other peels
- Avoid patients of Fitzpatrick IV, V skin types with acne scarring or other dermal problems. You will have to perform a deep peel to address the problem and this will risk dyschromia as a complication
- Avoid patients who work with chemicals unless they can take time off (painters, hairdressers and chemists).

PATIENT EDUCATION

I recommend writing the items below in one patient handout where each item is initiated.
- Confirm your patient has read both the prepeel and postpeel instructions before they have the peel done. They must be able to satisfy all the requirements such as no swimming for 1 week after the peel
- Confirm your patient has realistic expectations about what the peel will do and what the end result should look like
- Confirm your patient knows the number of sessions it will take to achieve the desired outcome and the cost of each session
- Confirm your patient knows there are companion cosmeceuticals that should be used to augment/maintain their result.

PREPEEL CARE

Skin priming with a skin lightener especially one that uses retinol may increase the effectiveness of your peel. 4–8 weeks is the standard time for prepeel priming.[1] Staged microdermabrasion (MCD) prior to peeling may help to remove stratum corneum

Chemical Peel Pearls

pigment and also increase the effectiveness. Active lesions of acne should be in resolution before doing mid-dermal peeling.[2]

PEEL PLAN

- Know what peeling agents are synergistic and what their neutralization needs are
- Know what peeling agents work best in a specific skin type, e.g., glycolic acid works better in Caucasian skin then African descendant skin for photoaging
- Know the typical number of peels needed for the indication being treated
- Know the companion products—for postinflammatory hyperpigmentation (PIH) secondary to acne you will want to have a take home with two basic qualities (1) folliculocentric cleaning such as salicylic/azelaic acid, and (2) brightening/lightening capability such as vitamin C, kojic acid, hydroquinone, arbutin, or another topical in this category.

PEEL PREPARATION TECHNIQUE

The preparation is traditionally used to prepare the skin for the peeling agent. It is usually alcohol or acetone based which degreases the skin by washing away superficial skin lipids/sebum and dehydrating the keratinocytes which may then absorb an increased quality of the peeling agent.

Before the preparation is done, protect the patient's lips, nares and earlobes with an occlusive like petrolatum to prevent seepage into these areas. A vigorous preparation may increase the strength of your peel and no preparation may severely limit your peel. For example, if you prep with acetone and apply it with woven gauze (4 × 4) and a heavy hand you can create superficial peeling in the absence of a peeling agent just from the exfoliation process. This effect may be desirable but most importantly may contribute to complications such as prolonged erythema and/or hyperpigmentation if the peeler is not aware of the compounding nature of prep and peeling.[3]

Another peel prep technique may be MCD, hydrafacial or other types of positive pressure exfoliation systems. I favor this type of mechanical prepping in the pigmentation group because the exfoliation removes dead keratinocytes, melanosomes and creates an easier path for the peeling solution to reach its target. If performing MCD prior to a peel on the same day you must be careful about the following:

- Keep the MCD superficial with gentle exfoliation. Do not repeat on treat problem areas
- After the MCD have the patients face washed so there are no crystal residues
- Make sure there are no other ingredients infused during the hydrafacial that could interfere with the chemical peel solution
- Be mindful of areas which have increased burning and may need earlier neutralization.

PEELING TECHNIQUE

I like to divide the face into two landscapes. The first is the active area. Where there are excessive rhytids, PIH, or whatever lesion you have planned this peel to treat. The second or inactive area is the area with the least pathology.

Roberts Spot Peel Technique

Utilizing this technique a mini treatment of the active zones is done prior to applying the peeling agent to the entire area. This works well on face, hands and buttocks. A small cotton-tipped applicator is used. The tip is soaked with the peeling agent and then it is manually rubbed into the lesion.

If it is a frosting agent you should wait for the lesion to completely frost. If it is a neutralization required peel then you can spot neutralize but will have to dry the area before applying the generalized solution. After the spot peel is completed you then use your peeling tool of choice to apply the rest of the peeling agent to the face or peeling site. The composition of the applicator and the pressure applied to the skin may change a peel from being a superficial refreshing peel to a deeper superficial peel, so be mindful a woven gauze rubbed over the skin with firm pressure will cause a deeper exfoliation then a cosmetic wedge or large cotton-tipped applicator.[4] Make sure the surrounding skin is covered especially when using a cotton-tipped applicator because the peeling agent may run down the sides of the face and neck to cause unwanted peeling.

POSTPEEL CARE

I tend to be quite conservative in this area. Favoring to let the peel act alone. To that end I do not recommend topicals with emollients. In deep peels occlusive may be needed if there are some barrier disruptions. With acne I have the patient begin using the 2–6% salicylic acid products after day 2 to take advantage of the open follicular ostia and promote follicular exfoliation. For peels addressing photo damage I wait until the skin has completely recovered to use topical cosmeceuticals. For pigmentation abnormalities I start the lightening agents as soon as erythema has disappeared and re-epithelialization has occurred to suppress melanocytic hyperactivity.[5]

Have proper written instructions about what the patient cannot do.

Do Not Do

- Overzealous face washing
- Use products other than the office has instructed you to use
- Swimming/Jacuzzi
- Painting/exposure to lacquer, chemicals, fumes
- Hair color, hair perming, keratin treatments
- Facials
- Heavy makeup
- Heavy athletic/physical activities
- Massage with face down
- Fillers or neurotoxin for 1 week
- Flying with air vents blowing on their face (increases risk of infection).

Follow-up appointments may be needed anywhere from 2 days for deeper peels to 2 weeks for superficial peels. The sooner you see the patient the more you can manipulate your result by adding a topical or starting them on a particular regimen so I favor early follow-up. Good luck!

REFERENCES

1. Tung RC, Bergfeld WF, Vidimos AT, et al. Alpha-hydroxy acid-based cosmetic procedures. Guidelines for patient management. Am J Clin Dermatol. 2000;1(2):81-8.
2. Landau M. Chemical peels. Clin Dermatol. 2008;26(2):200-8.
3. Matarasso SL, Glogau RG. Chemical face peels. Dermatol Clin. 1991;9(1):131-50.
4. Berson DS, Cohen JL, Rendon MI, et al. Clinical role and application of superficial chemical peels in today's practice. J Drugs Dermatol. 2009;8(9):803-11.
5. Rendon MI, Berson DS, Cohen JL, et al. Evidence and considerations in the application of chemical peels in skin disorders and aesthetic resurfacing. J Clin Aesth Dermatol. 2010;3(7):32-43.

Appendix 1

Consent Form for Chemical Peel

Patient name   : ....
Age and Sex   : ....
Contact Number   : ....
Address   : ....
                      ....
Type of peel used   : ....

I understand that chemical peeling is a treatment wherein application of chemical agents to the skin causes controlled wounding to a part or entire epidermis, with or without the dermis. This process stimulates the formation of newer healthy skin.

Multiple treatment sessions are required for optimal results. However no guarantee, warranty has been has been made to me as to the results that may be obtained. I understand that there is no way one can predict the final outcome and the number of sessions required. I also understand that this particular procedure may not always be successful, and there is no means to guarantee for successful outcome of the procedure.

I have also been informed of the alternative treatment methods including their advantages and disadvantages. I am fully aware of the possible side effects and risks involved in the procedure. It has been explained to me that during the procedure I might experience discomfort, stinging, burning and itching. My skin might appear pink and flaky following the treatment, and will return to its normal appearance in a week or so. There is also slight risk of scarring, textural/pigmentation changes following the procedure. These may also be permanent.

Topical, local, general anaesthesia may be required in a few patients. I am willing to take the appropriate form of anaesthesia.

I also consent for pictures taken of my treatment site which may be used for publication or teaching purposes. My name and identity will not be disclosed and complete confidentiality will be maintained.

By signing below, I acknowledge that I have been adequately informed of the risks of the chemical peel treatment.

I also agree to comply with the recommended aftercare instructions given to me.

Signature of patient/Thumb impression　　　　　　　　　Date: ....

Signature of parents/Guardian (For minors)　　　　　　　Date: ....

Witness : ....
Name   : ....　　　Date: ....
Signature:　　　　　　　　　　　　　　　　　　　　　　　　Date: ....

Signature of the doctor:　　　　　　　　　　　　　　　　　Date: ....

Index

Page numbers followed by *b* refer to box, *f* refer to figure, and *t* refer to table.

A

Acanthosis nigricans 88, 89*f*, 187, 261, 263*f*
Acetic acid 64
  black 181, 200
  peel 233
Acetone-soaked sponges 75
Acid 22, 23
  dissociation constant 22
  peels act 210
Acidic acid, pH of 6
Acne 39, 40, 42*f*, 43*t*, 60*f*, 64, 65, 73, 79, 82, 83, 84*f*, 85, 101, 134, 135, 158, 164, 165, 176, 181, 188*f*, 192, 194, 200, 203, 204, 223, 224, 236, 248, 261, 275, 282*f*
  active 126, 229, 236
  active inflamed 59
  adult 236
  comedogenic 158
  comedonal 59, 134, 184, 185*f*, 188
  complete subsidence of 89*f*
  effect on 103
  excoriée 73, 134, 236
  grading system, global 84
  indications in 225, 226, 229-233
  inflammatory 158, 161, 184*f*, 225, 289
  management of 40
  mild active 73
  noninflammatory 181, 289
  persistent 149
  reduction properties 223
  related conditions 59
  retention 310
  rosacea 173
  surgery 142
  treatment of 87
  types of 181
  wash postprocedure instructions 57*b*
  widespread 150
  with oily thick skin 236
  with peels, treatment of 234*t*
Acne prone
  patients 34
  skin 197
Acne scar 43*t*, 101, 110, 112, 117, 126, 129, 135, 141, 148, 150, 151*f*, 159, 181, 203, 204, 223, 225, 283
  box 142
  combination technique for 152*f*
  deep 124
  erythematous 183, 184*f*
  moderate-severe 117*f*
  regional 148
  severe 19*f*
  superficial 59, 134, 181, 192, 236, 261*f*
  technique for 152*f*
Acne treatment
  active 288
  with peels 233
Acne vulgaris 236, 275, 277, 282*f*, 286
  flare of 304
  grade II 231*f*
  management of 237
Acneiform eruption 47, 68, 304, 305
Actinic cheilitis 18*f*
Actinic keratoses 2, 14, 18*f*, 42, 64, 65, 82, 85, 97, 101, 110, 134, 314
Activa peel 197, 198
  forte 198
Acyclovir 98, 147
Adequate sun protection 93
Adnexal tissue 234
Advanced cardiac life support 147
Aesthetic indications 261
Aesthetic skin consultation 50
Afro-Caribbean woman 151*f*
Agents
  depth-enhancing 28
  priming 62, 74
Aging skin 74, 172
  changes 134
Allergic contact dermatitis 93, 248
Allergic dermatitis 61, 74
Allergic reaction 47, 68, 93
  contact 116
Allergies to resorcinol 91
Alopecia areata 110
Alpha ketoacids 192
Alpha-hydroxy acid 1, 5, 24, 37, 50, 52, 64, 72, 78, 87, 92, 98, 102, 103, 112, 143, 192, 212, 214, 232, 243, 252, 260, 276, 276*b*, 283, 287, 309, 312
  combination of 226
  peel 106, 210, 212
American Society for Dermatologic Surgery guidelines 61
American Society for Dermatosurgery 249
Amino acid 170
Amino fruit
  acids 279
  peel 171
Amiodarone 147
Analgesia 113
Anesthesia 136, 147, 266
  general 147

medications 147
monitoring 147
Angiogenesis 5
Antibiotic properties 79
Anticancer agent 104
Antidepressants 147
Anti-inflammatory powder 148
Antimicrobial effects 83
Antioxidant 104
  effect 104
Antipsychotics 147
Antiseptic 148
Antithyroid effects 93
Apocrine glands 5
Arbutin 28, 52, 90, 189, 210, 245, 319
Arginine 170, 193, 255
  gel peel 170
  party peel 255
Arginine peel 170, 171, 171t, 172, 172f, 173
  absolute 172
  chemistry 170
  complications 173
  contraindications 172
  formulations of 170
  indications of 171, 172b
  mechanism of action 170
  postpeel care 172
  prepeel precautions 172
  relative 172
Arrhenius acid 22
Arrhythmias 147
Ascorbic acid 164, 181, 187, 187f, 188f, 253
Ascorbyl glucoside 254
Ascorbyl linoleate 280
Asian and African skin 286
Aspergillus 256
Atopic dermatitis 52, 134, 248
Atopic eczema 303
Atrophic acne scars 97
Azelaic acid 52, 90, 103, 112, 181, 182, 184f, 186f, 188f, 193, 198, 245, 319
  cream 292
  topical 211
Azelan peel 188, 188f

B

Bacillus proteus 79
Bacterial infection 65, 69, 155, 304
Baker-Gordon
  formula 18
  solution 124
Baker's phenol-croton oil
  solution 11
Benzoin, tincture of 88
Beta-hydroxy
  acid 3, 25, 78, 87, 192, 243, 287, 309, 316
  peel 25, 212
  peels 165
Beta-lipohydroxy acid 279
Bio C 201
Bismuth subgallate 148, 155f
Black peel 193, 199, 233
  clear, application of 200
  indications 200
  ingredients 199
  procedure 200
  protocol 200
Bleaching 189, 190
  agents 90, 245
Blended peel 86
Blepharoplasty 61
Blood clots, reduces 104
Body dysmorphic disorder 159
Botulinum toxin 119, 134, 206
Brody' combination 109
Brody's peel 66, 133
Bronsted acid 22
Buffer capacity 23
Buffer solution 23, 24

C

Candida 139
Carbolic acid 122, 144
Carbon dioxide 83
Carboxylic acids 37, 265
Cardiac monitoring 147
Cardiac tests 146
Cardiotoxicity 146
Cardiovascular toxicity 20
Caustic chemicals, use of 108

Caustic effects 14
Centrofacial melasma 186f
Ceramide 196
Chemical agents, side effects of 290t
Chemical formulation, chemistry and 86, 96, 132, 260
Chemical peel 12, 22, 14, 15, 20, 25, 30, 33b, 35b, 79, 54f, 57, 131, 141, 156, 158, 176, 203, 207, 210, 218, 221, 237, 256t, 286, 297, 298, 301t
  agents of 120, 170
  and formulas, types of 143
  application of 53f, 54, 98
  choice of 250
  classification of 14, 15t, 108
  combination of 118
  complications of 284b, 302, 304t
  deep 17
  depth of 20, 20t
  different medium-depth 9
  efficacy of 78
  for acne 223, 280
  for melasma 210t
  for postinflammatory pigmentation 281
  formulations 210
  hyperpigmentation 219
  in acne 281b
  in dark skin 274
    indications for 275b
  in dark skinned patients 286
  in ethnic skin 297
  in melasma 209
  indications of 193
  medium-depth 16, 18f, 109
  of skin 267t
  procedure 53
  recent trend in 311
  superficial 15, 16, 58, 112, 132
  systemic effects of 306
  treatment with 183, 309
  use of 1, 72, 220
  with botulinum toxin 206

Index

with concomitant oral 311
with dermabrasion 206
with dermasanding 205
with fillers 206
with lasers 204
with microdermabrasion 205
with microneedling 206
with subcision 206
Chemical peel pearls 318
  patient
    education 318
    selection 318
  peel plan 319
  peel preparation technique 319
  peeling technique 319
  postpeel care 320
  prepeel care 318
Chemical peeling 2, 30, 35, 131, 140, 192, 202, 206, 259, 270, 274, 286, 301, 309
  agent 277b, 292
    medium-depth 109b
  complications 154
  for pseudofolliculitis barbae 283
  for scarring 283
  in dermatoses 264
  indications for 276t
  mother of 274
  of skin 170
  superficial 132
  to stratum papillare, middle-depth 132
Chemical peeling in sensitive skin 248
  complications 250
  contraindications 249
  indications 248
  patient preparation 249
  precautions 250
  priming 249
Cholecalciferol 196
Cholesterol, reduces 104
Chromatic tendency, individual 218
Citric acid 24, 37, 102, 175, 182, 185, 186f, 193, 198, 214, 229, 253

containing 1
party peel 253
peel 253
Citrus fruits 24
Claze peel 171
Cold aloe vera lotion 144
Coleman's combination 109
Coleman's peel 48, 66, 133, 158
Collagen
  effect on 240
  fibers 7
Colorimetry 219
Combination peel 16, 101, 132, 180, 183, 189, 193, 252
  common formulations 181
  in acne 183
  in melasma 185
  in nonfacial areas 187
  postpeeling care 190
  prepeel preparation 189
Combination therapies, list of 203
Comedolytic agent 6
Comedolytic properties 310
Cook's total body peel 266
Coronal brow lift 61
Corticosteroid 16
Cosmelan peel 193, 201
Cosmetic and cosmeceutical brands 270
Cosmetic dermatologists 56t
Cosmo peel 193, 199
  indications 199
  ingredients 199
  treatment protocol 199
Cotton-tipped buds 159
C-peel delivery serum 254
Cream 99
  formulation 52, 99
Cream-based retinoid peel, application technique for 99b
Crème-postprocedure skin relief, calming 196
Croton oil 18, 122, 123, 143, 144
  concentration 146
  phenol peels 141, 144, 146
Croton oil-free 125

phenol combination peels 120, 127
  indications of 126
Croton tiglium tree 288
Cutaneous macular amyloidosis 187
Cyclohexenyl ring 96

D

Dark skin 223, 274f, 275
  histologic features of 274
  morphologic features of 274
  peeling in 297
  types 120, 123, 125, 140, 166, 286
Deep peel 10, 34, 141, 244
  agent 123
  penetration 31
  to cheeks 300f
Demodex mite 44
Deoxyribonucleic acid 314
Dermaceutic solution 198
Dermal fibroplasia, reticular 12
Dermal necrosis, risk of 137
Dermal papillae 6
Dermal proteins 102
Dermal regeneration 5
Dermamelan peel 193, 201
  indication 201
  ingredients 201
  procedure 201
Dermatitis, contact 90, 93, 115, 155, 304
Dermatology 72, 144
Desonide 190
Diazepam 147
Distilled water 144
Dithranol 262f
Dizziness 306
DNA mutations, mitochondrial 240
Dry ice 144
  plus trichloroacetic acid peel 143
Dyschromia 42, 65, 101, 181, 241
  mild 241
  treating for 90

E

Edema 304
  mild 56
Elastic fibers 243
Electrocardiography 146
Electrolytic abnormalities 147
Endothelial growth factor, vascular 241
Enterobacter aerogenes 79
Enzyme
  peel 193, 233, 257
    advantages of 257
  tyrosinase 27
Epidermal appendages 5
Epidermal cell 224
  layers 7
Epidermal dyschromias 74
Epidermal edema 9
Epidermal exfoliation 277
Epidermal glycosaminoglycans 234
Epidermal growth 194, 261
  factor 313
Epidermal keratinization 72
Epidermal keratinocyte 143, 163
Epidermal melanin 163
  redistributes 27
Epidermal melasma 65, 185, 211, 213
Epidermal pallor 8
Epidermal proteins 102
Epidermal regeneration 12
Epidermal skin growths, benign 192
Epidermal sliding 10
Epidermal thickness, increased 6*f*
Epidermis 7, 30
  coagulation of 114
  thicker 96
Epidermolysis 47, 52, 148
Epithelioid cells 87
Erythema 33, 55, 56, 68, 83, 91, 102, 104, 127, 138, 173, 240, 284, 291, 304, 305
  and pigmentation 84
  endpoint of 55
  no 47
  pink 75
  prolonged 93, 124
Erythematous macules 231*f*
Erythromycin 147
Escherichia coli 79
Esterified solution 24
Ethnic skin 108, 123, 277*b*, 288, 297
  population 277
Ethyl macadamiate 280
Ethylenediaminetetraacetic acid 171
Exfoliate skin 3
Exoderm formula and technique 146
Extracellular matrix, density of 239
Extrinsic aging 239
Eye contact, accidental 91

F

Face peel procedure 53
Face towels 176
Facial dermatitis 134
Facial nerve blocks, use of 147
Facial pigmentation, improvement in 42*f*
Facial rejuvenation 172*f*
Facial skin 259
Facial warts 44
Facial wrinkles, erases 1
Fair skin 274*f*
Fentanyl 147
Ferula foetida 174
Ferulac peel 174, 175, 177, 177*f*, 178*f*
  application of 176*f*
  complications 177
  contraindications 176
  equipment required for peel 176
  formulation 175
  indications 175
  patient preparation 176
  peel technique 176
  postpeel care 177
  session of 177*f*
  system 177
Ferulic acid 174, 174*f*, 175, 193, 198, 255
  party peel 255
Fibroblasts 103
Fitzpatrick skin, type III 211*f*
Fitzpatrick's classification 32, 32*t*, 189, 275*t*
Fitzpatrick's skin 32, 92, 111, 180, 221
  type 176, 276, 286
Fluconazole 147
Fluorouracil 315
  peel 314
Fluticasone propionate 99
Follicular canal 224
Follicular hyperkeratinization 223
Folliculitis, reduction of 188*f*
Folliculocentric cleaning 319
Freckles 14, 134
Free acid 24
Frost 47, 114
Frosting, levels of 65*t*
Fruit acids 5, 102, 174, 175
Fungal infection 65, 69, 111, 115

G

Galactose 312
Gamma-hydroxypropionic acid 87
Gentle cleanser 113
Glogau classification 241
  of photoaging 32*b*, 241, 242
Glogau's score 159, 176
Glowing powder 254
Gluconic acid 312
Glucosidic form 175
Glutathione peel 313
  contraindications 314
  indications 314
  peel application 313
  postpeel care 314
  prepeel priming 313

Index

properties 313
side effects 314
Glycolic acid 8, 16, 37, 40, 44, 52, 55, 72, 90, 102, 108, 109, 117*f*, 120, 132, 142, 158, 159, 160*f*, 161*f*, 164, 181, 186*f*, 187, 187*f*, 189, 193, 210, 219, 227, 236, 243*f*, 249, 260, 263*f*, 276, 288, 309
  formulations of 38*t*
  full-face peel 282*f*
  gel 68
  regimens for 46*t*
  role of 9, 43*t*
Glycolic acid peel 7, 37, 40, 40*f*, 41*t*, 42*f*, 47*t*, 48, 57*b*, 102, 165, 171, 210, 211, 211*f*, 220, 221*f*, 224, 227, 234
  advantages of 39, 39*t*
  application of 46*f*
  classification of 38, 38*t*
  complications 47
  dermal effects 39
  disadvantages of 39, 39*t*
  epidermal effects 38
  equipment for 53*b*
  in melasma 41*t*
  mechanism of action 38
  preparing patient for 50
  preprocedure instructions 50*b*
  procedure of 50
  regimens 56*t*
Glycolic and citric acids 190
Glycolic peel 52, 228
  consent 51*b*
  effect of 228
  indications of 39
  serial 40
  session of 228*f*
Glycolic-hydroquinone cream 142
Glycosaminoglycan 7, 39, 96
Granulation tissue 5
Growth factor beta, transforming 241
Guinea pigs 12
Gylcolic acid 182

H

Habig peel 133
Hand rejuvenation 74
Hematoxylin 6*f*
Hepatic test 146
Herpes labialis 44
Herpes simplex 139
  infection 111, 154
  outbreaks 141
  virus 30
Herpetic infection 69, 111
Hetter's and Stone's formulas 146
Hetter's croton oil 19*f*
Hetter's formulas 18
Hetter's regions 146*f*
Hetter's-Heresy
  croton oil-phenol peel formulas 145*t*
  formulas 146
Hexachlorophene 144
Home care products 312
Human immunodeficiency virus 30, 61, 74
Human skin 253
Hyaluronic acid 254
Hyaluronidase 153
Hydrating and anti-inflammation 196
Hydrochlorothiazide 147
Hydrocortisone 99, 100, 206
  cream 57
Hydromorphone 147
Hydronutritional cream 201
Hydroquinone 27, 28, 52, 62, 66, 98, 136, 142, 189, 190, 210, 219, 319
  creams 211
  priming 299
Hydroxy acid 129
  cleanser 98*f*
  mild alpha 183
Hydroxy phenoxy propionic acid 280
Hydroxyl acid 24
Hygroscopic nature 65
Hyperemia 173

Hyperpigmentation, disorder of 209, 261
Hyperplastic epidermis 9
Hypoallergenic cream 149
Hypokalemia 147
Hypomagnesemia 147

I

Ice-pick
  acne scars 142
  scar 149, 150, 288
Idiopathic guttate hypomelanosis 110
Infection 69, 135, 139
Inflammation, effect on 241
Inflammatory acne, incidence of 275
Infraorbital nerve 136
Infrared radiation
  effect 241
  type A 239
Intralesional steroids 115
Intrinsic aging 239, 240
Irritant contact dermatitis 93, 262*f*
Irritation 68, 304
Isoflavones 254
Isotretinoin
  pills 142
  therapy 12
Itching 91

J

Jasmonic acid 181
Jawline comedonal acne 225*f*
Jessner's solution 212
Jessner's and resorcinol peels 86
Jessner's face peel 283*f*
Jessner's formula 198
Jessner's peel 86, 88*f*, 91, 93, 134, 137, 212, 226, 227, 232, 278, 282
  modified 215*f*
Jessner's plus, combination 144*f*

Jessner's solution 5, 6, 8-10, 16, 18f, 93, 109, 113, 113f, 114f, 120, 124, 132, 137, 214, 215, 224, 243, 244, 283, 287, 290, 298
   application of 134, 137
   coats of 137
   combination of 278
   component of 73
   dries 92
   enhanced 86
   modified 15f, 16, 17f, 18f, 278, 299f
   multi-coat 116f
   peels 7
   plus 109

K

Keloid 135, 138
   formation 189
   scarring 78
Keloidal tendency 207
   history of 65
Keratinocyte 6, 72
   discohesion 5, 163
Keratitis, superficial 168
Keratolytic agent 6, 224
Keratolytic effects 14
Keratosis
   absent 241
   pilaris 39, 44, 97, 187
Ketamine 147
Ketorolac 147
Kligman's formula 216
Knees, frictional melanosis of 262f
Koebner's phenomenon 33
Kojic acid 27, 28, 52, 66, 75, 90, 160f, 161f, 164, 182, 185, 186f, 189, 190, 198, 210, 245, 256, 319

L

Lactic acid 24, 28, 37, 50, 72, 87, 90, 102, 109, 137, 143, 164, 175, 181, 182, 185, 186f, 189, 198, 210, 212, 232, 245, 252, 277, 287
   amount of 1
   complications 232
   contraindication 232
   inhibits 277
   properties of 73
      antioxidant 73
      bacteriostatic 73
      comedolytic 73
      contraindications 74
      hydrating 73
      indications 73
      keratolytic 73
      patient preparation 74
      sebostatic 73
Lactic acid peel 72, 75f, 212, 224, 232
   chemical formulations 73
   chemistry 72
   complications 76
   postpeel care 76
   precautions 76
Lactic peel 72, 73, 75
Lactobionic acid 254, 312
L-ascorbic acid 253, 254f
Laser hair removal 112
Latin american skin 297
Latina woman with acne scars 150f
Lay peeler's formulas 146
Leaderma 171t
Leathery skin 137
Lemon extract 1
Lentigines 14, 131, 134
Leukoderma 293
Lewis acid 22
Lichen planus lesions 33
Lichen planus pigmentosus 110, 118, 127, 127f, 128f, 263f
   hyperpigmentation of 118f
Lichenoid disorders 158
Licorice 28, 189, 210, 293
Lidocaine ointment, topical 144
Life quality index 220
Lipohydroxy acid 78, 279, 309, 316
   chemical properties of 309
   complications 310
   contraindications 310
   indications 310
   side effects 310
Lipophilic nature 310
Luminous powder 254

M

Macular amyloidosis 261, 263f
Malar areas, bilateral 75f
Malar melasma 211f
Malic acid 24, 37, 102, 175
Mandelic acid 3, 24, 37, 43, 78-81, 102, 158, 181, 182, 184f, 187, 187f, 188f, 189, 193, 210, 277, 279
   chemical formula 78
Mandelic acid peel 78, 224, 230, 231, 277
   complications 80, 231
   indications 78
   peel technique 80
   pigmentary disorders 78
   postpeel care 80
Mandelic peel 158, 230
Mask peel 193, 199
   indication 199
   ingredients 199
   treatment protocol 199
Masson trichrome staining 6
Matrix metalloproteinases 240
Mela cream 197, 198
Mela peel 193, 197, 198
   forte 193, 198
      indications 198
      ingredients 198
      mechanism of action 198
      procedure, ingredients of 198t
   treatment 197
      indications 197
      protocol 198
Melanin grains 242
Melanocompetent 274
Melanostop peel 185, 186f
Melanotoxic chemical 122
Melasma 14, 40, 64, 79, 85, 88, 104, 120, 128, 134, 158, 185, 209, 213, 216, 293f

Index

and dark skin 276
area and severity index 41
quality of life scale 209
dermal-type 19
effect on 103
mixed 185
treatment of 103, 171, 277, 290, 292
Mental nerve 136
Mesoestetic hydra vital factor K cream 201
Metabolic effects 25
Meta-dihydroxybenzene 87
Methemoglobinemia 88
Methoxycinnamic acid 174
Methyl salicylate 65
Midazolam 147
Mid-reticular dermis 17, 123, 129
Milia 116, 134
 formation 34
Milk peel 193, 197
 treatment 197
  indications 197
  ingredients 197
  protocol 197
Molecular mechanisms 240
Molecules, novel 309
Monheit technique 226
Monheit's and Coleman's combinations 244
Monheit's combination 109, 117, 244
Monheit's peel 66, 133, 278
Monheit's technique 243f
Mono peel 252
Monocarboxylic acids 192
Monoprotic acid 23
Moy technique 92, 227
Mucopolysaccharide 7
 density 7
 synthesis 25
Mulberry extract 254
Myoinositol hexaphosphate 104
Myristoyl tripeptide-4 196
Myxedema 88

N

Natural moisturizing factor 72
Nausea 93
Necrotic coagulum 148
Neodymium-doped yttrium aluminum garnet 205, 236
Neostrata prosystem retinol peel 200
Nephrotoxic acid 265
Nerve blocks 136
Niacinamide 293
Nicotinamide 255
Nitrogen, liquid 144, 312
Nomelan fenol 125
 light peel 187, 187f, 188f
 medium peel 127f
 peels 125f
Nomelan peel 233
Noncomedogenic cream 149
Nonfacial skin 68, 259
Nonhydroquinone bleaching agents 287

O

Obagi's blue peel 133, 134, 193, 195, 279
Ocular complications 69, 116
Office peels 252
Oil massages 189, 190
Oily skin 286
Olive oil 144
Oral contraceptive pills 110
Oral isotretinoin 112, 223, 235
 therapy 61
Ortho-hydroxybenzoic acid 59, 87
Oxygen
 partial pressure 147
 species, reactive 255

P

Papillary dermis 6, 7, 30, 86
 level 205
Papillary reticular dermis 7
Papular acne 167f
Papular forehead acne 168f
Papulopustular acne 103
Party peel 201, 252, 254, 256t, 257
 advantages 252, 253, 255
 application technique 202
 indications 202
 ingredients 202
Patch test 52
Patchy erythema 47
 transient 106
Patient assessment and counseling 30
Peel 110, 135, 215, 235, 260
 additives 254
 anatomic site of 26
 anti-aging 173
 applications of combination 180
 before 110
 blue 137
 brands 271t
 classification 20
 combined 132
 common 224, 288
 combination 133
 complications of 302
 concentration of 26, 116
 contraindications of 194, 306
 cooling, next level of post 312
 day 8 of 150f
 depth of 15, 120, 301
 desired 266
 duration of contact with 26
 for acne 223
 for melasma 41t
 for photoaging 239, 242
 formulation, choosing 24
 freshening 252
 glycolic-based combination 180
 gold 15f
 histological classification of 192, 193t
 in acne scars, role of 234
 indication for 265
  medium-depth 110
 medium 7

medium-depth 10, 18f, 64, 69, 108, 110, 110f, 110t, 112, 117f, 120, 124, 131-133, 136, 137, 193, 244
  chemical formulations 132
  chemistry 132
  complications 138
  contraindications 134
  indications 134
  patient preparation 135
  postpeel care 138
mild 106, 250
name 256t
  argipeel 171, 256t
  azelac gel 256t
  cosderma gel party peel 256t
  easy phytic peel 256t
  lactipeel 256t
  mandelac C 256t
  mandelac L 256t
  mandelac T 256t
  pigment balancing peel 256t
  sesglicopeel K 256t
  ZO stimulator peel 256t
newer 193, 224, 233, 279
patch testing 120
phenol-based 130
phenol-croton 124
postauricular test 74
priming 172
product, specific 52
proprietary 102, 192, 195
protocol, optimum 120
pumpkin 257
radiant 133
right 235
safe combination 187
selection 142t
self-neutralizing 86
sessions and interval, number of 127
side effects 304
solution 195, 196
stand-alone 101
superficial 5, 6, 16, 32, 61, 67, 86, 165, 243, 298f, 299f, 306

depth 65
light 193
termination and duration 114
test 33, 52, 113
tray, typical 113
treatment
  intervals for 57
  repeat sessions of 314
types of 193
user-friendly 63
with properties and effects 182t
yellow 163
Peel agents
  advantage of combined 133
  medium-depth 110, 133t
Peel application 62, 113, 254
  sequence of 114
Peel complications
  factors influencing 302t
  handle 307
Peel procedure 66
  guidelines 200
  in general 194
  medium-depth 113f
Peel technique 62, 75, 91, 98, 136, 159, 266, 281t
  arrangements 136
  preparation 136
Peeling 31, 137
  at office 196
  effect 114
  excessive 284
  extra-facial 259
  frequency of 106
  ingredients, functions of 195t
  lack of 57
  materials required for 45f
  methodology of medium-depth 113
  modern era of 122
  off, starts 138
  procedure 219
  progressive 57
  safety of medium-depth 117 to deep 123
  steps of 45

technique for 45, 83, 315
treatment steps 310
Peeling agent 28, 33, 102, 122, 125, 174, 192
  classification of 192
  dependent factors 304
  newer 193, 193b
  superficial 171, 277
Peeling systems
  home-based 270
    chemistry 270
    contraindications 272
    indications 271
    postpeel care 272
    procedure of application 272
Penicillium species 256
Periorbital melanosis 65
Periorbital rejuvenation 172
Periorbital skin 180
Persistent erythema 47, 52, 69, 115, 139, 155, 207
Petrolatum, application of 54
pH 23
Pharmacology and chemical structure 37
Phenol 25, 108, 109, 122, 123, 129, 133, 139, 143, 146, 180, 183, 187, 187f, 188f, 226, 260
  application of 10
  based peels, timeline of 2t
  chemabrasion 151f
    technique 147, 150
  combination 127
    peels 125
  concentration of 123
  derivative 174f
  formulas 144, 146
  in skin of color 123
  low concentration 125
  properties of 123
  solutions, modified 122
  use of 108, 122
Phenol peel 122, 125, 146, 261, 262f
  combination 125
  contraindications to 125
  light 133

modified 123, 124
Phenol-croton oil 12, 288
  peel 126
    solutions 124t
Phloretin 174, 175, 175f, 255
  structure of 175
Phloridzin 175
Photodamaged skin 74, 110, 264
Photosensitizing drugs 30
Phototype
  adverse effects in higher 301t
  skin 197t
Phytic acid 37, 102-104, 106, 182, 186f, 187, 187f, 188f, 193, 253, 279
  combination peels 106
  effect of 103
  molecule 104
  on skin, effects of 103, 105
  precipitates 105
  solution 279
  structure of 104f
Phytic acid peel 79, 102, 104, 105f, 215
  complications 106
  contraindications 106
  drawbacks of 106
  indications 105
  postpeel care 106
  technique 105
Phytic peel 279
  easy 279
Phytin 104
Pigmentary abnormalities 115
Pigmentary changes, prevention of 52
Pigmentary complications 304
Pigmentary disorders 14, 78, 192, 193, 203, 204, 264, 310
  recalcitrant 205
Pigmentary dyschromias 110, 126
Pilosebaceous glands 31
Poikiloderma 134
Polyethylene glycol 298, 298f
Polyhydroxy acid 193, 254, 312, 316

party peels 254
Polyprotic acid 23
Pomegranate enzyme 233
Postacne
  complications 79
  hyperpigmentation 59, 60f, 73, 97f
  marks 203
  pigmented marks 164
  scarring 75f, 120
Postinflammatory
  hyperpigmentation 14, 25, 40, 41, 43, 64, 69f, 109, 110, 118, 141, 142, 153, 155, 188f, 218, 219, 220, 223, 236, 259, 262f, 275, 276, 286, 291, 297
  classification of 218
  etiopathogenesis of 218
  folliculitis with 188f
  risk of 28, 303
  treatment of 153, 219, 221f, 299f
Postpeel
  considerations 298
  erythema 34
  events, expected 115
  expectations 127
  guidelines 111
  hyperpigmentation 100, 168
  instructions 115
  photographs 33
  regimen for deep peels, alternative 153
  with Jessner's solution 293f
Postpeel care 27, 28, 47, 92, 99, 196, 220, 245, 257
  avoid scratching 29
  bland moisturizer 29
  broad-spectrum sunscreen 29
  cool water 29
  ice compresses 29
  mild cleansers 29
  regimen 127
Postradiation therapy 12
Potassium iodide 181, 200
Potential systemic toxicity 146

Precancerous and cancerous conditions 262
Prepeel 98, 266
  counseling 44
  priming 111
  regimen 280
  skin preparation 98f
  sun protection 52
Prepeel care 27, 28
  degreasing agents 28
  fluorescent additives 28
  topical anesthetics 28
Prepeel preparation 26, 98, 194, 286, 297
  immediate 53
Prophylactic acyclovir 61
Prophylactic antiviral medication 98
Propionibacterium acne 183, 227, 277, 288
Propofol 147
Protein oxidation, effect on 241
Proteolytic enzymes 257
Prototypical phenol solution 123
Pruritus 68
Pseudofolliculitis barbae 276, 286
Pseudofrost, white 81
Pseudohypopigmentation 155
Pseudomonas 139
Psoriasis 61, 74, 134, 303
  presence of 33
Pulsed-dye laser therapy 153
Punctate bleeding 148
Purulent exudate 19f
Pustular acne 105f
Pyruvic acid 82, 83, 85, 109, 133, 134, 137, 181, 182, 193, 215, 231, 244, 279, 300f
Pyruvic acid peel 82, 224, 231
  advantages 83
  complications 232
  contraindications 82, 232
  disadvantages 83
  formulations 82
  indications 82
  postpeel care 83

properties 82
side effects 83
Pyruvic peel 84, 84f, 232, 234

R

Red carpet peels 252, 257
Regen-D gel 115
Renal compromise 306
Renal test 146
Renal toxicity 146
Resorcinol 87, 103, 108, 139, 164, 186f, 198
  components 215
  metabolites 87
  peel 226
  toxicity 93
Resveratrol 293
Reticular dermis 10, 144
  lower 244
  upper 7, 30, 244
Retinaldehyde 96
Retinoic acid 15f, 66, 96, 181, 182, 187, 187f, 188f, 193
  peel 163, 224
Retinoid 97t, 174
  acid 96, 205
  boost 92
  creams, use of 142
  dermatitis 303
  topical 210
Retinoid peels 98, 99, 101
  yellow color of 99
Retinol 27, 101, 164, 255
  cream peel 99f
  crème 196
  ester 280
Retinol peel 96, 158, 164, 165, 167f, 278
  complications of 168
  formulations, combinations in 165
  response to 167f
  side effects of 168
Retinyl esters 96
Retinyl linoleate 280
Revitalize Personal Peel Program 257
Rhytidectomy 61, 146

Rhytides 9
  fine 261
Roberts spot peel technique 319
Rolling scar 150
Rosacea 43, 52, 61, 74, 181, 248
Rough skin texture 65
Rucinol 293
Rullan peel's postoperative regimen 153

S

Salicylate toxicity 93
Salicylic acid 3, 15, 27, 34, 43, 59, 63, 78, 86, 91, 104, 108, 139, 159, 160f, 164, 181-183, 184f, 186f, 187, 187f, 188f, 190, 198, 210, 219, 221f, 224, 236, 260, 263f, 277, 283, 287, 298f, 309, 316
  chemical peeling 136
  on pregnancy 272
  photomicrograph of 6
Salicylic acid peel 59, 62, 63, 84, 213, 221, 224
  complications 63, 225
  contraindications 61, 225
  indications 59
  patient preparation 61
  postpeel care 63
  practical tips 63
  precautions 62
  superficial 281
Salicylic mandelic acid 104, 184f
Salicylic peel 158, 225, 319
Salicylic-mandelic acid 41, 78, 80, 183, 228, 282f
Saline eyewash 176
Scabbing 47
Scar 33, 124, 176
  and striae 262
  hypertrophic 65, 78, 135, 150f, 153
  in males 165
  treatment 122
Scarring, superficial 73, 101
Sebaceous atrophy 12

Sebaceous glands 6, 32, 103
Sebaceous hyperplasia 14, 297
Sebaceous lighter skin 150
Seborrhea 158, 167f, 181, 225
Seborrheic dermatitis 52
Seborrheic keratoses 14, 65, 131, 134, 297, 314
Sedation 266
  and analgesia 144
Sensitive sites, protection of 113
Sensitive skin 172, 248, 303
  molecules for 312
Sequential peel 158, 161
  complications 160
  contraindications 159
  indications 159
  patient preparation 159
  postpeel care 160
  practical tips 161
Sesderma 171, 181, 185, 257
Sesglicopeel K gel 185, 186f
  peel 181
Skin
  and wound healing, histology of 5
  appearance 47
  barrier compromise 303
  defenses 241
  deodorization, effect on 103
  discoloration 93
  dry 303
  elasticity, improvement in 103
  extra-facial 264
  healing 34
  health care 1
  inflammation 196
  irritable 173
  lotion 103
  microcirculation 173
  peeling procedures 108
  phototype 275
  pigmented 134
  preconditioning 142
  proteins, coagulation of 25
  regeneration, stimulation of 52

Index

rejuvenation 2, 86, 79, 134
resurfacing 200
roughness 84
sensitivity 56
smoothness 84
structure, boosting 180
thickness 159, 176
treated 120
type 26, 32*t*, 111, 113, 141, 275*t*, 289
whitening 104
wound repair 12
Skin aging
  advanced 197
  mild-to-moderate 197
Skin burns 141
  blistering and 116
Skin care
  post-treatment 81
  pretreatment 81
  products, preprocedure 50
Skin layer
  ablation of 14
  target 15
Skin lightening
  agents 190, 210
  effect 103
Skin moisture 103
  effect on 103
Skin of color 122
  modifications for 122
Skin of neck
  after chemical peeling 133*f*
  before chemical peeling 133*f*
Skin priming 27
  prior 26
Skin scars
  chemical reconstruction of 68, 124, 133, 134, 142, 152*f*, 288, 291
  technique, reconstruction of 230
Slit-lamp examination 116
Sodium bicarbonate rinse 144
Solar lentigines 42, 64, 117, 118
Solar melanosis, treatment of 299*f*
Sour milk 24

Spillage, accidental 116, 136, 140
Spot peel technique 283
Spotty erythema 47
Staphylococcus 139
  aureus 79, 183
  epidermidis 183
Stellate cells 103
Steroid
  concomitant 303
  cream 93
    low potency 100
  damaged face, topical 248
  induced acne, topical 235
Stone phenol 124
Stone Venner-Kellson formula 261
Stratum basale, peeling to 132
Stratum corneum 163
  lower level of 72
Streptococcus 139
Stretch marks 97
Strip technique 266
Subsequent coats 126
Sulfur bonds, disrupts 123
Sulfuric acid 25
Sun protection factor 293
Sunscreen 50
Sun-tanned skin 187*f*
Superficial peels, combining 311
Supratrochlear nerve 136
Switch peel 158
Systemic steroids 115

T

Tachycardia 147
  risk of 147
Tartaric acid 24, 37, 102
  containing 1
Telangiectasias 34, 239, 241
Terfenadine 147
Terminative peels 165
Tetra-hydro-jasmonic acid 199
Thioctic acid 254
Tinnitus 93
Tissue
  dermal 131, 192

epidermal 131, 192
  radiated 12
Titanium dioxide 99
Tocopheryl linoleate 280
Tranexamic acid 315
Transepidermal water loss 180
Tretinoin 27, 50, 96, 97, 101, 142, 189, 210
  accelerates epidermal proliferation 27
  activates 96
  cream 12, 90
Tretinoin peel 165, 219, 233
  complications 233
Triazolam 147
Trichloroacetic acid 2, 8*f*, 15, 17*f*, 25, 28, 41, 64, 92, 102, 109, 117*f*, 122, 133, 133*f*, 143, 144*f*, 145*f*, 152*f*, 158, 164, 180, 187*f*, 188*f*, 192, 195, 204, 210, 219, 230, 243, 260, 263*f*, 277, 283, 291, 293*f*, 298, 300*f*, 304
  mechanism of action 64
  spot peel 283*f*
  technique 144
Trichloroacetic acid peel 48, 64, 67*f*, 68, 68*f*, 69, 70, 89*f*, 92, 145*f*, 213, 214, 214*f*, 224, 229, 229*f*, 263*f*, 278
  combination treatments 66
  complications 230
  contraindications 65, 230
  delayed effects 68
  formulations 64
  immediate effects 68
  indications 65
  method of application 66
  postpeel care 67
  preprocedure care 66
  side effects 68
  TCA cross 68
Trichloroethanoic acid 64
Tricholoroacetic acid 213
Triprotic acid 23
Truncal acne 261*f*, 264
Tyrosinase inhibitors 50
  preventive application of 52

U

Ultraviolet radiation 239
Uniform faint erythema 47
Unna's paste 87
Urticaria 47

V

Valaciclovir 61, 98
Vesiculo-bullae formation 144
Vi peel 279
Viral infection 111
Visual analog scale 220
Visual staging 267t
Vitamin
  A 163, 233
  C 93, 319
    peel 253
    properties of 178
  E 104, 201
    properties of 178
  K 201
Vitiligo 61, 74, 129

W

Warts 85
Watchful eye 173
Whitfield's ointment 224
Wiest-Walker peel 133
Wood's lamp
  examination 219
  visualization 28
Wound healing 5, 12, 112
  comparison of 9

X

Xanthelasma 64

Y

Yeast infection 155
Yellow peel 163, 164, 166, 168, 233
  chemical formulations of 163
  chemistry of 163
  complications 168
  contraindications for 166
  formulations of 164t
  indications for 164, 164t
  ostpeel care 168
  patient preparation 166
  photoaging 164
  pigmentation 165
  technique 166

Z

Zinc oxide 99

EU GSPR Authorised Reprsentative
Logos Europe, 9 rue Nicolas Poussin
1700, La Rochelle, France
Phone: +33 (0) 6 67 93 73 78
E-mail: contact@logoseurope.eu